Communication Therapy

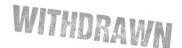

Communication Therapy

**An Integrated Approach to Aural Rehabilitation
with Deaf and Hard of Hearing Adolescents and Adults**

■ ■ ■ ■ ■ ■

Mary June Moseley
Scott J. Bally

Editors

Gallaudet University Press
Washington, D.C.

Gallaudet University Press
Washington, DC 20002

Cover design by Dorothy Wachtenheim
Text design by Alice Fernandes-Brown

Library of Congress Cataloging-in-Publication Data

Communication therapy : an integrated approach to aural rehabilitation with deaf and
    hard of hearing adolescents and adults / Mary June Moseley, Scott J. Bally, editors.
        p.   cm.
    Includes bibliographical references and index.
    ISBN 1-56368-054-8 (alk. paper)
    1. Deaf—Rehabilitation.   2. Children, Deaf—Rehabilitation.   3. Hearing
impaired—Rehabilitation.   4. Hearing impaired children—Rehabilitation.
    I. Moseley, Mary June.   II. Bally, Scott J., 1945–
    [DNLM: 1. Deafness—rehabilitation.   2. Communicative Disorders—therapy.
3. Hearing Loss, Partial—rehabilitation.   WV 270 C7366 1996]
    RF291.C63   1996
    617.8′9—dc20
    DNLM/DLC
    for Library of Congress   96-16866
                                                                                                         CIP

Contents

■ ■ ■ ■

Contributors

■ ■ ■ ■

Antoinette S. Allen, M.A., CCC-SLP
Speech-Language Pathologist/Aural Rehabilitationist
Department of Audiology and Speech-Language Pathology
Gallaudet University
Washington, D.C.

Scott J. Bally, M.S., CCC-SLP
Assistant Professor
Department of Audiology and Speech-Language Pathology
Gallaudet University
Washington, D.C.

Harriet Kaplan, Ph.D., CCC-A
Professor
Department of Audiology and Speech-Language Pathology
Gallaudet University
Washington, D.C.

Mary Ann Kinsella-Meier, M.S., CCC-A
Audiologist/Communications Specialist
Private Consultant
Montgomery County, Maryland

James J. Mahshie, Ph.D., CCC-SLP
Professor
Department of Audiology and Speech-Language Pathology
Gallaudet University
Washington, D.C.

Mary June Moseley, Ph.D., CCC-SLP
Professor
Department of Audiology and Speech-Language Pathology
Gallaudet University
Washington, D.C.

Maureen Nichols, M.A., CCC-SLP
Communications Specialist
Model Secondary School for the Deaf
Washington, D.C.

Janet L. Pray, Ph.D., LICSW
Professor, Chair
Department of Social Work
Gallaudet University
Washington, D.C.

Bobbi Redinger, M.S., CCC-A
Research and Development Audiologist
Decibel Instruments Inc.
Hayward, California

Susanne M. Scott, M.S., CCC-A
Audiologist/Aural Rehabilitationist
Department of Audiology and Speech-Language Pathology
Gallaudet University
Washington, D.C.

Mary Pat Wilson, M.S., CCC-A
Coordinator of Aural Rehabilitation
Department of Audiology and Speech-Language Pathology
Gallaudet University
Washington, D.C.

Preface

■ ■ ■ ■

The development of this book has been an evolutionary process. Over the years, the authors have developed the approach described here to facilitate the communication needs of adolescent and adult clients with varying degrees of hearing loss, who identify with differing cultures and use differing modes of communication. Throughout the developmental process, the authors have presented information about these clients at a variety of professional meetings (for example, American Speech-Language-Hearing Association, Self-Help for Hard of Hearing, Academy of Rehabilitative Audiology). Each audience was enthusiastic and genuinely concerned for more information about a functional approach to the needs of adolescents and adults with hearing loss, particularly those who consider themselves culturally Deaf. The material presented to these audiences became the basis for this book.

Several of the authors discussed the outline for this book and developed the format used here. In these discussions, three major emphases emerged:

1. *Elaborating on the functional approach to aural rehabilitation that we have refined over the past few years.* The integrated therapy approach has evolved through meeting the variety of needs of a given client in a functional manner while simultaneously working on several communication skill areas. This approach has helped the clients to become more effective communicators as well as increase their flexibility and independence in difficult communication situations. This model of communication therapy, using an integrated approach, is explained in the first part of this book and is expanded upon throughout. Although much of the communication therapy described in this book is appropriate for an individual therapy setting, some of the authors have chosen to emphasize the appropriateness of working on specific skills within a small group or classroom setting.

Each author describes the setting he or she discusses and provides alternative suggestions for other contexts.

2. *Emphasizing the needs of our adolescent and adult clients.* High-school and college-age adolescents and adults can participate in therapy programming in a way that young children cannot. In addition, adults who develop a hearing loss later in life have special needs that lend themselves to the integrated communication therapy approach. The involvement of these adolescent and adult clients in therapy decision making is a consistent theme through this book. The nature of some of the chapters may lead to an emphasis on one or the other of these populations.

3. *Presenting information about the unique needs of the culturally Deaf population.* These individuals may have different life experiences and communication needs than the "typical" adult seen in aural rehabilitation clinics around the country. Speech-language pathologists and audiologists need to be informed about the nature of Deaf culture and its impact on the services they provide. The discussions of communication therapy presented in this book are appropriate for the culturally Deaf population and may be modified for those who are hard of hearing.

The authors designed this book to be used as a text in college courses in aural rehabilitation. However, the information presented here will also be extremely useful to those practicing professionals who do not work exclusively with the Deaf and hard of hearing populations and who may have limited knowledge of the current practices in aural rehabilitation. Some of the chapters go into great depth in one area (for example, the methods for teaching vocabulary skills to adolescents). Other chapters present more introductory information that sets the stage for the reader to obtain more knowledge through other sources (for example, the chapter on technology introduces the reader to the various types of assistive technology currently available).

The book consistently discusses the use of sign language—referring to either American Sign Language (ASL) or "Contact" sign language—as a mode of communication with clients. Although ASL is a language unto itself, Contact sign language combines features of English and ASL. Contact sign language allows the user to sign and speak English at the same time, which cannot be done with ASL. Facilitating communication in clients may be accomplished more effectively using the mode of communication with which the clients are most comfortable (ASL or Contact sign). The book's intent is to encourage aural rehabilitationists to become fluent in sign language as a means of communicating with their culturally Deaf clients, for example, in presenting new information about a specific area (technology) or in discussing communication needs (strategies to be used in specific situations). The authors do not advocate teaching sign communication skills to a client, however. That is the role of the sign language specialist.

As with most authors in the 1990s, we have struggled with how to make this book reflect equal status for gender. Our choice has been to use nonspecific terms when possible. When this does not seem appropriate, we have varied the use of "he" and "she" through the different chapters of the book.

Finally, we would like to acknowledge the many people who have helped us in putting together this book. The collaborating authors worked diligently on their own chapters and provided excellent support and advice to us during the editing process. Colleagues and graduate assistants who have helped with the specifics (for example, conceptual development, graphics, typing, indexing, proofreading, referencing, and library research) include Fred Brandt, Melanie Lesko, Jamey Gitchel, Mary Hilley, Michelle Malta, Lynn Rowland, Melony Stanton, Carol Traxler, Jennifer Gardiner, and Stephen Lotterman. We are fortunate to have Ivey Pittle Wallace as our editor; she has continually provided encouragement and insight.

Mary June Moseley and Scott J. Bally, editors

.

PART

1

The Process of Communication Therapy

Introduction

This book is divided into four parts: (1) The Process of Communication Therapy; (2) Global Areas of Communication Therapy; (3) Communication Skills Areas; and (4) Integrated Therapy Case Studies.

The purpose of part 1 is to introduce students and professionals not experienced with the deaf and hard of hearing populations to the unique characteristics of individuals who may seek communication therapy services. Chapter 1 describes the characteristics of these individuals, with particular emphasis on culturally Deaf adolescents and adults. Culturally Deaf clients often make decisions regarding communication therapy from a cultural base different than later-deafened and hard of hearing individuals. Kinsella-Meier provides a description of Deaf culture and discusses how professionals in the fields of audiology and speech-language pathology might use this information to provide services to culturally Deaf populations.

In chapter 2, Wilson and Scott provide an overview of a model for communication therapy. This model is designed to integrate a variety of skill areas, depending on the client's individual needs and desires. The integrated therapy approach is one in which multiple aspects of communica-

tion are integrated in a given session or program into a meaningful, situationally based context. Greater carryover into real-life situations occurs with this approach as compared to an isolated skill-development approach. Each area presented in Wilson and Scott's overview will be discussed at length in the following chapters of the book.

1

Defining the Populations

Mary Ann Kinsella-Meier

■ ■ ■ ■

The purpose of this chapter is to describe the populations of individuals who are served by aural rehabilitationists and communication specialists. The discussion will focus on the characteristics of culturally Deaf individuals. Persons who are culturally Deaf possess unique characteristics that have a significant impact on the services provided by speech-language-hearing professionals.

Defining the Populations

Culturally Deaf Populations

The single unifying characteristic of culturally Deaf adults and adolescents is that they use American Sign Language (ASL) as their primary means of communica-

The following people have been instrumental in lending their viewpoints and support for this endeavor: Lee Ronis, Norma J. Sines, Bobbi Reddinger, Jerry Friedman, Beth Singer, Mary Hilley, Holly Roth, and the members of the Linguistics Department at Gallaudet University. I would like to thank the Department of Audiology and Speech-Language for providing the base from which I have grown. In addition, I would like to thank all the people—Deaf, hard of hearing, and hearing—who took the time to make the phone calls, write the letters, and share their perspectives; you have all taught me a great deal. Thank you to those organizations that chose to publish my request for feedback on terminology: the Bicultural Center, Silent News, TFA (Electronic Bulletin Board), Advance. I would like to thank Florence Vold (my guide through this journey) as the person who has always supported my work and encouraged me some ten years ago to keep a special "red notebook" of all my

tion (Kannapell and Adams 1984). (ASL will be discussed in more detail later in this chapter.) Members of this cultural group associate primarily with others who communicate in ASL. The culture of Deaf people involves not only their language, which is the root of their culture, but also values, beliefs, traditions, and technology (Kannapell and Adams 1984). There are social support systems within the Deaf community that are at the heart of their culture. The members of this community possess a variety of hearing levels, occasionally including persons with hearing in the moderate ranges (Kannapell and Adams 1984). Culturally Deaf people who seek out services from speech and hearing professionals tend to be interested in functioning biculturally and bilingually in ASL and in English. This may or may not include spoken English.

The term "*Deaf*," as used throughout this book, describes those persons who identify themselves as part of a cultural and linguistic group in which ASL is the primary means of communication. The use of this spelling to denote cultural and audiologic differences was first proposed by James Woodward in 1972 (Padden and Humphries 1988). The capitalization of the first letter differentiates its meaning when compared to the term "deaf," which is used by deafened individuals who do not affiliate with the Deaf community or refers to the actual audiologic levels the individual possesses (Levitan 1993).

Hard of Hearing

Hard of hearing refers to those persons who do not self-identify as part of Deaf culture. They communicate primarily with people who are hearing, relying on their oral/aural skills. This group includes persons with a wide array of hearing levels and configurations of hearing loss, such as people who are audiometrically deaf, with hearing in the profound range, but who still interact more with hearing persons through their oral and aural skills. Their speech may be intelligible or semi-intelligible. A person in this group may have become hard of hearing at birth or anytime during childhood. Further discussions of the terms hard of hearing and Deaf, from cultural and educational perspectives, can be found in Lane (1992), Padden and Humphries (1988), Sanders (1993), and "Be in the Know" (1993).

Late-Deafened

Late-deafened adults are those persons who became profoundly deaf after reaching adulthood. They developed spoken language skills and communicated in the

experiences. This notebook was of great service in writing this chapter. Without the family support of Tim and Michele, I would not have been able to get the quiet time to write, thank you. Most importantly, thank you to all the Deaf persons I have had the opportunity to work with throughout the years; you all have taught me so much about your world.

hearing world prior to becoming deaf. They may or may not elect to use sign language and may use either ASL or an English-based sign system. Most often they will experience significant receptive language problems and difficulty adjusting to the hearing loss. Additional information on this population may be found in Stone (1993).

The focus of the present chapter is those persons who consider themselves culturally Deaf. The perspective a culturally Deaf person may have on communication is often quite different than that which a hard of hearing or late-deafened adult might possess. Deaf people may not see themselves as having a hearing "loss," as most were born this way or became deaf early in their childhood. Therefore, they do not perceive themselves as *dis*abled, but as members of a unique community. This viewpoint can have a significant impact on the professional's successful service to this population. In order for services to be provided successfully, respect for an individual's identification as culturally Deaf needs to be maintained, and some aspects of therapy should be modified to meet needs within the culture as well as cross-culturally.

Characteristics of the Culturally Deaf Population

The following sections will discuss further the characteristics of culturally Deaf individuals and their perspectives on service delivery.

Language

The most important characteristic of Deaf culture is the language used by this population. In 1960 William Stokoe determined that American Sign Language, commonly referred to as ASL, was a language unto itself, containing all the necessary components of a language (Gannon 1981). He found that ASL was "the native and natural language of Deaf people (Gannon 1981, 365). It has its own set of rules for grammar and syntax, including regional signs, which are similar to spoken dialectical differences. It is full of the nuances of any language and, as such, is continually growing and expanding. Hypothetical thinking and all levels of abstraction can be expressed fluently through ASL. Because ASL has its own syntactical structure, it is impossible to speak English and sign ASL simultaneously and remain grammatically correct in both languages (Stokoe 1994). When a person combines spoken English and ASL, using them simultaneously, it then becomes a form of "contact signing." (Contact signing will be discussed later in this chapter.) There are adjectives, adverbs, and even lip movements, that do not correspond with English grammar or articulatory patterns of spoken English. Most signs have been found not to be iconic or picture representations (Bienvenu 1991).

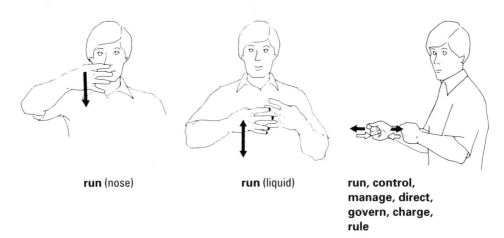

run (nose)   **run** (liquid)   **run, control, manage, direct, govern, charge, rule**

Figure 1.1.   Some signs used to convey the word *run*
Source: Shroyer 1982.

ASL was adapted from French Sign Language, a language first recognized by Abbé Charles Michel de l'Épee, who opened the first school for deaf children in Paris in the 1760s. Laurent Clerc, a graduate of and teacher in the Paris school, taught French Sign Language to Thomas Hopkins Gallaudet, a young American who had traveled to the Paris school to learn the teaching methods employed there. Gallaudet convinced Clerc to come to the United States with him to help establish a school for deaf children in Hartford, Connecticut. Together, they introduced this sign language to America in 1817. Approximately 60 percent of ASL signs have their origins in the French Sign Language (Gannon 1981). It was not until 1960, when Stokoe first published his findings, that ASL was identified as having all the necessary components of a language.

The specificity of the language and the grammatical rules that govern it are extremely complex. Brownlee (1989) states: "The word *look*, for example, can be changed to mean *gaze, stare,* and *watch* by making the sign for *look* while moving the hand in a circle, holding it still, or moving it back and forth" (86). Figure 1.1 demonstrates the complexity this language possesses in the number of signs available to convey the various meanings of the word *run*. Each conceptually distinct meaning has its own sign. "My nose is *running*," "the water is *running*," and "she is *running* the company," are all signed differently based on the context.

ASL is different from all of the artificially designed systems, such as Signing Exact English (SEE) or Manually Coded English (MCE). These systems attempt to make spoken English visible on the hands. They combine speech, some ASL signs, and newly created signs used to represent English morphemes. These systems are not designed to convey the concepts, but rather to attempt to convey the structural components of the English language.

When Deaf people come into contact with hearing people, they use a form of code switching called Pidgin Sign English (PSE). PSE combines features of both ASL and English. Lucas and Valli (1989) demonstrated that the code switching is based upon the perceived or known level of hearing of the other person. They state that the "code choice is thus sensitive to the ability vs. inability of participants to hear" (14). Stokoe indicates that there may be two PSE forms. The "PSE d" used by deaf signers is different from the "PSE h" used by hearing signers (Lucas and Valli 1989). "PSE d" follows more of the ASL grammar, whereas "PSE h" would hold more strongly to the English framework.

Lucas and Valli (1989) recommend that the term PSE be changed to "contact signing." It should not be referred to as a "pidgin" because it is not a separate language and is not evolving into another language, as other true pidgin languages do. Contact signing is a general term that represents the resultant communication mode used whenever a Deaf and hearing person communicate with each other. It has been found to be used in formal situations, such as during an interview, and in informal communication exchanges with a stranger.

Traditions, Values, and Beliefs

The pragmatics and other communication behaviors of Deaf people are different than those of hearing persons because Deaf people rely on vision as their primary channel for communication. Thus, some traditions have evolved, such as the pragmatics of beginning a conversation, which include tapping the shoulder/ knee, waving the hands, stomping the feet, and blinking the lights. Instead of clapping in applause, many Deaf people will shake their hands in the air to show their appreciation (Gannon 1991).

An introduction between culturally Deaf persons tends to progress as follows: when a Deaf person meets another Deaf person, the most likely exchange to occur first would be to introduce their full names and then to identify the name and type of school they attended (e.g., residential). In this way, a common bond can often be established quickly because the Deaf community is closely knit and there will often be connections made to the school they attended and people they know from that area.

One cultural tradition is commonly referred to as "the never ending goodbye." When parting ways at the end of a gathering, Deaf people tend to continue their goodbyes all the way out to the car, stopping and sharing one more story before they part company. Before the advent of TTYs, captioning, and computer communications, most Deaf people would see each other only on a Saturday night at the local Deaf Club. It would be difficult for these weekend conversations to end once a group got together. Still today, Deaf people can be seen leaving a party, taking small steps out to the car, but continually stopping to tell one more joke or one more tidbit of news. This behavior may also be seen in clinical service delivery situations.

A value that many Deaf people hold is a bilingual, English-as-a-second-language philosophy (Johnson, Liddell, and Erting 1989). Defining bilingualism with regard to the education of Deaf people is an evolving process. Quigley and Paul (1984) state that bilingualism is "exposure to ASL and English concurrently in infancy and early childhood" (165). They go on to state that such exposure needs to occur before the child is three years of age because this is the critical language learning period. Second language learning is where "ASL [is] developed first in a normal interactive manner and English [is] developed late" (165).

Supporters of ASL are striving for early immersion into American Sign Language so that deaf children can be exposed to a complete, visual language within the critical first three to five years of life (Johnson, Liddell, and Erting 1989). Their view is that once this language base has been established, then written English and possibly spoken English will follow. They believe, though, that the language base needs to be established first; for Deaf Americans, this would be either American Sign Language or written English. Once the language base is established and second language learning has begun, then other communication skills may be enhanced.

The Maryland School for the Deaf (MSD) is one of a growing number of schools that have developed a "Bilingual Education Policy Statement" (1993). This policy focuses on ASL acquisition as well as written English acquisition and states that the development of spoken English will be provided for all children when and if it is deemed appropriate. This policy for bilingual or English-as-a-second-language (ESL) education represents the trend toward which some schools for the Deaf are moving.

Rogers (1995) indicates that within culturally Deaf populations directness in communication is also valued. For example, a Deaf person may say to a friend or acquaintance, "Wow, you've really put on some weight," whereas a hearing person might be more circumspect and say, "You're looking healthy today." Another example might occur at a job interview where a hearing person might ask, "Is there a restroom on this floor?" whereas a Deaf individual might be more specific and say, "I need to go to the bathroom." When interacting with hearing people, Deaf people may ask an interpreter to interpret word for word or ask her to make cultural modifications as appropriate.

Given the unique characteristics of Deaf culture, the cultural framework from which the clinician is working may be different than that which the client has experienced. Therefore, it is important to look at the way services are provided and how well the needs and desires of culturally diverse clientele can be met most effectively. The native language of the client, the preferred language, and the mode of communication in which services will be provided are all important considerations. If the language, cultural values, and beliefs held by Deaf persons are respected and understood by the clinician, then services can be provided more successfully. Kaplan states (Hull 1992), "Most people who are culturally [D]eaf will meet hearing clinicians half-way [related to communication style] . . . if convinced of the genuineness of the relationship" (143). The Deaf person is likely to accommodate the hearing person by code switching to approximate English word order more closely if the hearing person is perceived to be willing to modify her own communication style.

Diversity within the Deaf Community

The Deaf community is a microcosm of the hearing community in that it also includes various racial, ethnic, physically disabled, and other groups. Persons within these groups often have fewer opportunities than other Deaf individuals, may be faced with additional difficult communication situations, and may experience decreased service support systems. An appreciation of the cultural aspects of Deafness as well as other diversity is the basis for the humanistic integrated therapy design presented and discussed in these first two chapters.

Racial and Ethnic Diversity

Davila (1992) indicates that the "American system of educating deaf students has been very successful in serving the bright, exceptionally deaf person, but it has been *much less successful* serving those who are less able academically" (49). He goes on to add that this second group comprises a significantly larger number of African and Hispanic Americans. For communication specialists, understanding the language used and the cultural nuances of the populations served is the key to becoming cognizant of the group, their culture, and their needs and interests. The clinician's cultural framework is most likely to be different from that which the client has experienced. The native language of the client, the preferred language, and the mode of communication in which services will be provided are all important considerations.

The country of origin for some Deaf individuals may have a significant impact on the service delivery process. The individuals seeking services in this country come from a variety of backgrounds. The communication behavior of some cultures is influenced by religious upbringing, cultural values, and economic and technological advancements different from those found in the United States (Lane 1992). For example, a passive nature may be viewed as demonstrating respect for others in one's home country, but may not be as effective in the United States. The classroom teacher or specialist may be revered and never questioned. Additionally, decisions regarding communication and educational options may be made by elders in a community, with very little input from the Deaf individual. These factors may result in a need to develop trust over a longer period of time before the person will feel free to discuss personal communication issues or disagree overtly with a professional's opinion or recommendation (Chough 1993).

Many cultures view a handicap or disability very differently than the majority culture does in the United States. There may be feelings of shame and guilt that the family must bear when a child is "different." Discussing genetic causes with a family of this background is often very difficult. Also, many cultures prefer to take care of their own people, shunning outsiders who may be perceived as interfering with their disabled family member.

In addition, technology in many countries is at a minimum or nonexistent for deaf persons. For example, while doing an initial communication evaluation on a student, this author placed a teletypewriter (TTY) in front of a student from India and introduced a simulation exercise. This simulation required the student to look at a drawing depicting the clinician lying down in the therapy room suffering a heart attack. The client was instructed to contact the appropriate emergency professionals for assistance. The client looked at the TTY and at the phone for a long period of time. She eventually said, "I don't know what to do with this computer. I have never seen this before, and I can't use the phone, so I don't know how to get the rescue people except to look for a hearing person to call for me." When it was explained what the TTY was and how it worked, she was amazed. She responded through tears "I never in my lifetime thought I would ever be able to use the telephone myself!"

Another factor that may present a challenge for international Deaf persons is the use of figurative language in English. For example, this author was asked to explain what is meant by the statement, "the student was in a car accident and is in *grave* condition." Several international clients interpreted this to mean that the student had died. Confusion over the figurative use of language can present a challenge for Deaf Americans, but is compounded for international Deaf persons.

Learning Disabled Individuals with Hearing Loss

Powers, Elliott, and Funderburg (1987) have found that the largest subgroup of deaf special needs students have a learning disability in addition to a hearing loss. The actual incidence of learning disabilities in the deaf and hard of hearing populations is difficult to determine. Rush and Baechle (1992) and Cherow (1985) estimate that as many as seven percent of the deaf population also have learning disabilities (LD). However, they suspect that given the major etiologies related to deafness, there may be a higher proportion of deaf and hard of hearing individuals who also may have learning disabilities. Seven percent is generally consistent with national statistics of hearing students with learning disabilities (Sikora and Plapinger 1994).

Historically, learning disabilities in the deaf population have gone mostly undetected, undocumented, and underserved (Rush and Baechle 1992). One of the primary reasons for this may be that they are "hidden disabilities" because the student's educational difficulties are often attributed to the deafness, not to the possibility of a learning disability. Professionals have not agreed upon a definition for deaf individuals who also have a learning disability (e.g., Learning Disabled Hearing Impaired—LDHI). In addition, there is a lack of professionals with training in both deafness and learning disabilities (Rush and Baechle 1992).

The speech-language and audiology professional can be an important service provider for this population. Diagnostic audiologic results and a complete communication assessment are important components for the LD specialist to consider when determining a diagnosis. However, because of the limited number of appropriate tests designed to identify the learning disabilities of deaf people, it is challenging to make an accurate diagnosis. Interdisciplinary teaming in this area can be beneficial to the client and the professionals involved.

The following example illustrates the successful efforts of teaming an LD specialist, a communications specialist, and a student diagnosed with a learning disability. The student had specific difficulties in verbal and social reasoning and memory. The LD specialist was able to discuss and provide strategies on how to cope with the aspects of the learning disability, while the communication specialist provided strategies for more successful communication exchanges. One of the outcomes of this work was to develop an office memorandum for the student to use for future employment opportunities. With guidelines provided by both professionals, the client developed the memorandum, which described strategies for hearing employees to use when communicating with a person who is Deaf and has an LD.

Physical Disabilities

This group includes those Deaf persons who also may have an accompanying physical disability, such as Usher's Syndrome, cerebral palsy, closed head injury, multiple sclerosis, cancer, stroke, HIV, and AIDS. These Deaf individuals may have additional communication needs, and/or their communication needs may change as the disease progresses. Augmentative communication technology and communication strategies are skill areas that can be very important to this group. These needs should be approached with an understanding of the unique communication desires of Deaf persons, most likely requiring a culturally sensitive approach, involving sign communication as part of the overall communication therapy needs. Teaming with allied professionals from the medical, counseling, and social work fields is vital to providing optimal services. This interdisciplinary approach is critical when providing services and support to Deaf persons with disabilities. The professionals involved should be those who understand the cultural implications for groups described in this section.

The following example illustrates this author's experience with a Deaf cerebral palsy client. While doing research on the type of augmentative communication devices on the market, it became evident that there is a wealth of options for the person with CP, but that adapting the equipment for a person who is deaf was very difficult. The establishment of an interdisciplinary team—hospital rehabilitation specialists, interpreters, equipment representatives, the communication specialist, and the client—provided the necessary professionals to determine the client's needs and desires and to make appropriate modifications related to the augmentative communication devices.

Clients with physical disabilities may seek or need additional information regarding their physical disability. For example, clients with Usher's Syndrome often seek out communication services. Many persons with Usher's Syndrome are unaware of its implications or of the connection between their hearing and their vision. The unique communication needs of this population are important for the communication specialist to recognize. Through interdisciplinary interaction the client may be educated about Usher's Syndrome, retinitis pigmentosa, and its genetic implications as well about as the range of communication strategies available.

Other Issues of Diversity

Sensitivity to other aspects of the client's life (e.g., sexual orientation or religious beliefs) may also affect the communication therapy process. For example, a Deaf Quaker woman was enrolled for communication therapy. The clinician had to modify his approach to assertiveness training based upon her strong religious beliefs (Bally 1994).

Cultural and Medical Paradigms

A paradigm represents the way one looks at a situation, the way one views the world, or the model or archetype used to describe a group of patterns (Webster's *New College Dictionary* 1975). The individual's view is based on how she perceives the world, often subconsciously. The paradigm we hold "shapes what we look at, and how we look at things. As educators, activists, researchers, professionals working with Deaf people, we are all influenced by the dominant paradigm, or by an alternative paradigm" (Kannapell 1993). For many professionals in speech and hearing, the prevailing paradigm for all persons with hearing loss is based on a medical or pathologic model. This viewpoint leads them to look at the Deaf person's condition as something that is diseased, lacking, deviant, broken, or in need of fixing. This approach focuses on the hearing loss and resulting "communication disorder," thus establishing a deficit-based model. This may be consistent with the view held by some hard of hearing and/or late-deafened adults, but it is a view not shared by many Deaf individuals.

An alternative paradigm for viewing the latter group is a cultural one. People with this perspective see a Deaf person as a person with a different language and culture, as a whole person, not disabled and not interested in "being fixed." Early detection is a "diagnostic" goal that Deaf persons support. But the "medicalizing" of deaf individuals begins once the child is found to be deaf, a practice with which Deaf people strongly disagree. Culturally Deaf people want early detection so that early language stimulation through ASL can be provided to the infant, thereby providing a full and complete language as early as possible.

As described in an earlier section of this chapter, Deaf individuals have values often different from those of hearing persons, particularly in the area of communication. To provide optimal services, their values, viewpoints, and desires need to be respected. This by no means negates the services that may be appropriate for these persons, but the importance placed on a particular communication skill should be considered. In reality, both the medical and cultural approaches may be held concurrently by professionals in the communication fields of audiology and speech-language. There is merit in this because the medical background needs to be fully examined and discussed within a cultural framework.

Factors Related to Successful Service Delivery

Factor 1: Approaching Clients with Honesty Regarding Their Communication Skills

Dr. J. Pachciarz, a medical doctor who is herself Deaf, explains how her speech-language specialists did not approach her regarding her communication skills with the honesty that should have been afforded her (Corbet and Madorsky 1991). She states, "One factor [was] that I had gone to all the interviews without an interpreter. I depended on my speech because I was programmed to believe that I could talk, that I could succeed in the hearing world. . . . There were people who were kind to me, too kind. They didn't just come out and tell me that my speech was not understandable by the general public. It takes a little time for a person to understand my speech, and for an interview, that's not good. Speech therapy never got me into medical school. Interpreters got me into medical school" (Corbet and Madorsky 1991, 517). Pachciarz is not alone. Many Deaf adults have described to this author that speech and hearing professionals would tell them their speech was good, but they would then go out to use their speech and would face embarrassment at not being understood.

Factor 2: Communicating Clearly with the Client

The lack of skilled signers in the speech-language and audiology professions is a very sensitive topic among Deaf persons. Both hostility and suspicion are apt to surface when members of the professions communicate in front of the Deaf person, without signing (Hull 1992). To illustrate this, Vold, Kinsella-Meier, and Singer (1990) asked Deaf adults to draw themselves communicating in both Deaf and hearing communities. The purpose of the activity was to ascertain their level of comfort in each community and to allow them to express this without the constraints of language to bind them. Deaf persons tend to be strong visually and less comfortable with rhetoric (Vold 1995). This approach capitalizes on their strengths to communicate visually and to tell their own stories through their

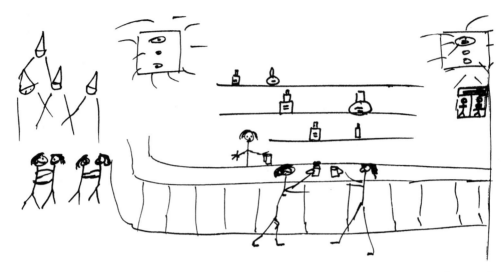

Figure 1.2. A Deaf adult's drawing of himself communicating in the Deaf community
Source: Vold, Kinsella-Meier, and Singer 1990.

drawings. The pairs of drawings are quite revealing in that they make clear the Deaf persons' attitudes while communicating in both groups. Figures 1.2 and 1.3 represent a sampling of these drawings as they responded to the questions "How do you feel when you are communicating in the Deaf community?" and "How do you feel when you are communicating in the hearing community?" respectively.

In figure 1.2, the Deaf individual indicated, "In the Deaf community I am happy, I have friends, we like to go to the Abbey [pizza cafe] and have fun and dance. Life is fun!" In figure 1.3, the same individual indicated, "In the hearing community I feel sad and alone, communication is too tough, I don't talk to many people." These two drawings indicate the vast difference in the comfort level this individual experiences in each community, with an emphasis on communication skills. Through this type of pictorial representation, other students have indicated they are nervous and/or "begin sweating" when they see professionals because those individuals cannot sign and, thus, cannot communicate easily (Vold, Kinsella-Meier, and Singer 1990). This would suggest a need for communication professionals to learn the language of the Deaf individuals with whom they interact.

Factor 3: Providing an Information Base for the Client

Fred Schreiber, past president of the National Association of the Deaf (NAD), addressing a group of audiologists, stated the following: "I sat down to assess what I knew about audiology and speech pathology, and it may not come as a surprise to most of you that the sum total of my knowledge added up to a little

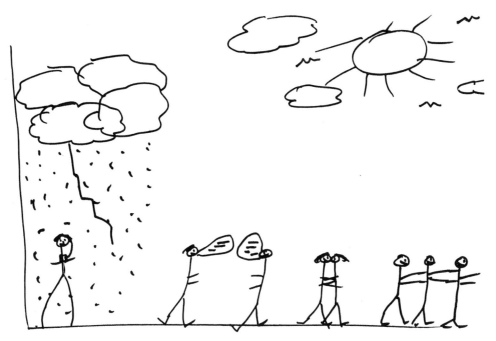

Figure 1.3. A Deaf adult's drawing of himself communicating in the hearing community
Source: Vold, Kinsella-Meier, and Singer 1990.

more than zero" (Schein 1981). One possible explanation for his comment could be that professionals do not provide sufficient information regarding their fields of expertise.

In addition, Deaf adolescents and adults appear to have insufficient information regarding their own communication skills and abilities. In an informal 1992 communication class survey, students were asked to describe the type of speech work they had done in speech therapy while growing up. The results indicated that the students were shocked to see that most of the other students also had been working on the same speech sounds. They had never known that their "errors" were common for Deaf persons to make. In addition, they had no understanding of the reasons why these were difficult sounds for them to produce. Ultimately, as a result of class discussions, there was the realization that their muscles *do* work in the larynx, that their minds are fine, and that there is a *reason* why these sounds are difficult. Following this type of discussion, some individuals inevitably seek out communication services. As one client seen by this author stated, "Now that I understand that my speech is similar to other Deaf persons, and I understand why this is so, I would like to see if I can improve it." These discussions occurred in a college level classroom and could easily occur in the elementary school classroom.

Table 1.1 Terminology

Current Usage	Projected Usage
hearing impaired, disordered, handicapped, disabled	Persons who are: deaf, hard of hearing, late deafened
hearing loss	hearing levels
prelingual postlingual	*Describe background:* age of onset; communication environment; age identified; additional needs of the child
patient	client, consumer
clinic	center

Factor 4: Becoming Aware of the Importance of Labels

Levitan (1993b) states, "Our long and bitter experience as an oppressed minority group has shown that labels can be very powerful weapons. Labels have caused us an immeasurable amount of damage—in terms of self-esteem, pride, and squelched potential as well as the more tangible economic sense . . . [and] called attention to our supposed deficits—never our strengths" (8). Bienvenu (1991) concurs: "How we label ourselves is very important. I don't know many deaf people who would define themselves as 'communication disordered,' yet that is the term many social service agencies and schools use to describe the deaf population with whom they work" (22).

In an effort to represent the most current viewpoints on which terminology is most acceptable to Deaf persons, an informal survey was conducted (Kinsella-Meier 1993b). Requests for feedback regarding terminology were sent out to various organizations representing Deaf, hard of hearing, late-deafened adults, and fellow professions. Table 1.1 summarizes some of the current terminology commonly used in the fields of audiology and speech-language pathology and the projected usage that would be more desirable in the Deaf community. Changing the words does not change the entire perspective a person has for a group, but it does allow the emergence of respect to grow.

Factor 5: Using Appropriate Evaluation Tools

Formal and informal evaluation tools tend to focus on what the client can't do instead of what the client can do. This fact may have an impact on the client's perception of services. When the clinician does not have the proper tools to work with Deaf people, Deaf people may not seek out the services. One possible way to adjust this perception is to provide ways to give the client positive feedback about what she can do as well as identify problem areas. For example, a diagnostic goal may be to perform an initial evaluation of a client's ability to sequence written English when provided with a picture story. A written language sample will then be evaluated for problem areas. The clinician may ask a Deaf client who uses ASL as her primary mode of communication to tell the story in ASL first. This approach helps the clinician evaluate the strengths of the client in formulating a story in the language with which she is skilled and provides a more comfortable environment for the client. In addition, clinical experience with Deaf clients indicates that formulation of written English may be facilitated by expressing a story first in ASL.

Integration of the Medical and Cultural Models

Ellicott and Ellicott (1993) state that "when it comes to succeeding in the profession, human relations skills are just as important as technical knowhow" (6). They continue, "The empathetic therapist will be able to quickly establish good rapport with his or her students" (6).

In an analysis of the ingredients needed for communication therapy services to be successful, one primary ingredient may be the *attitude* of the professional. The services of speech-language specialists and audiologists traditionally have been referred to as part of the *helping* professions. This view of the profession may be perceived by Deaf individuals as giving them very little control over their own communication needs, and so they view the professional as patronizing and oppressive. According to Whitehead and Barefoot (1992), the adulthood of the client needs to be recognized and the therapy approached from an adult model. This implies an equal role for both participants in the therapy process. It is important for the client to direct the sessions and to make the decisions based on increased awareness and understanding provided by the clinician.

In an humanistic/empathic approach, the Deaf adult helps decide the direction of her own communication goals, based on complete, realistic information and an understanding of her communication skills. The clinician may guide the client in the following ways:

1. He or she can be forthright with the client about actual communication skills. This establishes a level of honesty and trust necessary for successful enhancement of communication skills.

For example, in educating the client about her speech and in letting her know why parts of the body are making speech in this way, the clinician might say, "Your speech tends to be nasal, because you are able to monitor your speech better when you send sound through your nasal cavity. Try it, feel around your cheek area. That is your body's way of giving you feedback naturally." The person begins to realize that vocal chords do function and then can decide if work on

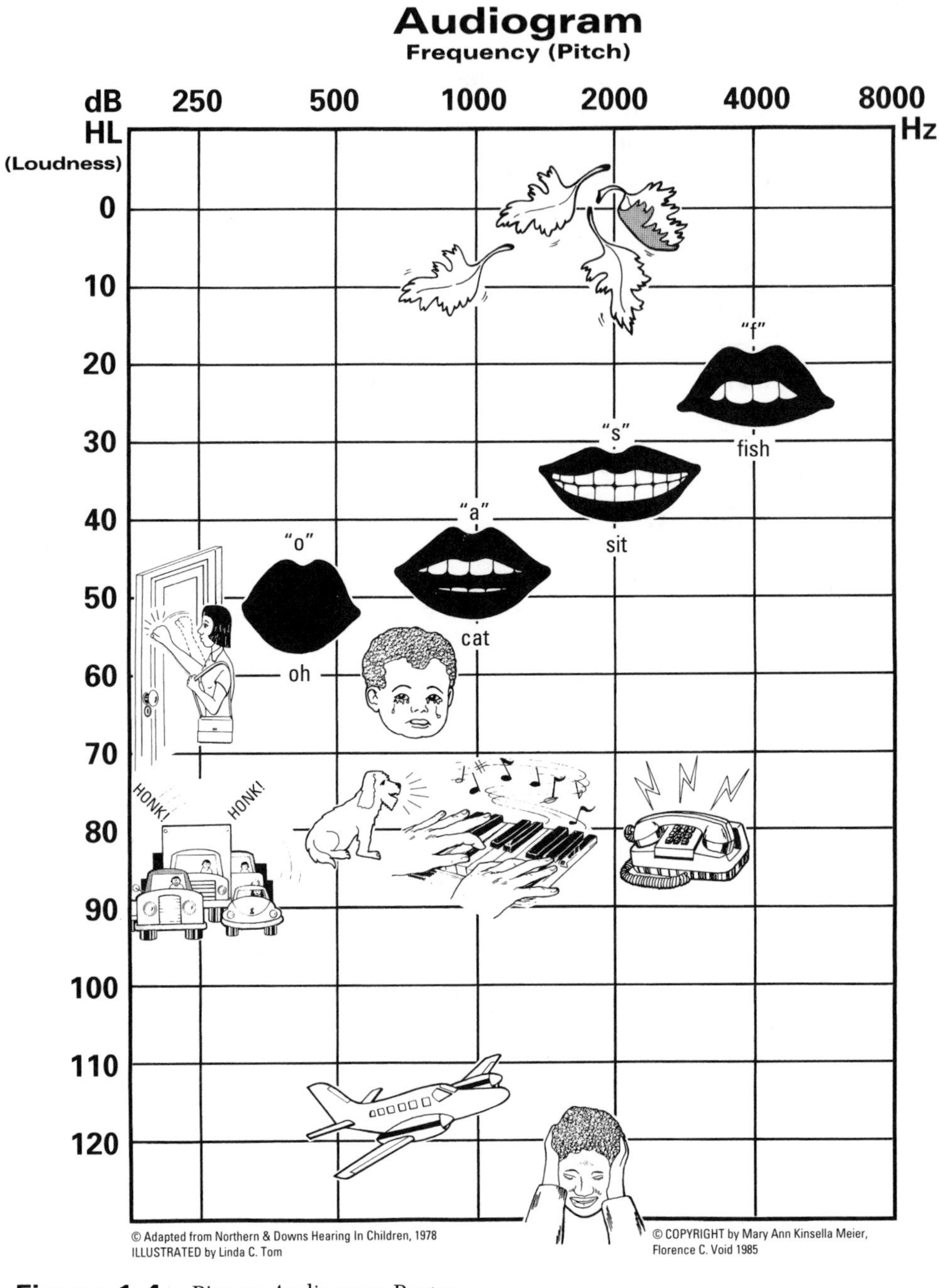

Audiogram
Frequency (Pitch)

Figure 1.4. Picture Audiogram Poster

Source: Kinsella-Meier and Vold 1985.

improving her voice or articulation is desired. When a client's maturity level is respected and appropriate teaching techniques are employed, he can gain a greater understanding of his own body and develop realistic expectations related to his communication skills.

2. He or she can modify information to ensure that it is visually clear and understandable to the Deaf client. The professional may choose to educate the client about her auditory system, including unaided and aided hearing levels, as well as the frequencies and decibels that can or cannot be heard. With this basic knowledge, the client can better understand how these results affect both receptive and expressive aural/oral communication skills. For example, this might include how the high frequency consonant components of speech may be missing and how this may impact expressive and receptive spoken language skills. The Picture Audiogram Poster (figure 1.4) (Kinsella-Meier and Vold 1985) was designed to provide more concrete examples of decibel (dB) and pitch. This audiogram enables clients and family members to better understand this important relationship.

In another example of how to change from a more auditory approach to an approach in which information is shared visually, the clinician begins to think of ways to describe the abstract concepts of frequency and intensity in ways that make them more concrete to the Deaf person. This author has found the use of paint sample swatches an excellent way to describe decibel levels. For example, 500 Hz may be represented with a gray swatch of color, the lightest shade being 0–20 dB HL and the darkest shade on the swatch being 90 dB HL or greater. Purple may be chosen to represent the high-pitched region of 8,000 Hz, with the shades of lavender to deep purple representing the variations in loudness or dB. This presents the information in a visual mode and in a way that the Deaf individual can understand.

3. He or she should include the client in the decision-making process. The client then becomes an active participant in the sessions and a decision maker. An understanding of the client's current level of skills leads to the establishment of a framework from which to build on or improve should the client choose to do so. It is necessary, and in the client's best interest, to establish first the "more medical" understanding in order to project the possibilities of what *can* be accomplished realistically on a short- and long-term basis.

Davila says it best in his discussion of deaf and hard of hearing persons: "Empowerment means providing persons with the knowledge and skills required to take control of their own lives and make their own decisions" (1992, 49).

Complete Communication Spectrum

The following section describes the humanistic-empathic approach through integrated communication therapy. This approach considers two parts to the process of communication therapy: (1) solving the needs of the client and (2) inte-

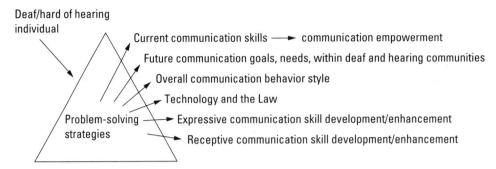

Figure 1.5. Complete communication spectrum
Source: Kinsella-Meier 1993a.

grating different skill areas into a communication therapy session. The first area will be discussed below. The second area is discussed at length in chapter 2.

The Complete Communication Spectrum (Kinsella-Meier 1993a) (see figure 1.5) visually demonstrates a problem-based, critical-thinking approach to services. Based on problem-solving scenarios most often provided by the client, the various spectrum of communication issues can be explored jointly by the client and clinician. The focus encompasses the communication interests of the client and need not be limited to spoken language or aural skills.

The triangle in the Complete Communication Spectrum represents the interaction of the client and clinician. The communication issues of deaf and hard of hearing individuals are brought to the therapy session. Discussion of these issues may have several outcomes, as represented by the arrows to the right of the triangle. The top three arrows represent discussion of communication needs and style. Discussion of current communication skills may lead to empowerment in communication situations. Future communication goals and needs, as well as overall communication style, of both Deaf and hearing communities will influence the progression of therapy.

The fourth arrow, technology and the law, represents the need for consumer information based on the recent innovations in the field, such as continual new technological developments and the passage of the Americans with Disabilities Act (ADA). (Technology will be discussed more in chapter 6 and the ADA in chapter 3.) The last two arrows represent the decisions made regarding specific areas of receptive or expressive communication that the client wants to include in the therapy process. Once decisions have been made regarding which skill areas to include in the communication therapy process, integrated therapy can occur. Throughout communication therapy, problem solving will continue to occur, as communication goals are reached and/or contexts change.

The Integrated Therapy Model, focusing on the skill areas, will be described in chapter 2 and will be discussed in depth in the remainder of the book.

Summary

This chapter has emphasized the unique characteristics of the culturally Deaf population and how the speech-language-hearing professional can best meet the needs and interests of this group. American Sign Language (ASL) and its impact on the linguistic and cultural development of the Deaf population were investigated. The diversity that exists within the Deaf community and how this diversity impacts the individual and clinical service were described. Several case examples were provided. Perspectives of Deaf consumers regarding the service delivery process illustrated the importance of communication and information for successful service delivery to be achieved. A model for meeting the needs of the client was discussed within the context of communication therapy. Aspects of the models discussed in this chapter will be further expanded upon in other chapters throughout this book.

References

Bally, S. J. 1994. Personal communication.

Be in the know: Your complete guide to terminology about hearing loss and communication access. 1993. *SHHH Journal* (January/February): 18–20.

Bienvenu, M. J. 1991. Can deaf people survive 'deafness'? *Perspectives on Deafness: A Deaf American Monograph* 41(2): 21–28.

Brownlee, S. 1989. The signs of silence: A deaf child's brain is primed to learn sign language easily. *U.S. News & World Report,* 16 October, 86–88.

Cherow, E., ed. 1985. *Hearing impaired children and youth with developmental disabilities.* Washington, D.C.: Gallaudet University Press.

Chough, S. K. 1993. The struggle to survive in America. Paper presented at Gallaudet University, Washington, D.C.

Corbet, B., and J. Madorsky. 1991. Physicians with disabilities. *Rehabilitation medicine: Adding life to years* [special issue] 154: 514–521.

Davila, R. R. 1992. The Black deaf experience: Empowerment and excellence. *Viewpoints on Deafness: A Deaf American Monograph* 42(3): 49–52.

Ellicott, B. A., and D. G. Ellicott. 1993. Addressing the psychological aspects of speech. *Advance for Speech-Language Pathologists and Audiologist* 3(10):49–52.

Gannon, J. R. 1981. *Deaf heritage: A narrative history of deaf America.* Silver Spring, Md.: National Association of the Deaf.

Gannon, J. R. 1991. The importance of a cultural identity. *Perspectives on Deafness: A Deaf American Monograph* 41(2): 55–58.

Hull, R. H. 1992. *Aural rehabilitation.* San Diego, Calif.: Singular Publishing Group.

Johnson, R. E., S. K. Liddell, and C. Erting. 1989. *Unlocking the curriculum: Principles for achieving access in deaf education.* Gallaudet Research Institute working paper 89-3. Washington, D.C.: Gallaudet University.

Kannapell, B. 1993. The power structure in the Deaf community. Paper presented at Studies III: Bridging Cultures into the 21st Century, 22 April, Chicago, Illinois.

Kannapell, B., and P. Adams. (1984). *An orientation to deafness.* Washington, D.C.: Gallaudet College.

Kinsella-Meier, M. 1993. Communication Spectrum Model. Gallaudet University, Washington, D.C.

———. 1993b. Terminology survey. Gallaudet University, Washington, D.C.

Kinsella-Meier, M., and F. C. Vold. 1985. Picture Audiogram Poster. Gallaudet University, Washington, D.C.

Lane, H. 1992. *The mask of benevolence: Disabling the Deaf community.* New York: Alfred Knopf.

Levitan, L. 1993. Why do deaf people use the term "hearing"? *Deaf Life* March: 8–9.

———. 1993. What do others call us? And what do we call ourselves? *Deaf Life* May: 2–29.

Lucas, C., and C. Valli. 1989. Language contact in the American Deaf community. In *The sociolinguistics of the Deaf community,* ed. C. Lucas. Boston: Academic Press.

Padden, C., and T. Humphries. 1988. *Deaf in America: Voices from a culture.* Cambridge: Harvard University Press.

Powers, A., R. Elliott, and R. Funderburg. 1987. Learning disabled hearing-impaired students: Are they being identified? *Volta Review* (February/March): 99–105.

Proposed Bilingual Education Policy Statement. 1993. Frederick, Md.: Maryland School for the Deaf.

Quigley, S. P., and P. V. Paul. 1984. *Language and deafness.* San Diego, Calif.: College Hill Press.

Rogers, P. 1995. Personal communication.

Rush, P., and C. Baechle. 1992. Learning disabilities and deafness: An emerging field. *Gallaudet Today* 22(3):20–26.

Sanders, D. A. 1993. *Management of hearing handicap: Infants to elderly,* 3rd ed. Englewood Cliffs, N.J.: Prentice Hall.

Schein, J. D. 1981. *A rose for tomorrow: Biography of Frederick C. Schreiber.* Silver Spring, Md.: National Association of the Deaf.

Sikora, D. M., and D. S. Plapinger. 1994. Using standardized psychometric tests to identify learning disabilities in students with sensorineural hearing impairments. *Journal of Learning Disabilities* 27(6):352–359.

Stokoe, W. C. 1994. Personal communication.

Stokoe, W. C., and R. Battison. 1981. Sign language, mental health, and satisfactory inter-action. In *Deafness and mental health,* ed. L. K. Stein, E. D. Mindel, and T. Jabaley. New York: Grune & Stratton.

Stone, H. E. 1993. *An invisible condition: The human side of hearing loss.* Bethesda, Md.: SHHH Publications.

Vold, F. C. 1995. Personal communication.

Vold, F. C., M. Kinsella-Meier, and B. Singer. 1990. Paper presented at the Academy of Aural Rehabilitative Audiology Summer Conference, Howie-in-the-Hills, Florida.

Webster's new collegiate dictionary. 1976. Springfield, Mass.: G&C Merriam.

Whitehead, B. H., and S. M. Barefoot. 1992. Improving speech production with adoles-cents and adults. *Volta Review* 94 (November): 119–134.

2

An Integrated Therapy Model

Mary Pat Wilson and Susanne M. Scott

■ ■ ■ ■

A familiarity with approaches to adult aural rehabilitation is of particular interest to the audiologist or speech-language pathologist working in the field of rehabilitative audiology. Although a variety of approaches are applicable to the individual with acquired hearing loss (Hull 1982; Alpiner and McCarthy 1993), limited information is available for providing services to the culturally Deaf adult.

The information in this chapter will provide professionals with a framework for a functional program of aural rehabilitation, including an integrated therapy model and overall assessment procedures leading to the establishment of rehabilitation goals. Although the approach presented is appropriate for a variety of populations, the focus will be on its application to hard of hearing and culturally Deaf clients.

Culturally Deaf individuals who seek aural rehabilitative services frequently want to function biculturally, by developing greater communicative independence in those situations where they need to interact with the "hearing world," such as in the workplace. This type of client presents a unique constellation of attitudes and motivational levels, existing skills, and communicative needs and interests. The integrated therapy approach presented in this chapter is designed to address the unique needs of this clientele through the development of functional skills for those communication situations that the deaf or hard of hearing client has deemed important in his career, social, and personal interactions.

Framework and Assessment

The professional who provides aural rehabilitative services to the hard of hearing and deaf client is faced with many challenges. Among these is the dearth of assessment tools developed for and standardized on deaf and hard of hearing populations, particularly in the adult and adolescent age groups (Horn et al. 1983). The limited number of assessment procedures that have been developed to evaluate the communication skills of the deaf and hard of hearing client have focused primarily on younger populations (Ling 1976; Moog and Geers 1979). Many of these tools can still be used with older populations as one component of the overall assessment process, as long as the results are used as a baseline for functional skills and not compared to the normative data.

Another related challenge is the need for determining a set of criteria for differentiating communication "needs" from the more traditional communication "disorders" or "pathologies." Barefoot (1982) has defined "speech needs" as "any aspect of speaking that is important for an individual deaf person to acquire and use in his or her own communication situations" (210). To apply and expand Barefoot's definition, "communication needs" could be defined as any aspect of receptive or expressive communication important for an individual deaf person to acquire and use in his or her own communication situations. These needs are practical ones chosen from the communication circumstances of each deaf person. Although some of these "needs" may coincide with the more traditionally defined "abnormalities," the deaf client and clinician may judge some "errors" as presenting no communication problems and some undeveloped skills as being unnecessary to acquire (Barefoot 1982). Thus, the need that the deaf client has for a particular skill in his or her *functional* communication interactions becomes the criterion for determining skill areas of focus in therapy, rather than the traditional comparison of the skill level to a standard norm.

Although a client may not always know the areas of concentration in therapy that would meet his particular needs, he can usually describe the communication situations in which those needs arise. For example, a client may express the desire to function more independently (without the help of a friend, parent, spouse, or interpreter) when he visits his doctor, dentist, or barber. Following the expression of the client's situational needs, the clinician may offer guidance in determining the most appropriate skill areas of concentration in order to facilitate meeting those needs. (For the above client, the stated needs may translate into focus on pronunciation of vocabulary related to specific situations, speechreading of situational vocabulary and phrases, and improvement in the use of communication strategies.)

A framework for determining communication needs and establishing therapy goals is depicted in figure 2.1. This model includes a system for assessing communication that allows for two outputs at the assessment stage: the client's perception and the clinician's perception. (For simplicity, the model depicts only one

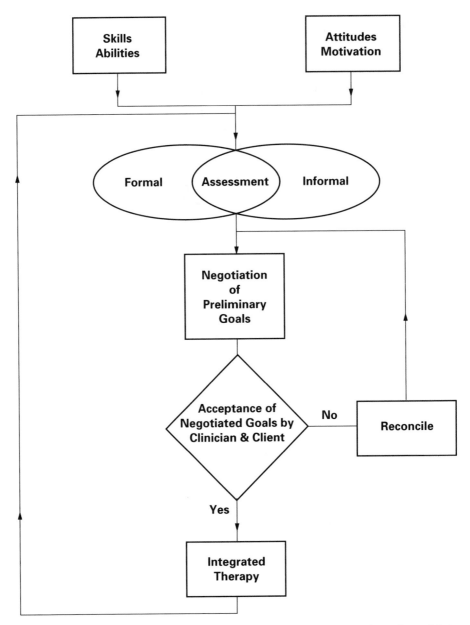

Figure 2.1. Framework for determining communication needs and establishing therapy goals

Revised Source: Wilson, Bally, Hughes, Kaplan, Kinsella-Meier, and Moseley 1990.

box each for skills/abilities and for attitudes/motivation. The following discussion, however, will describe how the client's perception of his skills/abilities and attitudes/motivation are integrated with the clinician's perception through the assessment and negotiation processes.) The client's perception of his communication skills is often based on communication experiences, as well as on feedback received from family, friends, and previous clinicians. When real-life experiences have been in conflict with feedback received about communication, the client may have developed unrealistic expectations about his communication abilities, either overestimating or underestimating these skills. The clinician's perception of the client's communication skills is based upon the interview, observation, and formal and informal assessment. A major goal of this approach to assessment and negotiation of therapy objectives is to help the client develop a more realistic view of his skills and become better able to self-evaluate in communication situations.

Assessment

The top portion of the model depicts *Assessment* as an interaction of formal and informal evaluative measures. A system for assessment should include an information gathering interview—skill assessment using traditional tools, role play, and analysis of the individual's overall communicative competence (Horn et al. 1983). Although traditional assessment tools and procedures are included in this framework, the results should be interpreted cautiously as they may not be an accurate indicator of how an individual functions in real-life situations.

An information gathering interview is an effective means of gaining insight into the client's *Attitudes and Motivation* (upper right-hand box of figure 2.1). As the initial contact between client and clinician, the interview provides a means of establishing rapport and affords the clinician an opportunity to assess the client's motivation for therapy and attitude towards oral/aural communication. Through this interview, the client can provide background information (i.e., age of onset, etiology, hearing threshold levels/stability, amplification/assistive technology use, educational history, and career goals) and prioritize those skill areas he is most interested in improving based on the kinds of communication interactions he regularly encounters. As part of the interview, the clinician may be able to make some initial judgments about the client's speech intelligibility (if voice is used), discourse skills, and overall effectiveness during oral/aural communication.

A client questionnaire is another means of assessing attitudes and motivation and is an important component of the information gathering process. (See appendix 2A for a sample of a questionnaire that has been used at the Gallaudet Aural Rehabilitation Clinic.) The client's responses on the questionnaire provide information about the reasons for current interest in communication therapy and insight into his self-perceptions of overall communication skills. Additionally, because the questions require a written response, the questionnaire provides the clinician with a means of informally evaluating the client's reading and writing skills.

Evaluation of the client's communication *Skills and Abilities* (upper left-hand box of figure 2.1) is accomplished through the use of both formal and informal assessment tools. In this chapter, formal assessment tools are defined as those tools that have been standardized on either a hearing or on a deaf and hard of hearing population. Informal assessment tools are those tools that have not been standardized. In the absence of normative data for the adult deaf and hard of hearing population for most of the formal tools, assessment results are interpreted cautiously within the context of the individual's communication needs and interests, as opposed to being compared to individuals who may be dissimilar in age and/or hearing ability. The primary value of assessment for this population is to establish a baseline of skill level competence for comparison purposes at a future time following intervention. (Assessment tools and procedures, as they relate to specific skills and abilities, will be discussed in later chapters devoted to the individual skill areas.)

Although assessment of specific communication skill areas provides important diagnostic information, it fails to provide information about other factors that have a significant effect upon the client's communicative competence. In order to determine the client's ability to integrate communication skills during difficult communication situations, the clinician must assess those skills through observation of the client during interaction in a functional environment. The use of role play may provide a means of assessing this interaction of skills and abilities with attitudes and motivation in a simulation of a functional setting. Examples of settings that can be used in therapy for the role play of communication encounters include visiting a physician's office, a restaurant, the dry cleaners, the ticket counter at an airport, etc. During role play, the clinician may gain some insight into the client's ability to integrate and generalize his or her skills and abilities, observe how attitudes and motivation may affect communication, and determine the kinds of communication strategies he currently employs. The results of role play, in conjunction with traditional assessment results, enable the clinician and client to make a better judgment about the client's overall communicative effectiveness.

Negotiation

Following the process of information gathering and assessment, the client and clinician arrive at the point of *Negotiation of Preliminary Goals* (middle of figure 2.1). When establishing functional goals for therapy, the clinician must consider the relationship between the assessment results and the client's communication needs, as well as his motivation, attitudes, and interests. Having considered those factors, the clinician can then present the suggested preliminary goals to the client for discussion and revision. When agreement has been reached between the client and clinician through mutual acceptance of the negotiated goals, they are ready to proceed with the *Integrated Therapy* process (bottom of figure 2.1). The client, satisfied that the goals are designed to meet personal communication needs, will take a more active role in the process of integrated therapy. If the perceptions of goal areas are not the same for client and clinician, further discussion and negotiation must occur in order to reconcile the perceived differences and establish a set of preliminary goals that are mutually agreeable (middle right-hand box of figure 2.1).

Integrated Therapy Model

Integrated therapy is an approach in which all aspects of communication are integrated in a given session into a meaningful, situationally based context. Communicative effectiveness in a variety of problem situations is enhanced through skill development and the use of appropriate communication strategies. The potential for greater carryover into real-life situations exists with this approach as compared to an isolated skill-development approach.

A visual representation of the integrated therapy process is shown in figure 2.2. As depicted in the model, all therapy areas are integrated, meaning that the focus of therapy is rarely on one receptive or expressive area only. Instead, work with the client in therapy focuses on those skill areas established as important during the negotiation process previously described. The skill areas are linked by focusing on the difficulties encountered during oral/aural communication as described by the client, with communication strategies, technology, and informational counseling supporting the process.

Global Areas

The model (figure 2.2) shows three concentric circles surrounding integrated therapy: Communication Strategies, Technology, and Informational and Adjustment Counseling. These represent global areas that are supportive to many aspects of skill development. In order to facilitate acquisition of new skills and/or modification of existing skills, it is beneficial to incorporate the global areas into the therapy process, as appropriate. For example, if a client wanted to acquire skills to increase success with the use of the voice telephone, it would be appropriate to include the global area of Technology, specifically exploration of appropriate telecommunication devices, in the therapy process. Each of these global areas will be described briefly here and covered in greater detail in later chapters devoted to each topic.

The innermost concentric circle represents *Communication Strategies,* defined as behaviors that allow an individual to avoid communication breakdown or resolve that breakdown when it occurs during oral/aural communication encounters. The use of appropriate anticipatory, maintenance, and repair strategies in situationally based communication encounters may contribute to a client's sense of confidence and control during those encounters. Anticipatory strategies are behaviors that occur prior to a communication event—that is, planning ahead

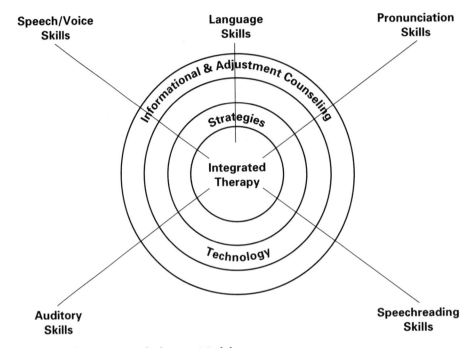

Figure 2.2. Integrated Therapy Model
Source: Wilson, Bally, Hughes, Kaplan, Kinsella-Meier, and Moseley 1990.

to prevent difficulty. Predicting dialogue and vocabulary, as well as analyzing potential environmental problems, are examples of anticipatory strategies. Maintenance strategies are behaviors that occur during a communication event to facilitate the continuation of a conversation. Maintaining appropriate eye contact and turn taking are examples of maintenance strategies. Repair strategies are behaviors that attempt to resolve communication breakdown when it occurs. Many repair strategies, such as repetition, can be used both receptively and expressively: the deaf or hard of hearing individual may ask the talker to repeat something more slowly (receptive), or he may repeat his own statement more slowly when it is clear that the listener did not understand (expressive).

The next concentric circle encompasses the area of *Technology*, which may be supportive to many aspects of expressive and receptive skill development. Included in the area of technology are feedback systems used for speech production, augmentative communication systems, conventional hearing aids, assistive listening devices, alerting devices, and telecommunication devices. Appropriate use of technology should be considered early in the therapy process, following needs assessment and negotiation.

The outermost circle on the model represents *Informational and Adjustment Counseling*, an integral part of the overall intervention process. Informational guidance is an activity during which the aural rehabilitationist provides information about tests and their results, the nature of the hearing loss and resulting communication difficulties, the need for amplification and/or assistive devices, consumerism and advocacy, and the various types of remediation. For a culturally Deaf client, this activity may be confined to providing information on the latest technology and the implications of the Americans with Disabilities Act (ADA), for example. Adjustment counseling is an activity during which the aural rehabilitationist assists the client in accepting the reality of the hearing loss and creates a climate in which solutions to the resulting communication difficulties can be found (Sanders 1980). Although this activity would not be appropriate for a culturally Deaf client, adjustment counseling may be very important for a client with a recent onset of deafness who is struggling to accept the reality of the changes that have occurred in his life. Informational and adjustment counseling are ongoing processes that may begin at the outset of therapy and resume again during the course of therapy as the need arises.

Skill Areas

In addition to the concentric circles surrounding Integrated Therapy, the model also depicts spokes that represent specific skill areas. The expressive areas include *Speech/Voice Skills* and *Pronunciation Skills,* and the receptive areas consist of *Auditory Skills* and *Speechreading Skills.* The *Language Skills* area encompasses both receptive and expressive modalities. The degree to which each of these skill areas will be incorporated into the integrated therapy process will have been determined during assessment and negotiation, previously discussed. Each area will be described briefly below and covered in greater detail in the chapters to follow that are devoted to the individual skill areas.

The upper left spoke of the model represents *Speech/Voice Skills,* which include articulation, voice characteristics, and intelligibility. In this model, articulation refers to the production of individual sounds in isolation and in connected discourse (coarticulation). Voice characteristics include resonance, voice quality, pitch, loudness, coordination of respiration and phonation, rate, and the prosodic features of blending, stress, and inflection. Speech intelligibility, a measure of the degree to which a segment of speech is understandable, can be evaluated through subjective or objective means. One subjective means for evaluating speech intelligibility is through the use of a rating scale by a trained listener or group of trained listeners (Frisina and Bernero 1958).

In the process of integrated therapy the relative emphasis placed on speech/voice skills is determined by a variety of factors, many of which have been determined through the interview, assessment, and negotiation stages. The most important factor for determining the emphasis placed on speech/voice skills, as well as all skill areas, is the communication preference of the deaf client. If the client chooses to use writing rather than voice in all communication interactions with hearing people, then speech/voice skills would not be selected as an area of focus in therapy. However, a client who is generally unintelligible in connected discourse may still demonstrate semi-intelligibility for a limited set of words or core vocabulary. For this individual, speech instruction may afford the opportunity to develop skills to facilitate improved communication in a variety of everyday encounters. Ultimately, the decision to focus on speech/voice skills should be made by the deaf client based on his communication preferences, abilities, needs, interests, and future goals.

The upper right spoke of the model represents *Pronunciation Skills,* which include knowledge of the rules for sound/symbol or phoneme/grapheme relationships and the ability to apply them to the pronunciation of unfamiliar vocabulary (Pschirrer 1980a and Bally 1984). Skills taught through pronunciation training include the functions of the phonemic (sound) and graphemic (letter) systems as well as their interrelationship; rules that determine what one says versus what one sees, including rules for letters that represent more than one phoneme, silent letter rules, and rules for past tense, plurals, and possessives; and dictionary symbols, such as vowel diacritical marks.

The deaf client for whom pronunciation skill training is appropriate is usually one whose preference is for oral communication, in at least some communication situations. Often the individual has previously experienced difficulty in independently learning the pronunciation of new vocabulary (Barefoot 1982) and may have avoided certain situations due to unfamiliarity with the correct pronunciation of key words specific to that situation or topic. Although overall intelligibility of the client's speech is not required for pronunciation training, an adequate speech base or semi-intelligibility is needed (Pschirrer 1980b).

The lower left spoke of the model represents *Auditory Skills,* which include suprasegmental and segmental speech-perception abilities, as well as perception of nonspeech sounds. The suprasegmental, or prosodic and temporal, features of speech include intonation, rhythm, stress, and duration (Stein et al. 1976). The segmental features of speech are the individual phonemes that comprise a syllable or word (Stein et al. 1976). Nonspeech sounds would include environmental sounds and music.

In determining the importance of auditory skill training for a given client, the clinician must first ascertain if there is sufficient auditory potential so that training will improve understanding of speech, with or without speechreading. If the auditory channel is the primary receptive mode, auditory skill training can focus on comprehension of connected speech in a variety of situations varying in complexity, both face-to-face (in quiet and in the presence of background noise) and on the telephone. The use of appropriate amplification and/or assistive listening devices is an integral part of this training.

For some individuals, auditory potential may not be sufficient for understanding of speech through audition alone, but may be sufficient for understanding of speech when combined with visual information. In these cases, auditory skill training would be combined with speechreading training to maximize the integration of visual and auditory cues for the perception of speech. Other individuals may not have sufficient auditory potential for understanding speech but may have sufficient residual hearing for awareness to environmental sounds, particularly warning signals. For these clients, auditory skill training might focus on the detection and discrimination of a variety of environmental sounds.

Auditory skill training also may be incorporated with speech and voice training to facilitate a client's ability to monitor and modify speech production, or it may occur as part of an individual's adjustment to hearing aid use, particularly for a new hearing aid user. As with the other skill areas, the clinician must be guided by the client's communication preferences, as well as his skills and needs, in determining the focus in the area of auditory skills.

The lower right spoke of the model represents *Speechreading Skills,* which include the use of visual information, as well as linguistic and situational clues. Visual information important for the reception of speech includes movements of the lips, tongue, and jaw; facial expression; body language; and gestures (Kaplan, Bally, and Garretson 1985). Comprehension of a message is aided by the integration of linguistic clues, including syntactic, semantic, and phonologic aspects (Stein et al. 1976) and by familiarity with vocabulary and dialogue related to a particular situation.

Speechreading skill training may be considered as a supplement to auditory skill training for the individual with sufficient residual hearing to rely primarily on the auditory channel. For this client, training may focus on learning to make maximum use of available clues to increase the likelihood of understanding a message under conditions in which auditory information may be incomplete or distorted. For the individual who must rely on visual information as the primary mode of reception, training may include analytic elements of viseme perception in addition to the synthetic training.

The center spoke of the Integrated Therapy Model represents *Language Skills,* which encompass both expressive and receptive modalities. Among the language skills that may be incorporated into the integrated therapy process are: vocabulary development, figurative language, morphology and syntax, pragmatics, and written expression. Vocabulary development may include work on basic vocabulary skills, job-related vocabulary development, or vocabulary enrichment. Figurative language development may include training in the following categories: multiple meaning words, similes, two word idioms, phraseological idioms, well-established sayings and proverbs, puns, and plays on words (Hughes, Brigham, and Kuerbis 1988). Language training in morphology and syntax may include work on sentence construction and forms of words and their formation by derivation and inflection. Language training in the area of pragmatics may include practice with discourse rules and taking the receiver's perspective. Written expression may be a component of the integrated therapy process when the client uses writing for communicative purposes, such as when communicating with salespeople, doctors, or waiters.

The language skill area is usually incorporated into most aural rehabilitation programs to some extent, regardless of whether the client communicates with hearing individuals through oral/aural or written expression. In the area of figurative language development, for example, a client may work on receptive understanding of idioms to improve his ability to understand everyday conversation and/or to improve his ability to comprehend newspapers, magazines, and other written materials. Expressively, the client may wish to improve his own use of idioms in either spoken language or written expression, depending upon his communication preference when communicating with nonsigners.

The focus of integrated therapy is to develop functional skills for those communication situations (employment, social, and personal) deemed important by the deaf or hard of hearing client during the interview and assessment process. This is accomplished by enhancing existing skills or developing new skills needed for communication success in those core situations. This may involve work in all or some of the skill areas listed in the model as communication problems are identified and analyzed. Although this concept will be demonstrated through case presentations in other chapters, a brief example will be described here.

Sample Case

A deaf college senior has enrolled in aural rehabilitation to prepare for good communication on the job after graduation. He will be working in an environment where he will have some contact with hearing employees. He currently has fairly intelligible speech, but demonstrates pronunciation difficulties with some multisyllabic words and unfamiliar vocabulary. Receptively, he is able to follow most conversations in quiet environments, when the topic is known, through the use of amplification and speechreading.

Following the process of assessment and negotiation, the client and clinician have agreed to focus on the following areas in therapy: pronunciation of job-related vocabulary, use of receptive and expressive communication strategies, understanding of common idiomatic expressions, exploration of assistive technology that might provide benefit on the job, and discussion of consumerism and advocacy issues. These skills will be developed and enhanced within the context of the situational constraints of his workplace and with the language and vocabulary specific to his intended vocation. Through the integrated therapy approach, the client can focus on the pronunciation of his job-related vocabulary, as well as speechreading that same vocabulary in the context of phrases and sentences that are likely to occur in his work environment. In addition, he can analyze challenging communication situations that might occur at work, such as small group meetings of three to four employees, and determine what strategies and/or technology would assist in improving communication in those environments. Through discussion of the ADA, he can be made aware of the types of accommodations that he would be entitled to in a particular work setting.

Over the course of therapy as skills are acquired or refined, they may be applied to additional situations that are considered important by the client. For example, he may choose to apply his knowledge of pronunciation rules and dictionary skills to the pronunciation of words related to his hobbies. Additionally, he may begin to analyze other situations in his social and personal life to determine if use of communication strategies and assistive technology could prove beneficial.

Summary

In this chapter, the process of integrated therapy has been described and schematically represented. In addition, a framework that includes the interview process, assessment procedures, and negotiation preceding the initiation of integrated therapy has been thoroughly described. The essential element of this integrated therapy approach is the focus on the individual as he interacts with others in a variety of communication encounters and environments, and as he assigns relative importance to those situations in regard to his lifestyle, goals, and values.

Appendix 2A
Gallaudet University Department of Audiology and Speech-Language Pathology Aural Rehabilitation Questionnaire

NAME: _____

DATE: _____

1. Why are you interested in improving your communication skills?

2. What are the communication areas *you* feel particularly weak in?

3. Have you ever had speech therapy/communication training before? What did you practice? (for example, using the telephone, saying long words, lipreading sentences, etc.)

4. Do you feel you improved because of this previous therapy/training?

5. Did you enjoy therapy/training?

6. Do you use a hearing aid?

7. How often do you use the hearing aid?

8. Do you usually use your voice on campus?

9. Do you usually use your voice off campus?

10. How do you usually communicate with hearing people who do not know sign language?

11. Where do you communicate with hearing people who do not know sign lan-

12. When you go out to restaurants, stores, bars, etc., do you make sure that you have a friend with you to help you communicate?

13. When *you* communicate in restaurants, stores, bars, etc., do you have problems communicating?

14. How do you feel when you have problems communicating?

15. What do you do when you have problems communicating?

16. Rate your communication skills in the areas listed below using this rating scale from 0 to 10.

0	1	2	3	4	5	6	7	8	9	10
no skills					average skills					excellent skills

Write in a number for each skill area:
ASL (American Sign Language) ـــــــــــ
PSE (Pidgin Sign English) ـــــــــــ
Speech ـــــــــــ
Speechreading ـــــــــــ
Understanding speech by listening ـــــــــــ
Voice telephone use ـــــــــــ
Understanding magazines and newspapers ـــــــــــ
Repairing communication breakdown ـــــــــــ

Source: Hughes and Wilson 1987.

References

Alpiner, J. G., and P. A. McCarthy, eds. 1993. *Rehabilitative audiology: Children and adults.* Baltimore: Williams & Wilkins.

Bally, S. J. 1984. *Pronunciation Skills Inventory.* Unpublished assessment tool, Gallaudet University, Washington, D.C.

Barefoot, S. 1982. Speech improvement by the deaf adult: Meeting communicative needs. In *Deafness and communication: Assessment and training.* Baltimore: Williams & Wilkins.

Erber, N. P. 1988. *Communication therapy for hearing impaired adults.* Victoria, Australia: Clavis Publishing.

Friedman, J. L., J. E. Hastings, D. Langholtz, and M. Hughes. 1989. Services for the culturally Deaf adult: Professional and consumer perspectives. Paper presented at the Annual Convention, American Speech, Language, and Hearing Association, St. Louis, Missouri.

Frisina, D. R., and R. J. Bernero. 1958. A profile of the hearing and speech of Gallaudet College students. *Volta Review* 60:316–321.

Horn, R., J. Mahshie, M. P. Wilson, and S. Bally. 1983. Audiologic habilitation with the hearing-impaired adolescent/adult: An integrative approach. Paper presented at the Annual Convention, American Speech, Language, and Hearing Association, Cincinnati, Ohio.

Horn, R., J. Mahshie, M. P. Wilson, S. Bally, and H. Kaplan. 1984. Assessing communication skills of the hearing-impaired adolescent/adult: A comprehensive approach. Paper presented at the Annual Convention, American Speech, Language, and Hearing Association, San Francisco, California.

Hughes, M. C., and M. P. Wilson. 1987. Aural Rehabilitation Questionnaire. Unpublished clinical questionnaire. Gallaudet University, Washington, D.C.

Hughes, M. C., E. T. Brigham, and T. L. Kuerbis. 1988. Approaches to teaching figurative language to hearing impaired students. Unpublished assessment and intervention materials. Gallaudet University, Washington, D.C.

Hull, R. H., ed. 1982. *Rehabilitative audiology.* New York: Grune & Stratton, Inc.

Kaplan, H., S. J. Bally, and C. Garretson. 1987. *Speechreading: A way to improve understanding.* 2d ed. Washington, D.C.: Gallaudet University Press.

Ling, D. 1976. *Speech and the hearing-impaired child: Theory and practice.* Washington, D.C.: Alexander Graham Bell Association for the Deaf.

Moog, J., and A. Geers. 1979. *CID grammatical analysis of elicited language.* St. Louis: Central Institute for the Deaf.

Pshirrer, L. 1980a. *Pronunciation training for students with poor hearing discrimination* (internal report). Rochester, N.Y.: National Technical Institute for the Deaf.

————. 1980b. Using imagery to teach independent pronunciation skills to deaf college students. *American Annals of the Deaf* 125:855–860.

Rohland, P. A., and B. Meath-Lang. 1984. Perception of deaf adults regarding audiologists and audiologic services. *Journal of the Academy of Rehabilitative Audiology* 17: 130–150.

Sanders, D. A. 1980. Hearing aid orientation and counseling. In *Amplification for the hearing impaired,* 2d ed., ed. M. C. Pollack. New York: Grune & Stratton, Inc.

Stein, D., G. Benner, G. Hoversten, M. McGinnis, and T. Thies. 1976. *Auditory skills curriculum.* North Hollywood, Calif.: Foreworks.

Wilson, M. P., S. Bally, M. C. Hughes, H. Kaplan, M. A. Kinsella-Meier, and M. J. Moseley. 1990. Current aural rehabilitative approaches for deaf and hard of hearing individuals. Paper presented at the Annual Convention, American Speech, Language, and Hearing Association, Seattle, Washington.

2

Global Areas of Communication Therapy

Introduction

Chapters 3 through 6 provide detailed information regarding areas that pertain to all aspects of the communication therapy process. In chapter 3, Bally discusses communication strategies that support receptive and expressive communication between two individuals. These strategies include information about environmental variables and ways to maintain and repair communicative interactions. Chapter 4 presents informational needs and adjustment counseling appropriate for aural rehabilitationists. Kaplan discusses how attitudes and motivation may be assessed and how this may affect the communication therapy process. Chapter 5, by Pray, further discusses adjustment needs by looking at the psychosocial factors involved in hearing loss, particularly with adults who become deaf later in life. The chapter provides information for the clinician on how individuals may cope with the onset of hearing loss. Pray also discusses some factors that may affect the culturally Deaf individual. In chapter 6, Kaplan presents technical information about available technology. The purpose of this chapter is to discuss the various kinds of technology that may be used to enhance the communication process.

3

Communication Strategies for Adults with Hearing Loss

Scott J. Bally

■ ■ ■ ■

Communication strategies may be broadly defined as anything a communicator does that facilitates, enhances, or repairs the communication process. These may include modifications in both expressive or receptive communication as well as in the communication environment. Such strategies may be employed in anticipation of a communication event to help prepare for it, during a communication event to help maintain it, or in a communication breakdown to help reestablish the process.

The objective of teaching communication strategies is to help persons with hearing loss increase communication effectiveness by using such strategies more efficiently and effectively. Intervention should result in a systematic increase of the number of strategies available and the frequency with which they are used appropriately.

Background

Expressive communication strategies are used to increase the efficiency and effectiveness of conveying information to a receiver. This may include oral or manual

Thanks to Mary Hilley, for conceptual development and strategy hierarchies, and to Fred Brandt, for graphics.

communication, including formal sign systems or the use of gesture, body language, and facial expression. Strategies may be used to help effectively convey or clarify information. Some may more specifically focus on directing or educating the communication partner as to how to better meet the needs of the person with hearing loss.

Receptive strategies are employed to increase the efficiency and effectiveness of speechreading or the comprehension of sign language. Kaplan (chapter 8) describes the components of speechreading (Sanders 1971) or speechreading to include lipreading; audition (residual hearing, use of amplification, vibrotactile information); nonverbal communication (body language, gesture, and facial expression); situational clues; and linguistic information. Linguistic information includes the primary visual, auditory, and cognitive information that, when integrated, composes our receptive communication. Therefore, the term *speechreading* in this chapter will refer to all receptive communication for the receipt of information through speech as experienced by persons with hearing loss. The term *lipreading* will refer to the analytic training of visual receptive skills only.

Although the environmental strategies to be discussed later in this chapter may vary based on the extent to which an individual is dependent on either the auditory or visual mode, other receptive strategies remain surprisingly similar. Because it is a natural process to integrate auditory, visual, and cognitive information, it is logical to assume that communication strategies should not isolate or emphasize one mode over the other. The most effective strategies are likely to be those that maximize the amount of information received, regardless of mode.

The Impact of Hearing Loss on Receptive and Expressive Communication

Because hearing loss limits or deprives an individual of one of the two predominant input modes used in today's society and environments, individuals who sustain such a loss are at a distinct communication disadvantage when functioning in the world at large. Hearing loss impacts on both receptive and expressive skills. The loss itself limits auditory input for speech and language and, in turn, often limits the feedback necessary for the development of effective articulation, voice, pronunciation, and expressive language ability. These limitations are further exacerbated by confounding environmental factors such as auditory and visual noise and poor lighting. It is necessary for persons who are deaf or have a hearing loss to develop behaviors that enable, enhance, or repair communication to compensate for such limitations.

Because of the varying degrees of hearing ability as well as an individual's communication abilities and preferences, the clinician may help the client identify and develop the most relevant and effective strategies. A mildly hard of hearing person might merely eliminate background noise to affect successful communication whereas a person with a more severe hearing loss might need a full range of repair strategies as well as environmental modifications.

For persons who identify themselves as hard of hearing and view their hearing loss as a disability, the challenges of overcoming the handicap may be perceived differently than by individuals who are culturally Deaf. As described by Pray in chapter 5, acceptance of the hearing loss may be a difficult process. It may be especially difficult for individuals who are hard of hearing to overcome the perception that they must assume exclusive responsibility for their hearing loss and its ramifications in the area of communication.

Hard of Hearing and Late-Deafened Individuals Onset of hearing loss may have an impact on how a hard of hearing individual views and responds to intervention. Individuals with progressive loss may be more likely to develop strategies naturally and over time. However, these strategies still may not have the depth and breadth needed for successful communication and may include counterproductive strategies that may or may not be helpful. By contrast, persons with sudden-onset hearing loss may find themselves with limited coping mechanisms, including strategies that work for hearing persons but are no longer successful given the diminished auditory input. Such individuals with reduced hearing ability, even with amplification, may be responsive to guidance in developing new and more effective approaches to communication. From either perspective, individuals may perceive themselves as handicapped and wanting to overcome barriers to communicating in their primary oral/aural language.

When seeking professional intervention, hard of hearing people may deny that they are able to speechread at all. The ability to lipread may not be recognized, but can be demonstrated in several ways. For example, the ability to acknowledge when a foreign film has been dubbed or the sound track is off on an English film is dependent on lipreading ability. Most people have experienced and can relate to either of these situations. Lipreading a few simple words within a limited set, such as days of the week or the numbers between one and ten, may also provide proof of lipreading ability for individuals who remain skeptical.

Deaf Individuals Deaf individuals, although successful communicators within their own culture and language, may find communication with hearing people a daunting prospect at best. Communication behaviors for communicating with hearing people modeled by family, teachers, and friends may have proven to have limited success. Communication strategies designed to meet an individual's specific skills and abilities may help her effect successful cross-cultural communication with hearing persons. This enables Deaf individuals to interface with "the hearing world" for vocational, economic, or educational purposes. The professional may wish to help these individuals approach communication with hearing individuals as "learning to access English as a second language." This demonstrates a respect for ASL and Deaf individuals' ability to communicate successfully, using appropriate communication strategies in their primary language. Additionally, it places the need for oral communication (receptively, expressively, or both) in an appropriate perspective (Andersson 1995).

The majority of strategies designed to foster more successful aural communication also have the result of improving visual communication (either lipreading or sign communication). The importance of this fact is relative to the varying degrees to which persons with hearing loss are dependent on oral or visual receptive ability. Regardless of an individual's degree of visual or auditory dependency, the use of communication strategies can be effective. For example, asking a person to speak more slowly may be as helpful to a hearing person making the request as it is to a deaf person who is almost completely dependent on lipreading. Similarly, asking a person to slow down manual communication (i.e., sign language) may also result in increased intelligibility of the message.

From a cultural perspective, these considerations provide a basis from which culturally Deaf individuals may see that the use of communication strategies is not exclusively their "burden." Individuals who are "culturally hearing" (sic) also routinely encounter difficult communication situations such as those where there is competing auditory or visual noise and in which they are forced to rely on combined visual and auditory modes as well as communication strategies.

Culturally Deaf individuals are frequently surprised to realize that hearing persons routinely use lipreading skills for reception (Andersson 1995). A hearing person's reliance on this ability can be demonstrated to deaf and hard of hearing individuals by describing the frustration of a hearing person when trying to communicate at a rock concert or sports event. The knowledge that the development of such receptive skills is not exclusively the domain of persons who are deaf or have a hearing loss may foster a greater acceptance of these therapy processes.

This chapter will focus on communication therapy that emphasizes anticipatory, maintenance, and repair strategies that may enhance the communication abilities of persons with hearing loss. Discussions will include impact of culture and onset of therapy, assessment of communication strategies, and therapy protocols for teaching communication strategies.

A Systematic Approach

Systematic training in the use of communication strategies may be fostered by helping clients to analyze communication situations and to apply appropriate receptive and expressive strategies specific to the identified problems (Erber and Greer 1973; DeFilippo and Scott 1978; Owens and Telleen 1981; Kaplan, Bally, and Garretson 1987; Erber 1988). To help clients learn an organized and manageable approach, two models may be applicable to understanding inherent structures of the communication process. These include (1) the Communication Model (figure 3.1) and (2) the Communication Event Time Continuum (figure 3.2).

The Communication Model

The Communication Model is a modification of traditional communication process models (Zimmerman, Owen, and Seibert 1977; Garretson and Jordan 1982).

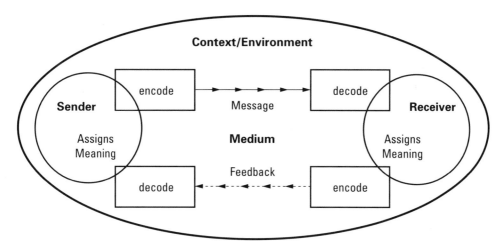

Figure 3.1. The Communication Model
Source: Horn, Mahshie, Bally, Kaplan, and Wilson 1984.

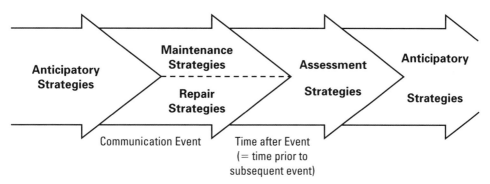

Figure 3.2. Communication Event Time Continuum
Source: Bally 1987.

(See figure 3.1.) It identifies the key elements in the communication process. These include:

1. *Sender*—the person who initiates or sends (encodes) the information through a given communication mode or modes (speech, sign, nonverbal communication, writing, etc.)

2. *Encode*—the cognitive process through which an individual assigns meaning by changing a thought into a language form that the receiver will understand (sign, speech, etc.)

3. *Message*—the verbal and/or nonverbal behaviors providing the information

4. *Medium*—the physical medium through which the information travels (e.g., air, water)

5. *Decode*—the cognitive process by which the message, having reached the receiver through auditory or visual modes, is interpreted as meaningful information

6. *Receiver*—the person who receives and interprets (decodes) the information (i.e., assigns meaning to the message)

7. *Feedback*—the response to the sender's message (verbal and/or nonverbal) sent from the receiver back to the sender

8. *Environment/Context*—the circumstances in which the communication exchange takes place, including such related factors as the physical surroundings; background, emotional state, and expectations of the communicators; time; place; culture; as well as sensitivity to the appropriate means of transmission.

During the communication event, the roles of the sender and receiver alternate.

The Communication Event Time Continuum

A second model illustrates the Communication Event Time Continuum. (See figure 3.2.) In the continuum, communication strategies are categorized along a time line as *anticipatory, maintenance* or *repair* and *assessment strategies.* Anticipatory strategies include anything an individual does to prepare for a given communication situation. This may include modification of the communication environment, of the individual or interpersonal behavior of the communicators, or of the linguistic structures and approaches that are used. Maintenance strategies, mostly functional in nature, are those things that are done to sustain the communication process, such as confirming information when it is understood. Repair strategies, as the name implies, are those approaches used to reestablish communication when it has broken down (e.g., asking someone to say something again). Finally, the use of assessment strategies is an evaluative process used to determine reasons for the success or failure of a communication situation. This provides the basis for adding or modifying anticipatory, maintenance, and/or repair strategies. The evaluation process may also be considered as an anticipatory strategy in an ongoing strategy cycle as shown in figure 3.2.

The two models may be used in tandem for understanding and teaching communication strategies. If each of the components of the Communication Model is examined with respect to the Communication Event Time Continuum, a thorough, systematic inventory of possible strategies may be developed. For example, the receiver may wish to anticipate a communication event and consider environmental suitability and modifications, ways in which the sender's appearance and/or behavior might be changed, and the potential of unfamiliar vocabulary or language structures. All of these areas could be reviewed to effect better communication.

In the following section, the four strategy areas of the Communication Event Time Continuum (anticipatory, maintenance, repair, and assessment) will be discussed in the context of the communication therapy process. Assessment and therapy approaches will be described for each.

Anticipatory Strategies

As stated earlier, individuals develop strategies to sustain communication in the native environments they occupied before they sustained a hearing loss or in those they occupy subsequent to sustaining the loss. Culturally Deaf individuals may develop such strategies to effect communication with hearing individuals as the need arises. The advent of a hearing loss or change in context may require adaptations to (1) the environment (*environmental strategies*), (2) the communication-related appearance and behaviors of communicators (*interpersonal strategies*), or (3) linguistic usage (*linguistic strategies*). Each of these three anticipatory strategy areas will be discussed below. Culturally Deaf individuals may benefit from learning similar strategies for use when communicating with hearing people as well as with members of their own ASL-based community.

Environmental Strategies

Communication success may be hindered by environments incompatible to good communication, such as restaurants that are too dark and rock concerts or sporting events that foster significant decibel levels. Both verbal and nonverbal communication may be impacted negatively. Of all the strategy areas, making changes in the environment often seems the most tangible to the client. Therefore, the clinician may wish to focus on environmental strategies early in the therapy process in order to achieve an immediate degree of client success.

There are four areas of consideration when assessing and modifying environments to meet communication needs: (1) vision, (2) audition, (3) spatial relationships, and (4) comfort. Home, work, and social environments as well as public places visited by clients should all be assessed in terms of communication function and adapted as possible (Kaplan 1982; McCall 1984; Kaplan, Bally, and Garretson 1987).

Vision Two components of the visual field may impact communication: poor lighting and *visual noise*.

Home lighting is often designed for aesthetics rather than practicality. For effective speechreading, the light should be on the face of the speaker without blinding her. For manual communication, the sign field—from waist to forehead—should be illuminated. A vast variety of lighting options may be considered when illuminating a home for communication purposes. One can take advantage of natural light by arranging furniture in such a way that it maximizes light where it is needed on communication areas and more specifically on the faces of senders. Table lamps should have opaque shades, which allow light toward the speakers' faces rather than limiting it toward the table surface and ceiling. Generalized indirect lighting and overhead lighting including overlapping broad beam spots (recessed broad beam parabolic reflector 60-watt halogen bulbs at 3½-foot intervals provides clear bright light without shadows 18 inches from ceiling level and below) should also be considered so as to minimize shadows on faces (Bias 1995).

Work environments are often designed without consideration of the communication needs of individuals, especially those with hearing loss. Lighting may be uniform throughout a variety of work settings, regardless of the function or communication need. In some settings, lighting may focus on work surfaces rather than on workers, creating the potential for communication difficulties.

Visual noise includes anything that interferes with communication on a visual plane. This may include things that affect distracting movement such as TV, active pets, too many people, or an otherwise busy environment. Many of these factors, when identified, can be reduced or eliminated.

Natural light in outdoor situations may also hinder effective communication. Lighting directed to the sender's face may help the receiver but may be construed as glare by the sender. Moving into light shade or standing sideways to the source of light may be helpful.

Homes in which deaf and hard of hearing persons live may also be designed or modified to include assistive devices. Such technology may substitute light or vibration for sound to alert occupants to fire or smoke alarms, door bells, a telephone ringing or a baby crying. (See Kaplan, chapter 6.)

Audition In today's world many environments have excessive ambient noise—traffic, increased technology in the home and work place, background music. Persons with hearing loss are at a great disadvantage, sometimes unable to use amplification in noisier situations because the competing signals are amplified along with the primary signals of communication. When the noise is dampened or eliminated, better communication results. Work, social, and home settings should be inventoried, and objectives and strategies established for modifications that may improve audition. For example, use of absorbent materials such as draperies, carpets, and acoustic tile may be considered. Additionally, stereo systems and radios should be used judiciously. Use of the mute function on remotes can instantly eliminate competing noise and, therefore, may be a valuable tool supportive to unhindered communication.

Personal amplification—hearing aids and cochlear implants as well as group listening systems (FM, infrared, loop, hard-wired)— are important options for increasing auditory input for many persons. Both wired and wireless systems bring the signal directly to the listener's ear, thereby reducing or eliminating competing signals. Such systems may be especially effective for deaf and hard of hearing persons in meetings, at plays and concerts, in restaurants, and when they are watching TV. Trial use of such systems in critical communication environments may be assessed for effectiveness and comfort by the client with the guidance of the professional. (See chapter 6 for a description of these devices.)

Spatial Relationships For effective communication, either verbal or nonverbal, it is important for the sender and receiver to have an unobstructed view of one another. Living and work spaces should be reviewed for ease of communication. Often, the spaces in which individuals function have odd shapes (e.g., L-shaped or multilevel rooms) and barriers such as columns, large furniture units, room dividers, or table lamps. The furniture in a given room may be arranged to be pleasing to the eye or to focus on a particular point such as a TV or fireplace. When work or social facilities are designed and built, structural and aesthetic considerations often supersede a need for a barrier-free communication environment. As part of the communication strategy process, clients may be encouraged to assess work and social environments in terms of their communicative needs and set goals for modifications to such facilities to help meet those needs. Arranging furniture into more communication-supportive conversation groupings may be helpful. Meeting rooms should be arranged for full visibility (e.g., arranging chairs in a circle rather than in rows) whenever possible.

Comfort The importance of the comfort level of an environment and its impact on communication is often overlooked. The right temperature, comfortable seating, and a comfortable number of participants at a particular communication event are among the considerations a client should examine.

Garstecki and Alpiner (1982) describe effective proactive therapy approaches in which simulated environments can be modified. Home or office inventories are made and evaluated for ease of communication. Then modifications are made to the space and the results are assessed to see if communication is more successful. In addition, Kaplan, Bally, and Garretson (1987) suggest that diagrams of both problematic and communication supportive rooms that show seating, lighting, and sound sources may be helpful in developing analytic skills with clients.

All environments in which communication occurs should be assessed, and modifications in the four areas described above should be made or requested whenever possible. When such modifications cannot be easily made, the client should learn to consider the necessity of sustaining communication in such an environment and the effort it would take to effect changes, and should then act accordingly.

Two additional therapy areas relevant to environmental strategies are assertiveness and consumerism. Supportive to the modification of shared environments as well as the acquisition and use of assistive technologies is the incorporation of assertiveness training into communication therapy. In addition, an understanding and use of the basic principles of good consumerism may make acquisition of assistive technologies feasible and practical.

The provision of appropriate facilities and auxiliary aids supportive to communication on the job and in public places falls under the domain of the first three titles of the Americans with Disabilities Act (ADA). Communication therapy objectives may include informational counseling. This may include familiarization with the provisions of this law, determination of which provisions are applicable for a particular client's situation, and ways to effect compliance with this legislation (these are described later in this chapter).

Interpersonal Strategies

The appearance and behaviors of speakers may interfere with effective communication, thereby compounding the difficulties related to limited hearing. Interpersonal strategies are those a receiver develops that may effect a change in the speakers' appearances or behaviors. Asking speakers to modify their appearance or behavior relative to communication is perhaps the most intimidating aspect of strategy use for the client. Careful assessment of a communication situation must precede this strategy use.

Clinical experience has demonstrated that it may be helpful for the client to generate a list of those characteristics they feel impact negatively on communication function. These may include the speaker's speech behaviors (talks too fast, slow, loud, soft; mumbles; has an accent; doesn't move lips, etc.) and external characteristics and behaviors (untrimmed mustache, gum chewing, eating, smoking, moving, obscuring mouth, etc.). These characteristics should then be assessed in terms of how easily and realistically change can be effected, and efforts should be directed toward changing what is most readily changeable. For example, asking someone to speak more slowly is realistic and may be readily achieved with periodic reminders, whereas asking someone to trim a beard depends heavily on the sender-receiver interpersonal relationship. In contrast, a request to change an accent would probably be considered unreasonable under most circumstances.

Supportive to asking another person to change their behavior, the professional may wish to develop a therapy component on assertive approaches. This will be discussed later in this chapter.

Linguistic Strategies

Linguistic strategies are those the receiver develops or selects that utilize language (i.e., vocabulary, language sequence) and language structures to effect more successful communication in the absence of adequate auditory input: "One can provide . . . clients with directed practice in anticipating the form and content that others are likely to produce in response to specific verbal stimuli" (Erber 1988, 111). These strategies may be used by both hard of hearing and Deaf populations and may supplement auditory or visual input. They may include *receptive strategies*, such as anticipating vocabulary and dialogue, and *expressive strategies*, such as preparing "limited-set" questions or structuring a conversation. Linguistic strategies such as the use of association drills, constellations, and scripting as well as communication structuring, including the use of limited-set questions, will be described in this section.

Anticipating Vocabulary and Language for Improved Receptive Ability To increase the likelihood of comprehension, individuals may consider key vocabulary and language structures of communication situations before they occur (Erber 1988). The overall structure of some situations are easy to predict, such as the question-answer format of a job interview or the exchanges that occur at a bank. Social conversations may be more erratic and, therefore, less easy to anticipate. However, the receiver may be encouraged to examine the social commonalities of the sender and the receiver. For example, if one goes to the dentist, the primary language structure will be question and answer ("Do you have an appointment? Have you been flossing regularly? Where does it hurt?") and will mostly focus on the oral adventure. However, if the dentist is also your neighbor or member of your golf club, the discussion may also include neighborhood issues or golfing events (Watzlawick, Bavelas, and Jackson 1967).

Association Activities for Improved Receptive Ability A hierarchy of activities known as *association activities* (Kaplan, Bally, and Garretson 1987) may be used to help develop greater associative thinking for use in communication situations. As a result the client may be able to anticipate more readily vocabulary and language relative to a specific communication situation—discussing a football game, conversing at a specific family gathering (wedding, birthday, etc.), or going to the dry cleaners. Such activities enable an individual to predict vocabulary as well as key words and may be supportive to audition and speechreading (see the discussion of "Repair Strategies") (Erber 1988). The following procedure includes such activities and may be used to enhance association ability through speechreading:

1. The professional may present words within a concrete or abstract category (family names, numbers, emotions, etc.) or topic area (visiting the post office, a trip to Santa Fe, etc.). Initial presentations may be made without informing the receiver of the category or topic. Each word may be presented twice before moving to the next word. The receiver is instructed to try to identify the topic.

2. Once receivers have identified two or more words, they will probably identify the category or topic. At that point they should be encouraged

to think actively about the topic. This should result in a significant increase in the number of correct responses. (Bally, Goffen, and Scott 1995.)

3. After all the words in a category are presented, the speaker should repeat the words that were presented before the receiver guesses the category or topic.

4. The professional should place the words in a short sentence or phrase context. Additional linguistic context should help the receiver build on the known key word.

5. Next, the sentences may be put in connected discourse as a continuous discourse tracking activity (see the discussion of "Assessment"), which more nearly simulates normal connected discourse.

Materials for the above activity may be designed to simulate problem situations identified by the receiver.

Constellations and Scripting to Improve Receptive Ability The use of the constellation configuration (see figure 3.3) may be helpful for structuring receptive vocabulary and dialogue. Constellations can work in tandem with the previously described activity:

1. A horizontal line surrounded by a series of radiating lines gives a visual base for this receptive language activity (Kaplan, Bally, and Garretson 1987).

2. A key word or topic (a situation or place—job interview, bank) is put on the horizontal line.

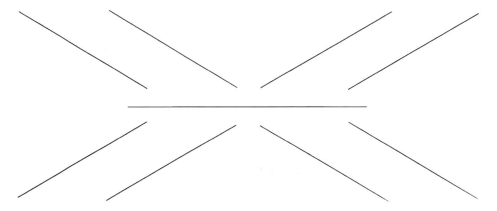

Figure 3.3. Constellation configuration
Source: Kaplan, Bally, and Garretson 1987.

3. Related vocabulary or phrases are brainstormed by the receiver and placed on the radiating lines.

4. Receptive practice using auditory and/or visual modes for the related vocabulary is initiated.

5. Next, the words and phrases are replaced with sentences using the key words and phrases. These should be utterances that other people might say to the receiver. For example, at a supermarket the checkout person may ask, "Paper or plastic?"

6. Practice in comprehending these sentences visually or auditorally would then be initiated.

7. After determining the topic-related sentences, the sentences should be put in an estimated chronological order. For example "Good morning, may I help you?" would come first whereas "Thanks, I'll see you next week!" would probably be last. Additional sentences that would complete a script could be added (Mayo and Waldo 1986).

8. The speaker and speechreader could then role play the situation, at first just following the script.

9. Given the unpredictability of many conversations, the speaker may then vary the discourse from the script to simulate real life and give the receiver the opportunity to use maintenance and repair strategies.

Research in Linguistic Strategy Use In the context of synthetic lipreading approaches for effecting improved receptive comprehension, Tye-Murray (1992a,c) has challenged professional thinking about the effectiveness of some anticipatory efforts. She has demonstrated that brainstorming and practicing familiar words may not increase speechreading success nor help the client to be less anxious during communication events. Further, Tye-Murray (1994) speculates that a reason for this lack of success "lies in the nature of communication; except for occasional ritual and phatic interactions, conversation is dynamic—unexpected twists and remarks occur and these cannot be anticipated or predicted" (201).

Given these assertions, the benefit of increasing lipreading ability as a component of receptive ability might be greatest when conversation is highly structured by the receiver/speechreader so that a limited set of utterances or, more specifically, responses is evoked. The benefit of knowing a topic can easily be demonstrated by asking clients to lipread words without knowing the topic. When the topic is revealed, lipreading ability increases dramatically. Teaching effective pragmatic skills for guiding conversation and asking specific questions that evoke responses within a limited set would then be indicated.

Bally, Goffen, and Scott (1995) demonstrate that the strategy of introducing unfamiliar vocabulary prior to a communication event results in a significant increase (60 percent) in word identification scores in structured situations. In this study the speaker presented familiar direction-giving constructs ("Take the {name of community} exit" or "Follow Route 22 to {name of community}"). The names of communities were constructed from generic or recurring components of town names. For example, *river, lake, ridge, town, view, ville,* or *mont* were combined to form Rivertown, Lakeridge, Lakeview, Ridgemont, or Riverview. Subjects demonstrated an increased ability to speechread these directions an average of 50 percent greater after reviewing for two minutes a map on which the communities were highlighted. These studies may suggest that therapy will have greater effectiveness when directed toward unfamiliar but relevant vocabulary and are analytic in nature.

Structuring and Guiding as Expressive Strategies Expressively, communication may be enhanced by structuring and guiding a conversation. The receiver may plan to introduce topics when appropriate and ask questions that will guide the conversation in ways that will be understood more easily (Erber 1988). For example, the use of limited-set questions such as "What days is the clinic open? Is the clinic open on Fridays? What hours will the clinic be open on Friday?" is preferable to a more open-ended question such as "When is the clinic open?"

Considering the information desired in a given exchange and planning the questions may put the receiver at an advantage. However, care must be taken by the receiver not to control or monopolize a conversation completely.

Ways of integrating therapy for the development and use of linguistic strategies with auditory training and speechreading are apparent in the previous discussion. Similar strategies may be modified to develop or enhance receptive and/or expressive language skills. For example, auditory training may emphasize the recognition of common linguistic constructs for inquiry relative to specific communication events—"Who is coming for dinner?" or "What is the balance of my savings account?" This refined questioning limits the auditory information that may need to be interpreted. Additionally, learning to construct such specific questions may develop skills in vocabulary use and syntax. Finally, speech, voice, and pronunciation skills may be reinforced in both word and connected-speech contexts during such activities.

Assessing Anticipatory Strategies

Anticipatory Strategies may best be assessed using interview or inventory formats. An in-depth interview focusing on a cross section of communication situations may help identify problems. The professional may then ask questions regarding the ways in which the client prepares for specific communication events, including methods that are successful and those that are not. Linguistic, environmental, and interpersonal factors should be inventoried. Responses from the Communication Scale for Deaf Adults (CSDA) (Kaplan et al. 1994) may be useful in identifying problem situations and in developing an inventory. (See chapter 4 for further discussion of the CSDA.)

Maintenance Strategies

In the following section the use of maintenance strategies will be discussed. These strategies are used to support or to help communication flow smoothly with a minimal number of breakdowns. Discourse among hearing people is characterized by pragmatic skills learned at an early age (Deyo and Hallau 1984; Erber 1988). These include such skills as getting the attention of the listener, turn taking, and confirming, among others. Deyo and Hallau (1984) describe use of such conversational skills as limited among many deaf children, especially those from culturally Deaf environments. This may be explained by variations in pragmatic skills within Deaf culture or by a lack of receptive input in hearing situations.

Discourse Skills

Some discourse skills are particularly effective and supportive to communication for persons with hearing loss and may be taught as maintenance strategies because they effectively help maintain conversation. These may include initiating or terminating a conversation, turn taking, summarizing, and confirming. In *Ring/Flash,* Deyo (1984) outlines exercises for developing specific discourse skills within the context of learning to use the telephone or a telecommunication device for the deaf (TDD or TTY). These exercises may be readily adapted for older Deaf or hard of hearing populations and generalized to face-to-face communication situations. The skills areas will be discussed below.

Initiating a Conversation Strategies to initiate conversations are those that alert the other person of the deaf or hard of hearing person's presence and get his attention to begin a conversation. Both nonverbal and verbal strategies to initiate a conversation should be included in communication therapy. Nonverbal strategies are useful for all persons with hearing loss and may include making eye contact, raising the head, leaning forward as if ready to speak, or gesturing with the hand or a finger. Physical contact is appropriate in many contexts after a rapport has been established and may include a light tap on the back, shoulder, or arm (Andersson 1995). Within some culturally Deaf environments, especially learning institutions, flashing lights and a substantial tapping of a common surface such as a desk, table, or the floor with a hand or foot may be considered acceptable and appropriate behaviors ("For hearing people only" 1994). Professionals may wish to consult their respective clients for their cultural views and preferences. Verbal strategies to initiate a conversation may be taught to include some attention-getting phrases such as "Good Morning, Hi, Excuse me," etc. or the individual's name.

Turn Taking Turn taking refers to alternating the roles of sender and receiver in a smooth and equitable way (Clark and Clark 1977). This allows conversation to proceed without interruption and in a timely manner. "Turns are taken and relinquished according to social conventions as well, such as: eye contact, facial expression, gesture, posture, voice level and pitch, pause, prompting and so forth" (Erber 1988, 111). For persons who depend on lipreading, turn taking is a necessity as well as a courtesy. Frequent turn taking facilitates receptive ability in that it reduces the quantity of information to be interpreted.

Interrupting a Conversation Sometimes a receiver needs to interrupt the flow of the speaker's message to confirm information or ask for clarification of a message. Individuals may also have reason to interrupt a conversation between two other parties. When interrupting a conversation already in progress, clients may be advised to stand at the periphery of the conversation but within the peripheral vision of the individual with whom they wish to converse. In urgent situations, a polite "excuse me" may be used to interrupt the conversation. In either situation, some explanation as to the reason for intervening should be forthcoming.

Confirmation and Summarization Both confirmation and summarization are used to ensure that information has been received accurately by the receiver and to verify this to the sender.

The frequent use of *confirmation* may be among the most effective maintenance strategies that can be developed by a person with hearing loss because the receiver assumes the majority of the responsibility for maintaining the conversation. For example, the receiver may use nonverbal strategies such as nodding of the head or saying "uh-huh" during a dialogue. Or, the receiver may also repeat key words or information (a specific time, amount, direction, etc.) at intervals or at the end of a conversation. This strategy not only confirms the information that is received, but also demonstrates to the sender that the receiver is actively listening and making an effort to understand. It is interesting to note that Nitchie (1912) embraced the use of *verification* as opposed to *repetition* as an important factor in a synthetic approach to lipreading in receptive communication. This reflects an early understanding of the shared nature of the communication process relative to persons with hearing loss.

Summarization is another strategy used by the receiver to indicate understanding. The receiver reviews in an abbreviated form the most important information points at the end of a conversation (e.g., "Tuesday at 2 at Union Station . . . Okay!"). This may be a slightly less effective alternative to confirmation in that it requires the receiver to retain information for a longer duration of time. It also may cause some confusion if the sender identifies several points of misunderstanding. Both confirmation and summarizing may be effective and should be emphasized in strategy training.

Terminating a Conversation Conversations are generally closed using a variety of socially accepted protocols such as summarizing or expressing the need to move on to another activity (Deyo and Hallau 1984). As described by Kinsella-

Meier (chapter 1), these protocols may be somewhat different within Deaf culture (e.g., the "long goodbye"). The professional may wish to direct therapy toward an understanding of cultural differences and the inherent messages projected to individuals outside that culture. Individuals may wish to modify their approaches with respect to members of the other culture or mainstream population.

Careful attention to carryover should be emphasized in the aural rehabilitation process. An increasing number of target situations in which strategy use is monitored by the client and/or others may be helpful. These may start out as small, relatively structured tasks (e.g., asking someone for directions or for the time) in close proximity to the clinical setting. Initially, the clinician may wish to accompany the client to monitor strategies and success. Later, the client should assume greater responsibility for self-monitoring, assessing, and reporting communicative success in nonclinical settings.

Nonverbal Behaviors as Maintenance Strategies

Nonverbal behaviors such as gestures, facial expressions, and body language may be universally helpful in both spoken and manual languages to maintain conversation by giving feedback to the sender or receiver. Raised eyebrows may signal the receiver that a question has been asked. A shocked or puzzled look may signal a reaction to a sender.

The increased use and quality of gesture and body language by persons who communicate with deaf and hard of hearing persons may be incorporated as necessary. Although it is probably a natural tendency for persons who experience hearing loss to develop their nonverbal skills, it cannot be assumed that this is uniformly true. For some aurally oriented or auditory learners, these skills may need to be taught and practiced. Using nonverbal communication in tandem with verbal communication, especially when speech is not completely intelligible, should be encouraged in deaf, Deaf, and hard of hearing populations and may be a primary focus in initial integrated therapy programming.

The use of role playing to practice use of gestural communication should focus on problem solving or communicating information in everyday situations that may be problematic (going to the bank, cleaners, or a restaurant). This may range from the use of pointing to a menu in a restaurant to the use of more sophisticated gesturing to a tailor when having clothing altered. The use of nonverbal communication is a natural part of American Sign Language and may already be used extensively by Deaf individuals. Often, the receiver with hearing loss must model or demonstrate appropriate communication behaviors when communicating with hearing people to help them understand how to utilize nonverbal communication effectively.

It should be noted that some culturally Deaf individuals may have difficulty in distinguishing which gestures are signs unique to ASL and which are more generally universal gestures that occur both in American Sign Language and English. For example, the ASL sign for *baby* would be almost universally recognized in that it mimes cradling a baby in one's arms and rocking it. In contrast, the sign for *girl* is made by moving one's thumb along the chin line (derived from the line of a bonnet string), a gesture that would not be generally recognized by people unfamiliar with signing (Baker and Cokely 1980; Sternberg 1994). In such circumstances, individuals may not always convey the intended concepts or attitudes. The appropriate and effective use of gesture should be assessed and developed with the client as part of an integrated approach to therapy.

Cued Speech as a Maintenance Strategy

"Cued Speech is a phonemically-based system used in conjunction with speech-reading [which is] comprised of eight handshapes representing groups of consonant sounds and four positions about the face representing vowel sounds. Combinations of these hand configurations and placements synchronized with natural speech movements make spoken language clearly visible and understandable to the Cued Speech recipient" (Kipila and Williams-Scott 1990). (See figure 3.4.) Cued speech allows a deaf or hard of hearing person to "see-hear" precisely every spoken syllable that a hearing person hears. Because this visually based system is used simultaneously with connected speech, communication is less likely to break down because of confusions between homophenous words—words that look the same on the mouth. If both parties in a conversation are fluent at cueing, communication is more likely to be fluid and breakdowns will rarely occur (Cornett 1972; Williams-Scott 1994). Williams-Scott (1994) notes additional benefits to using Cued Speech: "A further significance of the phonemic basis for the Cued Speech system lies in its benefit to spoken language development and reading comprehension" (1). Thus, Cued Speech may be considered as an effective maintenance strategy with secondary benefits.

The limiting factor is that cuers are dependent on the system and there will be a marked decrease in comprehension when senders do not use the system. In addition, the number of skilled Cued Speech interpreters or teachers is very small on a per capita basis and access to such skilled personnel is therefore very limited.

Assessing Maintenance Strategies

Maintenance strategies may best be evaluated by observation and role play. A clinician-guided analysis of a videotaped communication interchange may be effective. Observation may include interaction with clinic or facility personnel, family members, and friends or with the clinician outside of the therapy room. A tendency may be noted for the client to utilize these strategies in the therapy room and discontinue their use outside of the therapy context.

This author has found the giving of directions or instructions to be a particularly effective construct for assessing and reinforcing the use of maintenance strategies. These situations require frequent confirmation or summarization. For

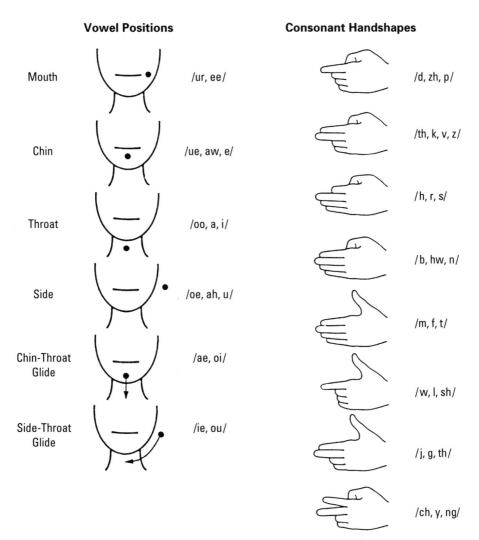

Vowel Positions

Mouth /ur, ee/

Chin /ue, aw, e/

Throat /oo, a, i/

Side /oe, ah, u/

Chin-Throat
Glide /ae, oi/

Side-Throat
Glide /ie, ou/

Consonant Handshapes

/d, zh, p/

/th, k, v, z/

/h, r, s/

/b, hw, n/

/m, f, t/

/w, l, sh/

/j, g, th/

/ch, y, ng/

Figure 3.4. Cued Speech configuration
Source: Kipila and Williams-Scott 1990.

clients whose experience and skills in using these strategies are limited, visual representation in writing on the TDD, with a print-out feature, may be helpful. Highlighting, underlining, or restructuring may aid the client in the identification of key words and concepts for confirmation and summarization.

In addition, role play may be an effective therapy as well as an assessment tool. Role plays should be based on problem listening situations as reported by clients or identified on the communication scales. Advantages to group therapy are that role plays may be more spontaneous, more closely related to the client's real-life experiences, and that some group members may act as observers and suggest alternate solutions to those acted out by the participants.

Counterproductive Strategies

When unsuccessful in either manual or verbal communication, an individual may adopt strategies that may not prove successful and may even prove to be counter-productive. These *maladaptive strategies* are those that an individual may use to compensate for or hide the fact that she has not successfully received the information (Demorest and Erdman 1986; Kaplan, Bally, and Garretson 1987; Hallbergh and Carlsson 1991; Tye-Murray 1994a). Although there is no reported research relative to training that eradicates these negative-result strategies, one may reasonably conclude that when the communication cycle (sender-message-receiver-feedback) has not been completed successfully, communication is *not* successful.

Maladaptive strategies may include, but are not limited to, the following:

1. *Avoidance.* The individual may avoid interactive communication situations.

2. *Bluffing.* The individual may smile or nod his head, feigning comprehension.

3. *Ignoring or looking away.* The individual may pretend that she was not paying attention or didn't realize that she was being addressed by the speaker.

4. *"Huh?" or "What?"* The individual says "huh?" or simply shrugs without further explanation or direction. The sender may, therefore, get errone-ous messages—the receiver is not interested, the receiver is not paying attention, the receiver is not too smart. The receiver must assume the responsibility of repeating the entire message.

5. *"Say it all again."* The individual may consistently ask the sender to re-peat the entire message whether or not she understood some of it. This imposes unnecessary efforts on the sender. When possible the receiver should in some way let the sender know what was understood and what information is needed.

6. *Monopolizing.* The individual may monopolize a conversation so that the risk of not understanding others is eliminated.

The use of such strategies may have adverse effects on communication in that the consequences may be embarrassing or even dangerous (bluffing: "I hear you . . . I'll be there in a minute!"; meanwhile, the house may be on fire). In some communication situations such strategies may be appropriate. The professional may wish to help a client identify use of maladaptive strategies and substitute more appropriate strategies when deemed necessary.

Assessing Counterproductive Strategies

The clinician has a responsibility to help the clients self-assess the effectiveness of the communication strategies they use. The Communication Scale for Deaf Adults (CSDA) (Kaplan, Bally, and Brandt 1991) and the Communication Scale for Older Adults (CSOA) (Kaplan et al. 1994) may help the clinician identify the use of such counterproductive approaches. They may further be revealed in general conversation between the clinician and the client. Once they are identified, it may be useful for the client to self-monitor her use of these techniques and the results they have. Alternate strategies that have more positive results should be explored. Again, role playing may be useful.

Repair Strategies

When communication breaks down during a communication event the receiver should: (1) inform the sender, and (2) instruct the sender as to what she should do to help reestablish the communication cycle (Tye-Murray et al. 1994). Communication is reestablished by using a variety of different repair strategies that will be discussed in the following section. Results of several studies show that repair strategies can effectively remedy communication breakdowns (Gagné and Wyllie 1989; Tye-Murray, Purdy, and Woodworth 1992). Repair strategies may be equally appropriate when receiving either oral or manual communication.

Repair strategies may seek to modify either the sender's communication behavior *or* the structure and content of the message. Modifying the sender's communication behavior may include asking the sender to speak/sign more loudly or quietly, more slowly, more clearly, incrementally or in shorter increments. Often, individuals with hearing loss become frustrated when a friend or partner fails to modify his or her speech behavior after repeated reminders. The receiver should be made aware that such communication behaviors may be habitual, having been established over decades, and may not be easily changed. Some of the anticipatory strategies discussed earlier may also be employed as behavioral repair strategies during a conversation (e.g., remove gum, face the speaker, etc.).

Repair strategies that ask the sender to modify the content or format of her message appear to be more successful than requests to modify behavior because they require a short rather than long-term change in behavior (Tye-Murray et al. 1990). Given the time and motivation, repair strategies, when used effectively, may result in almost complete understanding of a message. However, "how willingly and how effectively a person uses repair strategies appears to vary with the conversational setting, the familiarity with the conversational partner(s) to the client, the client's personality and willingness to signal a communication break-down, and the client's judgment concerning how well the partner might follow the repair strategy directive" (Tye-Murray et al. 1994, 108).

The objective of therapy should be to increase the number of strategies em-ployed and the flexibility with which they are used. Two different strategy hier-archies may be useful in helping clients to improve strategy use. The first may be used when *none of the message is understood*. The second hierarchy may be used when *some of the message is understood*. Together, they demonstrate the hierarchi-cal relationship of the repair strategies described below.

Relative to the two hierarchies, there are considerations (see table 3.1) that the sender should review before selecting a specific strategy for a specific com-munication event (Erber 1988; Hilley and Bally 1990). Although some clients express some discouragement because the process appears time consuming in its graphic representation, the professional may assure them that these considera-

Table 3.1   Repair Strategies Hierarchy

Considerations for Feedback

A. Assess importance of obtaining information.
  B. Assess why breakdown occurred
    C. Assess time considerations
      D. Consider options
        E. Select option
          F. Choose most appropriate strategy

Options

Bluff
  a. smile and nod   Use repair strategies to try to
  b. answer using your "best guess."   understand what was said.

Give up

Ignore

(Fast . . . but effective?)   (Takes more time.)

            Understood none   or   *Understood some*

1. Select appropriate repair strategy

2. Remember: Use an *assertive* approach!!!!
    a. courtesy
    b. explanation (once may be enough)
    c. direction/education

Source: Hilley and Bally 1990.

tions are likely to come quickly and naturally after practice. These considerations include:

1. Assessing the relative importance of receiving the information

2. Assessing why communication broke down and if it can be realistically repaired

3. Assessing the time available, given the circumstances, to repair the breakdown

4. Assessing the psychosocial implications of the subsequent behavior

Based on these considerations an individual can determine which option is most likely to be effective. If the individual opts to use repair strategies, a specific strategy or series of strategies may be selected.

Both hierarchies require the listener to identify the reason for communication breakdown as either (1) the speaker's behavior (too fast, slow, soft, gum, etc.) or (2) the listener's inability to receive the message. In the former circumstance, the listener asks the speaker to modify his behavior. In the latter, the listener evaluates the potential of the following strategies designed to get some information regarding the communication utterance and selects the one likely to achieve the best results.

Understood None of the Message

If the receiver has understood none of the message (figure 3.6), she should ask the sender to repeat, rephrase, or give a key word.

Repeat Asking the sender to repeat the entire message is the most frequently used repair strategy and often results in successful repair of the communication. However, subsequent to a given communication breakdown, the likelihood of success in speech recognition is in inverse proportion to the number of requests for repetition (Tye-Murray 1994a). Using the repeat strategy twice seems likely to exhaust its effectiveness. Then, alternative strategies should be selected.

Although often effective, the repeat strategy may also be the most overused of all repair strategies. Clinical experience indicates it is frequently the only repair strategy a person with hearing loss employs. In this case, habitual requests for repeating an entire message when part has been understood should be diminished as a therapy objective and alternate strategies should be increased as appropriate.

Rephrase This strategy requires the listener to ask for the sender to use *alternate wording* or *different words* to say the same thing: "Could you please say it again using different words?" The listener may be more specific in asking for rephrasing by specifying whether the speaker should *elaborate, increment,* or *synthesize.* Asking the speaker to elaborate or expand the information—"Tell me more about that" or "Could you tell me a little more about what you want to know?"—may provide the listener with additional information and may facilitate the identification of key words or phrases. Asking the speaker to increment the information—"Could you break that up into smaller sentences"—may reduce the utterances or signed phrases into more manageable units that may more easily be recognized. For example, "Turn right on Moorland Lane, go three blocks, passing Kurt's Video and the community hospital on the left, and bear right onto Arlington Road at the fork" may become "Turn right on Moorland Lane. Go three blocks. Watch for Kurt's Video and the community hospital on the left. Bear right at the fork. You will be on Arlington Road." Finally, asking the individual to synthesize—"Give me that information in as few words as possible"—may result in the identification of key words or phrases.

Key Word Clients are often able to comprehend an entire utterance once they have determined the topic or a key word. The listener may ask the speaker for the topic or a key word ("Could you tell me the most important word in the sentence?"). If this is not successful, the listener may ask for the second most important word in the sentence, a synonym for the key word, or for the spelling of the key word. Once the key word has been identified, the listener may proceed to ask the sender to repeat the original sentence. (See table 3.2.)

Understood Some of the Message

The second part of the repair strategy hierarchy (table 3.3) assumes that the receiver has understood some of the message. This information may be used to structure a request or response that secures the missing information. The following hierarchy demonstrates a variety of ways to repair the breakdown.

Repeat Part The listener may facilitate the repair by indicating an understanding of some of the information based on what was already comprehended and request some repetition. This may include a specific word or words ("What was the last word of the sentence?" or "What was the word after 'forfeit'?") or a specific part of the sentence ("Could you repeat the end of the sentence, please?").

Some individuals may be inclined to ask for repetition of the entire sentence although they understood some of the message. As stated before, this may give the sender mixed signals and requires the speakers to do more than their share in the communication process. When alerted to the option of asking for partial repetition, clients enthusiastically embrace this strategy (Owens and Telleen 1981).

Rephrase This is the same strategy described above (expand, increment, or summarize). However, in the context of "understood some," the receiver asks for a synonym or different phrasing of only the part of the message that she did not understand.

Table 3.2 Repair Strategies, Part 1

PART 1: Understood None of the Message

Strategy	Request	Response
1. Repeat	"Excuse me, what did you say?"	Usually will repeat all of what was said in the same way.
	"Could you say that again, please?"	
	"Please repeat that slowly."	
2. Rephrase	"Could you please say that in a different way?"	Usually will repeat all information in a different way.
	"Could you please rephrase that?"	
3. Key word	"Could you please repeat the important words?"	Usually will repeat part of message with emphasis on important words.
	"Please tell me the topic of this conversation."	
4. Proceed to appropriate level of part 2.		

Source: Hilley and Bally 1990.

Key Words The use of key words in this context should focus on words or phrases not understood by the receiver. The receiver may get this information by asking the sender a specific question. For example, "Which building did you say I should go to for that information?"

Spelling If a particularly elusive word cannot be understood, the client can ask for it to be spelled *letter by letter*. The receiver asks the sender to spell a word letter by letter. This strategy may be effective because the responses consist of a limited set of twenty-six (mostly V-C and C-V) combinations (i.e., /bi/, /si/, /əf/). They are relatively easy to understand through auditory and visual modes, especially if an individual is familiar with the viseme groups (sounds that look alike

Table 3.3   Repair Strategies, Parts 2 and 3

PART 2: Understood Some of the Message

Strategy	Request	Response
1. Repeat part	"Could you repeat that date, please?"	Usually will repeat what is needed.
	"I understood what you said but could you please repeat the end of the sentence?"	
	"Where are they from?"	
2. Rephrase	"I keep missing that last word (or phrase). Could you please use a different word (or phrase)?"	Usually will reword.
3. Key word (ask a specific question)	"What day did you say you're leaving?"	Usually will give only information needed.
	"What is that address?"	
	"Where were you at 9 A.M. yesterday?"	
	"Will you buy one?"	
4. Spell		
key word	"Could you please spell that last word?"	Usually will spell requested word.
proper nouns	"Could you please spell her last name?"	"S-M-Y-T-H-E."
numbers	"Could you spell that apartment number?"	"T-W-E-N-T-Y."
5. Code word	"Was that 'F' as in Frank?"	Usually will confirm letters.
6. Alphabet	"Could you start at letter 'A' and stop at the letter where my seat is located?"	Usually will reply "that's A,B,C,D,E,F,G . . . row G."
7. Air or palm writing	Trace desired spelling in the air or opened palm	Usually understood.

Table 3.3 *Continued*

Strategy	Request	Response
8. Numbers		
digits	"Could you please say each of the numbers individually?"	"4-2-1-9 Montclair Drive."
counting	"Could you please start at '0' and stop when you get to each digit of her address?"	"0-1-2-3-4, "0-1-2, . . ." etc.
spelling	"Could you spell that number?"	"E-I-G-H-T-Y."
fingers	"Could you please hold up the correct number of digits for each number?	Usually understood.
9. Writing	"Could you please write that word (or number)?"	Usually will write.

PART 3. You Understood Everything (or You Think You Did!)		
Confirm/ summarize	"That's Thursday at eight at Sam's. Right?"	Will confirm . . or correct if inaccurate.

Source: Hilley and Bally 1990.

when lipreading) or with which graphemes are homophones. Asking for spelling of a key word, proper noun, or number may be especially helpful.

Code Words Spelling can also be facilitated by the receiver asking the sender to use *code words* such as "B as in boy," "D as in dog" (Castle 1980). Seniors are often familiar with the military-based "Abel, Charlie, Baker" series popularized by its use during World War II. Using environmentally based code words is also effective ("D as in desk," "C as in clock," the sender simultaneously pointing to the stimulus object).

Air or Palm Writing Another spelling strategy is for the receiver to ask the sender to use *air or palm writing,* using the index finger to draw successive letters in the air or on the outstretched or upheld palm of the other hand.

Numbers The essential function of numbers in our society is evident in everyday life. Telephone numbers, dates, time, schedules, course numbers, credit card numbers, social security numbers, pin or account numbers, addresses, and flight numbers are but a few. Numbers are included in most conversations and, by their very nature, are often critical to comprehend. Some numbers within conversational contexts (e.g., eight, nine, and ten) are homophenous, and others are frequently so long they defy comprehension through speechreading. Five number strategies may be selected:

1. *Digits.* For long series of numbers, the receiver can request that the sender say the number digit by digit—"One-one-four-nine" rather than "one thousand one hundred forty nine." This strategy utilizes a limited set: only ten numbers (zero to nine) need to be identified.

2. *Counting.* A further modification of the digit strategy would have the receiver ask the sender to count up to each number.

3. *Spelling numbers.* Numbers that are homophones are not so when spelled. The receiver can ask the sender to spell out each digit (n-i-n-e, e-i-g-h-t, etc.).

4. *Fingers.* This is another modification of the digit strategy in which the receiver asks the sender to hold up the appropriate number of fingers for each digit.

5. *Writing.* The receiver asks the sender to write or summarize the message on paper. Writing is usually a reliable repair strategy if the receiver has good writing skills. This strategy, also an alternate communication mode, will be discussed further below.

The clinician should encourage the receiver to confirm *all* important information to be sure it has been received accurately.

The strategies described above may also be valuable when taught to the communication partners of persons with hearing loss or of deaf individuals. Partners knowledgeable in use of strategies may initiate appropriate strategies, even when not asked. The Repair Strategies Hierarchy for Communication Partners in appendix 3A parallels the Repair Strategies Hierarchies (tables 3.1, 3.2, and 3.3) and the Maintenance Strategies for Partners in appendix 3B outline strategies for which the communication partner can take the initiative. This is especially effective in situations where a knowledgeable hearing "partner" communicates with an untrained or unskilled sender or receiver. Ideally, communication partners will be active participants in the aural rehabilitation process.

Measuring Repair Strategy Use

Four components of repair strategy use may be examined. First, an individual needs to be cognizant of the fact that communication has broken down. Second, she should understand why communication has broken down (sender, receiver, message, or feedback problem). Next, the individual should be able to identify and assess repair strategies that might be successful in a specific situation. Finally, she should be able to employ the strategy to repair communication. The ability to use the first three components may be assessed by using brief case studies in which the professional describes a situation wherein communication has broken down. The client determines if communication has broken down, identifies the source of the problem, and enumerates appropriate repair strategies. Actual application of strategies may be assessed using the continuous discourse tracking procedure (DeFilippo and Scott 1978; Owens and Telleen 1981; DeFilippo 1988).

The continuous discourse tracking procedure uses connected material that provides linguistic information. It is a time-based measurement of words-per-minute identification of materials spoken by the clinician (sender) and repeated verbatim by the client (receiver). Progress is measured by comparing words-per-minute scores, usually for five or ten minutes, over a series of sessions (DeFilippo and Scott 1978). It should be noted that neither the frequency and diversity with which the strategies are used nor comprehension are examined.

The following steps are used in the continuous discourse tracking procedure. The clinician:

1. introduces and describes the tracking procedure and its objectives.

2. demonstrates the procedure in unambiguous practice with easy introductory text material.

3. reads from appropriate age-level texts (book, magazine, newspaper, prepared texts) for a timed period of five or ten minutes. Duration of utterance may be by sentence, phrase, or word, depending on the perceived ability of the client.

4. pauses at intervals (end of phrases or sentences) she feels are appropriate to allow the client to repeat the text verbatim.

5. continues to the next part of the text if the repetition is exact. If the message is not repeated correctly, the clinician repeats the information, modifying the presentation (duration, articulation, rate, intensity, stress, etc.), to help the client receive the message more accurately. The process continues until all parts of the message are repeated accurately.

6. calculates the words-per-minute tracking score.

Modifications of continuous discourse tracking may be employed as a within-subject measure of the ability to increase the number and variety of strategies used (Tye-Murray et al. 1988). Such modifications require the client to assume responsibility in identifying and directing the clinician as to the specific modifications she wishes to have used. Robbins et al. (1985), Owens and Raggio (1987), Owens and Telleen (1981), and Erber (1982, 1988) describe other modifications to the procedure in which the sender must follow a hierarchy of strategies (i.e., repeat, rephrase, ask for key word). The receiver instructs the sender as to which strategy to use, choosing from a list of acceptable options. To encourage practice and greater flexibility in using a greater number of strategies, strategy options may be limited or changed during practice sessions. Tracking results may then reflect range and flexibility. A further advantage is that the speechreader is not required to repeat verbatim. Instead, the speaker reads on when she understands the gist of the message. Finally, Erber (1982, 1985) describes use of tracking for providing listening practice for the telephone.

There are several limitations to the continuous discourse tracking procedure. First, written materials differ syntactically from spoken discourse. Also, results reflect the ability of a speechreader to receive information from a specific speaker. Results may be influenced by a particular speaker's speaking style or readability. Continuous discourse tracking is discussed further in chapter 8.

Assessment Strategies

Following a communication event, clients may be encouraged to assess that event. This approach may be helpful in analyzing the cause(s) for communication breakdown relative to the sender, receiver, environment, or feedback. Once the problems are identified, professionals may help clients to identify viable solutions and to implement them. In addition, it is equally important for clients to consider the reasons why communication was successful in events where communication achieved the intended objectives. This may give insight into which strategies may be most successful for the individual. Clients should then be encouraged to increase the use of those particular strategies in subsequent situations.

Other Communication Strategies

Several other systems may prove effective in facilitating the communication process. These include writing, signing, and fingerspelling and will be discussed below.

Writing as a Communication Strategy

Within the Deaf community and among deaf and hard of hearing persons a pad and pen are standard equipment when venturing into hearing environments. For many hard of hearing, deaf, or Deaf individuals writing may be the most efficient or least stressful method of interfacing with hearing people. However, writing skills of culturally Deaf individuals are often weak (Kretschmer and Kretschmer 1978). Inappropriate content and poor formatting of notes may render them unintelligible to readers. Therapy may support the use of writing as a communication strategy and focus on the production of clear, concise, and functional notes. Skills should be assessed and developed using role play situations.

Writing may also be viewed as a confirmation strategy. Factual information including numbers (time, dates, phone numbers, addresses, flight numbers, etc.), names, directions, or schedules may be written. Therapy objectives should include skills such as writing quickly and concisely, summarizing telegraph style, using abbreviations and relating to previously established information (Palmer, Bement, and Kelly 1990). Nichols and Moseley discuss assessment and development of writing skills further in chapter 11.

Sign Language as a Communication Strategy

The introduction and development of sign language skills may provide nonverbal skills that enhance communication ability in a variety of circumstances. Introducing sign systems to deaf and deafened individuals who do not function primarily in culturally Deaf environments has more applications than one might anticipate. Manual systems learned by these individuals and their primary communication partners can be used when use of the repair strategy hierarchy is not practical because of time limitations, when it is impossible to eliminate background noise, when a noncompeting communication mode to assist in group communication situations is needed, and when other situations arise specific to individual needs.

Late-deafened adults who have had little or no exposure to sign may look toward learning sign as a panacea for their problems. However, such enthusiasm seldom reflects the reality that most of their friends and family members do not know or are not motivated to learn a sign system. Some late-deafened adults may find that learning and using a limited sign vocabulary can be helpful in communicating with frequent communication partners in the home or in social situations, especially when background noise is significant. A single sign may act as a key word in establishing a topic or concept. When a spouse or other communication partner knows that sign, information may be provided during group conversations or meetings without the disruption caused by an oral request for clarification or repetition.

Deaf youth who come from hearing families and are mainstreamed will often have picked up some elements of sign to facilitate communication with Deaf peers. These are learned through a variety of sources, including Deaf friends in the community, instructors and other professionals, relatives, and school or interschool activities. The result may be that the individual develops a mixed sign system, part signed English (or other English-based sign system) and part American Sign Language (ASL). The result may be communication that is sometimes successful, but sometimes inaccurate. An individual may not be successful in communicating with those who use straight ASL or those who use signed English.

It would be reasonable to assume, therefore, that training in a single sign system would be warranted. Circumstances should dictate the value of such learning and help clients to determine which system would be of greatest benefit.

An additional benefit of the use of sign language for the populations discussed above may be an increased ability to conceptualize and communicate through gestural modes. Anecdotal information from audiologists and speech-language pathologists working with deaf and Deaf populations suggests that professionals who know sign tend to integrate signs into their everyday gestural systems. One might project that the same peripheral results would occur with more orally oriented deaf clients even if signing would not be a primary or preferred mode.

In addition, professionals working with deaf populations may find the use of sign languages as useful tools in communication therapy. Speech-language pathologists sometimes find it easier to clarify or explain concepts related to articulation or voice using a visual-gestural mode. Use of signs while a client is practicing oral skills may provide a noncompetitive signal to help the client modify efforts during trial productions.

Professionals should assess their own skill level before incorporating such training into the therapy or before deciding to make a referral to an appropriate training program. Formal sign classes may be considered to help facilitate sign skills in the most appropriate system for the individual.

Various sign systems may be examined in selecting an appropriate system for an individual. Among individuals whose primary language is oral/aural English, a signed English system may be effective. Using oral communication simultaneously with signing may utilize whatever residual hearing an individual may have.

Within culturally Deaf environments and communities, American Sign Language and "Contact Language" are more routinely used. American Sign Language, described in chapter 1, is culturally based within the Deaf community (Baker and Cokely 1980). However, Contact Language more closely describes the type of communication used cross-culturally by hearing persons. "Contact" describes the simultaneous use of voice and sign in which both ASL and English sign structures are used and an abbreviated English is voiced simultaneously (Bally 1991). The extent to which ASL structures are used depends on the preferred language of the receiver as well as the sender's ability to modify signing in favor of more ASL structures.

Other systems include Signed English, Signing Exact English (SEE II), the Linguistics of Visual English (LOVE), and the Rochester Method (fingerspelling everything). Student communication self-assessments reflect that these systems seem to be declining in use.

ASL may be the most effective language in which to conduct therapy or assessments with culturally Deaf populations. Attitudes of Deaf students (Rohland and Meath-Lang 1984) reflect that lack of communication skills (sign) was the primary cause of negative attitudes toward audiologists. Students mostly favored audiologists who knew sign language and had an understanding of Deaf culture. On a more practical level, sign skills can facilitate easier professional-to-client communication in test site situations.

The communication strategies described earlier in this chapter can be applied equally well to receptive communication through manual modes. Creating an effective communication environment, improving receptive language skills, and modifying the sender's communication behaviors are all skills that can be taught or enhanced in signed communication. Maintenance strategies, especially the use of confirmation, and repair strategies are easily adapted to ASL and other nonverbal (and verbally supported) signed modes.

Fingerspelling as a Communication Strategy

The use of a system of unilateral handshapes representing the letters of the alphabet is known as *fingerspelling*. (See figure 3.5.) As an adjunct skill, fingerspelling may have greater applicability to orally oriented deaf students or adults than to culturally Deaf individuals who would already have these skills. Within a family or an immediate peer group—classroom, sports team—fingerspelling may be taught quickly and reinforced through immediate application. It can be used as an adjunct to receptive understanding as a means for establishing a topic or as a repair strategy in situations where a particular word might be elusive. Owens and Telleen (1981) incorporated fingerspelling into the tracking procedure, demonstrating its effectiveness when clients were stuck on difficult or unfamiliar words. Similarly, speechreading teachers have reported that they find fingerspelling useful in analytic exercises to give a first letter or syllable in lipreading drills. In addition, it may help the receiver differentiate between viseme groups. The use of fingerspelling between communication partners may provide a quick (nonverbal) channel thorough which key words or important information may be communicated.

Strategies for Group Communication Situations

Group communication situations may be among the most difficult for individuals with hearing loss and may call for somewhat different strategies in addition to those already discussed in this chapter. Professionals may introduce different pragmatic approaches for anticipatory, maintenance, and repair strategy use, and a variety of assistive devices (see chapter 6) may be employed to enhance the communicative functioning of the group. For example, anticipatory strategies may include approaching group leaders or the group as a whole to discuss the communication needs of an individual who is deaf or hard of hearing. The communication environment may be modified or changed to one in which all participants have a clear view of one another. Lighting may need to be inclusive of all

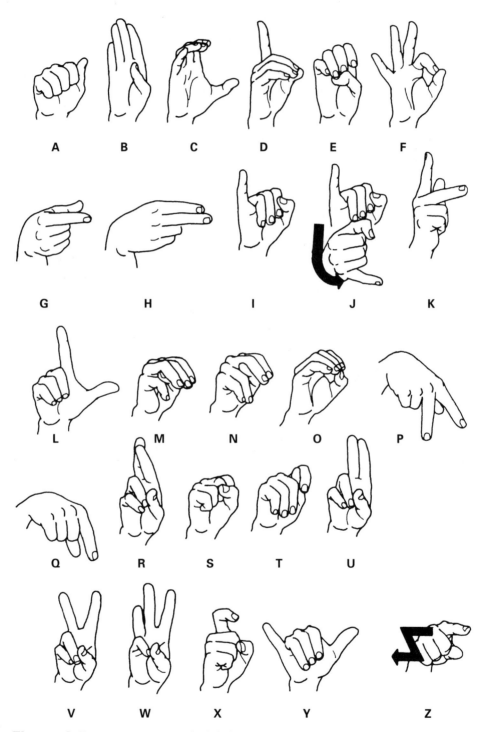

Figure 3.5. American Manual Alphabet

communicators. Public address and other group amplification systems may need to be considered. Manual notetakers or computer-assisted notetaking may be helpful.

In addition, some protocols may need to be established to modify group discourse. Individuals may need to identify themselves visually (coming forward or raising hands) before addressing the group or to ask the leader to repeat questions from the floor. Turn taking may be essential; rules against more than one person talking at a time may need to be enforced. An agenda or outline may be requested. These protocols may be established with the group as a whole or in meetings with group leaders prior to the event.

Knowledge of the tenets of the Americans with Disabilities Act related to public access, private entities, or employment may be helpful to clients in group contexts. Aspects of the law require that reasonable accommodations be made for persons with disabilities, including those who are deaf and hard of hearing.

Effective Behavioral Approaches: Assertiveness Training

The use of communication strategies requires two abilities that may be developed or enhanced in the therapy situation. The first is the development of realistic expectations. The second is the ability to effect successfully modifications in another individual's communication behaviors or in shared communication environments.

Developing Realistic Expectations

The professional may want to help individuals objectively examine the modification of communication and communication behavior. The axiom "Change what you can, don't frustrate yourself trying to change what can't be readily changed" may be a valuable reminder to clients to assess how readily things may be modified and to help them direct their energies most efficiently.

Assertiveness Training Supportive to Strategy Use

The use of effective assertive approaches to support strategy use may be a skill included in the communication therapy process for both culturally Deaf and hard of hearing persons. Assertiveness training may result in a more successful effect or approach when the receiver wishes to modify the language or behavior of the sender.

Clinical experience demonstrates that traditional assertiveness training often leaves clients feeling there are three alternative behaviors or approaches that they may employ in problem solving: passive (does nothing), aggressive ("slow down, damn it!"), assertive behavior ("please talk more slowly!"). On that basis, clients may be asked to select the behavior that they deem most appropriate in a given situation. As discussed in chapter 5 individuals vary in their capacity to effect assertive behavior.

Given that the primary focus of communication strategies is changing the behavior or environment of others, these changes must be achieved in an effective way. Erdman (1993, 401) presents definitions and characteristics of passive, assertive, and aggressive behaviors as well as various types of reactions to communication difficulties experienced by adults with hearing loss. The professional may help clients examine their behavioral approaches and the consequences of such approaches. If the desired consequences are not forthcoming, clients should be encouraged to select more effective approaches for most communication situations. Clients should be able to meet their own needs without violating the rights of others. However, circumstances wherein passive behavior is appropriate should be noted. In addition, *perceptions* of people's behaviors should be discussed.

Assertiveness may be better explored relative to a continuum of behavior. Examples of varying degrees of behavior may be elicited from the client. For example, an individual may be having difficulty understanding a lecturer who keeps turning her back to write on the chalk board while continuing to lecture. The following strategies may be possible:

1. *Passive*

   Drop out of the class. (passive-aggressive)

   Suffer through it.

   Complain to class mates, hoping they will do something about it.

2. *Assertive*

   Raise your hand and inform the lecturer of your needs.

   Speak to the lecturer during break time or after class informing her of your needs.

   Get a small representative group together and meet with the lecturer and explain your needs.

   Speak to the lecturer's supervisor informing her of your needs.

   Complain to the lecturer's supervisor.

3. *Aggressive*

   Pass a petition around the class and send it to the lecturer.

   Stand up in class and demand that the lecturer respect your rights.

   Complain to the administration, demanding that the lecturer be fired.

File a law suit because this is a violation of your right to equal access under the Americans with Disabilities Act.

Drop out of the class. (passive-aggressive)

Once it has been established that there are a variety of *choices* within the realm of assertiveness, problem solving may be initiated. The problem should be defined, the solutions enumerated. Selection of the best solution should be based on a perception of the probable consequences and of the *comfort* of the client in initiating that particular strategy. As in the previous example, some clients would have had no difficulty in interrupting a lecture if their needs were not being met, whereas others would not be able to initiate such an approach. They might be more inclined to pass a note to the instructor or make an appointment and discuss it in privacy at a later time. The objective of this aspect of communication therapy is to empower the client to initiate changes that meet his or her needs as long as the rights of other people are not violated.

Some individuals may have more difficulty in assuming a more assertive stance than others. It is unrealistic to expect major changes in a client's behavioral affect but movement toward a more assertive approach may be encouraged (Bally and Pray 1990). It may be useful to have the client pinpoint her perception of her assertiveness level on the 10-point Behavioral Continuum (figure 3.6) and select a nearby point on the continuum toward the aggressive range but still within the assertive range as a realistic individual objective in improving assertiveness. Then, some realistic objectives toward effecting a more assertive approach may be identified and plans made to implement this change.

Clients may benefit from incorporating three essential features into their assertive approaches for greater success: *direction, explanation,* and *courtesy.* A clear description of the specific communication behavior that would be most effective (direction) may be critical for communication success. Asking an individual to "speak a little more slowly" (specific) may be more helpful than repeatedly asking a person, "What did you say?" (nonspecific) (Erber 1988).

An explanation of why an accommodation is needed helps one to understand why the person with hearing loss is making the request. Usually the explanation need only be stated once—"I have a hearing loss, so could you please . . . ?"

Finally, basic courtesy may result in an improved willingness on the part of others to accommodate communication needs (Gagne 1991; Tye-Murray 1994a). The use of simple, courteous phrases such as "please" or "it would be helpful if . . ." may change the perception of a sender so that he perceives a request as

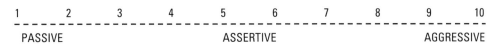

Figure 3.6. Behavioral Continuum

asking for help (assertive) rather than demanding it (aggressive). Many individuals may use a courteous tone of voice to achieve the same results. Here are some examples of the three components:

> *Direction:* "Face me when you are lecturing."
>
> *Explanation:* "I depend on lipreading, so face me when you are lecturing."
>
> *Courtesy:* "I depend on lipreading so please face me when you are lecturing."

Therapy should focus on the identification of effective, yet comfortable approaches for improving communication situations. The use of the continuum model, anecdotal problem solving, and role playing are among the techniques for improving the use of an effective assertive approach.

Cultural considerations need to be examined when working with minorities such as culturally Deaf populations. A more succinct and direct approach in asking for behavioral modifications is generally more acceptable within the Deaf community, especially with the younger members who are not as aware of social nuances (Becker 1987; Anderson 1995). The professional may wish to discuss the cultural implications of requests for behavior changes with the client if there is any doubt.

Stress Management and Relaxation as Coping Strategies

Trychin (1987a–g, 1988a,b and 1990) has developed the Coping Strategies Series. This comprehensive series is designed to teach clients and their families to understand the physical and psychological reactions to hearing loss and to learn effective techniques for dealing with the inherent problems. Techniques related to the reduction of stress and relaxation exercises may be useful when working with clients who have such difficulties in coping.

Using an Effective Consumer Approach

Clients who are considering the use of assistive devices or modification of a communication environment may also find some background information in the area of *consumerism* helpful. The Seven Steps for Effective Consumerism (Bally 1991) may be helpful in the acquisition of goods or services:

1. *Identify needs and preferences.* Individuals need to consider what they would like to have and the features that they need as opposed to those they desire. For example, in selecting a telephone amplifier, the greater power and consistency of a telephone handset may be preferable to the battery power of a portable amplifier unit. For others, however, the por-

table aspect of the unit may be preferable to the power of the handset. Another example of this process would be in selecting a speechreading class. Needs might include close proximity to public transportation, an instructor who can sign, or a reasonable cost, whereas a preference might be a group situation or location near one's place of business. One person's need may be another person's preference.

2. *Prioritize needs and preferences.* A product or service will rarely meet all the needs or preferences of an individual. Therefore, an individual should prioritize her needs. For example, she may wish to have a portable TTY and one with a printer. Because portable TTYs do not have printers, an individual would need to decide which feature was more important. Selections for purchasing goods or services can then be made based on the number and priority of features desired.

3. *Research.* Clinical experience shows that many clients report a random approach to obtaining information on products or services. For some the process starts and ends at the most convenient store or the Yellow Pages. The professional may provide guidance in how to get accurate and reliable information on products and services. All of the following may provide helpful and reliable information: research-oriented publications such as *Consumer Reports* or *Consumer Digest*; professional organizations and the local Better Business Bureau; and consumer organizations such as Self-Help for Hard of Hearing People, Inc. or the National Association of the Deaf. (See Resource List, appendix 3C.)

4. *Evaluate.* Once priorities have been made and the above information has been collected, it should be reviewed and the most appropriate products or services identified.

5. *Negotiate.* Prices for goods and services are often negotiable. Payment plans vary and at times provide discounts for cash. Some clients may not be aware of these options. Some comparison shopping on the telephone/TTY/relay or by visiting stores or offices may help consumers get the best value and service for their money.

6. *Initiate.* Individuals who are contracting or purchasing the products or service may need clarification of the terms of purchase, service contracts, warranties, etc. before paying or signing a contract.

7. *Follow-up.* Once a purchase has been made or contract for services established, consumers sometimes fail to carry through with their inherent responsibilities. The consumer's responsibilities may include reading product literature (e.g., directions for product use), as well as understanding and following up on the terms of purchase, warranties,

and guarantees. Follow-up on services may include following the directions of professionals (e.g., having prescriptions filled, completing tests, attending classes and doing homework, and making follow-up appointments).

Identifying Integrated Services

Clients often describe major difficulties in finding appropriate services and professionals who are experienced in working with persons with hearing loss. Many report that aural rehabilitation often consists of single-session hearing aid orientation presented by the dispenser, or enrollment in community classes, taught by noncertified, nonlicensed "lipreading teachers" who may use dated materials and focus solely on an analytic approach. Even with listings of certified members obtained from the American Speech-Language-Hearing Association, consumers may have difficulty identifying sources for integrated programs that include communication strategies as a primary or secondary focus. Clinicians may wish to conduct a survey to be sure that referral sources (ENTs, the Vocational Rehabilitation Administration, Hearing Aid Dealers, etc.) are aware of the services they provide. Referral sources may be provided with literature that describes the breadth and depth of the clinical services being offered as well as the experience and qualifications of the professionals who offer the services.

Global Assessment and Therapy for Communication Strategy Use

In the previous discussion of anticipatory, maintenance, and repair strategies, specific means of assessment and therapy have been discussed. Communication strategy use may also be assessed globally and general steps to therapy recommended.

Global Assessment

Several tools for global assessment are available. Most are designed for assessing hard of hearing or postlingually deafened individuals, including the Communication Profile for the Hearing Impaired (CPHI) designed by Demorest and Erdman (1986, 1987). The Communication Scale for Late Deaf Adults (CSDA) (Kaplan, Bally, and Brandt 1991), based on the CPHI, was developed to assess strategy use, identify difficult communication situations, and identify attitudes related to communication and hearing loss with culturally Deaf populations. More recently, the Communication Scale for Older Adults (CSOA) (Kaplan et al. 1994), a modification of the CSDA, was developed to explore communication attitudes and strategy use within senior populations.

The Denver Scale of Communication Function for Senior Citizens in Retirement Centers (DSSC) (Zarnoch and Alpiner 1977), the Nursing Home Hearing Handicap Index (Schow and Nerbonne 1977), and the Communication Assessment Procedure for Seniors (Alpiner and Baker 1981) were designed for institutionalized populations. Although all three lack standardization, they may provide information helpful to the clinician and client in designing therapy protocols. These scales identify areas relevant to institutional living in which communication strategies are used effectively, not used, or used ineffectively or inappropriately.

The above scales provide a basis for determining which areas of intervention are appropriate for a client. Because these tools identify problem *areas* somewhat generically, the aural rehabilitationist must help clients relate test results to their respective life situations, evaluate their communication approaches, and find successful alternatives when communication is not successful. (See chapter 4 for detailed information on communication scales.)

Additional diagnostic information may be gained from such informal approaches as monitoring informal conversations, role playing difficult communications, videotaping for in-depth analysis, observing clients in clinical and nonclinical interactions, and modifications of the tracking procedure (Erber 1988; Owens and Telleen 1981; Tye-Murray et al. 1988).

Steps For Integrated Therapy

The professional may guide a client through the following steps in the therapy process:

1. help the client achieve a global understanding of the communication process. The communication model and the strategy time continuum may be helpful in explaining the theoretical basis for therapy.

2. explain to the client what test procedures will be used and why.

3. explain the results of the diagnostic evaluation in terms of the communication models. Clients should have a clear understanding of their own communication skills and abilities.

4. guide the client into making appropriate decisions for intervention— given stimulability, motivation, and cultural considerations.

5. guide the client into setting clear therapy objectives with increments that can be quantified.

6. develop activities in which the client becomes empowered to analyze both successful and unsuccessful communication situations.

7. guide the client toward the identification of anticipatory, maintenance, and repair communication strategies that will facilitate success in previously unsuccessful communication situations.

8. guide the client toward an effective assertive approach that will facilitate implementation of communication strategies.

9. identify quantitative and qualitative measures that will help the client calculate progress toward effective communication strategy use.

10. help the client learn to self-monitor strategy use effectively.

The clinician may employ an extensive variety of activities to facilitate strategy use. These may include but are not limited to: role play and videotaping; scripting and the use of constellations (Kaplan et al. 1987); analysis of case studies or written samples of dialogues; brainstorming; discussion and problem solving; use of models and hierarchies; and use of questionnaires, daily logs, diaries, and elicited narratives as well as oral and written examinations.

Sources for Materials

A wide range of materials is available for improving communication strategies. These include such diverse approaches as one-on-one "therapy"; group "classes"; intensive programs (the "Hearing Loss in Later Years" Elderhostel, Elderhostel National, Inc., offered by Gallaudet University, Washington, D.C.); videotapes (New York League 1990); waiting room based videotapes (Abrahamson 1991); workbooks (Kaplan et al. 1987; Mezei and Smith 1993; Trychin 1987a–g); consumer-oriented guides (Rosenthal 1978; Rezen and Hausman 1985; Bally and Trychin 1989; Shimon 1992; Tye-Murray 1992a, 1994b); interactive computerized videodisc training exercises (Sims et al. 1979; Tye-Murray 1991); structured programs (QUEST?AR* [*Quest*ions for *A*ural *R*ehabilitation], Erber 1985b; ASQUE [*A*nswers/*S*tatements/*Que*stions], Erber 1985c); and self-help workbooks (Kaplan et al. 1987; Marcus 1985; Mezei and Smith 1993). Some materials may focus on specific skill areas, whereas others integrate therapy areas. For example, Deyo (1984) and Castle (1980, 1988) integrate language skills and auditory training with telephone training. Each of these materials needs to be evaluated for its usefulness with an individual client based on the established objectives.

Training Communication Partners

The value of including family and friends who most frequently interact with a person in the (re)habilitation process has received increasing attention during the past few years (Erber 1988, 1993, Tye-Murray and Schum 1994). Ideally, communication partners will participate actively in the entire process, attending sessions and participating in activities. In the Gallaudet University Elderhostel programs (Bally and Kaplan 1988) partners have long been encouraged to attend. They participate in most activities along with their friends or spouses. They also have sessions specifically designed to meet their needs, including rap sessions where they can discuss their concerns with social workers and with aural rehabilitationists, simulations of hearing loss (Kemp 1989), and conversation training from the perspective of the communication partner that emphasizes strategy use (see appendix 3A and 3B). Erber (1988, 1993) suggests using samples of everyday conversation to illustrate that they have inherent commonalities and individual differences. These differences and similarities may be used to help clients analyze reasons for communication breakdown and design individualized approaches for successful communication between partners.

Partners training may also include:

1. Understanding of the communication process

2. Fostering empathy for the impact of hearing loss on communication

3. Identifying and reducing behavioral and environmental distractions

4. Identifying and utilizing optimum speaker behaviors (verbal and nonverbal)

5. Structuring conversation to maximize comprehension

6. Utilizing personal adjustment counseling (see chapter 5)

Case studies, structured communication interactions, strategy hierarchies, role plays and simulations, questionnaires, logs and diaries, and elicited narratives are all techniques to use with partners. Intradisciplinary approaches to partner training, such as teaming with professionals in the counseling areas, may prove highly effective.

Summary

This chapter has explored, in a systematic way, the principles and techniques for assessing and improving the use of communication strategies supportive to more effective receptive and expressive communication. The Communication and Time Continuum Models were used as a theoretical base. A discussion of anticipatory strategies included assessment and training in the use of environmental, interpersonal and linguistic strategies. Training and assessment of both verbal and nonverbal maintenance strategies were described including the use of Cued Speech. By contrast, the assessment and reduction of counterproductive strategies were characterized. Hierarchies for the use of repair strategies were put forth and assessment techniques described. Other approaches include the use of writing, sign language, and fingerspelling. Therapy approaches, reflecting cultural differences for Deaf and hard of hearing individuals, were discussed. These included self-assessment and global assessment, group strategies, partner training, and effective behavioral and consumer approaches. Finally, sources for materials were enumerated.

Appendix 3A
Repair Strategies Hierarchy
for Communication Partners

CONSIDERATIONS FOR FEEDBACK

    A. Assess importance of relating information.
      B. Assess why breakdown occurred.
        C. Assess time considerations.
          D. Consider your options.
            E. Consider options with respect to partner.
              F. Select your option.
                G. Choose the most appropriate strategy.

REASONS FOR BREAKDOWN

Communication Style	*Communication Environment*	*Communication Content*
Slow down	Modify environment	Use repair strategies
or	or	*Understood none *Understood some
Speak louder or Speak more clearly	Change environments	

REPAIR STRATEGIES

Part 1: Understood None of the Message

Repeat	Repeat the message in the same way.
Rephrase	Give the same information using different words or format. May be incremented.
Key Word	Give the topic and most important words; then give the message with emphasis on the key words.

Part 2: Understood Some of the Message.
    Ask the listener to confirm what was understood, then:

Repeat	Repeat ONLY what the speaker-listener has requested.

Rephrase	Use a different word or words for the ones that were not understood. May use fewer words or elaborate more extensively.
Spell	Spell the requested word. This may include the key word, proper nouns, and numbers.
Use Code Words	Confirm letters: "F as in Frank."
Give Digits	Say numbers individually: "4-2-1-8 Hill Street."
Counting	Start with "0" and count up to each digit: "0-1-2-3-4, 0-1-2, 0-1-2-3-4-5, etc."
Air or Palm Spell	Use your finger and writer letters or numbers in the air or on your palm.

Part 3: Ask for Confirmation.
Source: Bally and Hilley 1992.

Appendix 3B
Maintenance Strategies
for Communication Partners

I.   *Use Effective Communication Behaviors*
   A. Speak slowly

   B. Speak clearly (but don't over exaggerate!)

   C. Speak with adequate volume (but don't yell!)

   D. Use gesture, facial expression, and body language

II. *Ask for Needs*
   "What can I do to help us communicate better?"

III. *Confirm Information*
   Summarize and confirm to show you understand

IV. *Ask for Confirmation/Summary*
   Make sure your partner understands you

V.   *Structure Communication*
   A. Use familiar vocabulary at a comfortable level

   B. Answer questions specifically (before elaborating)

   C. Increment information

   D. Sequence information

   E. Make topic changes evident

Appendix 3C
Resource List

American Speech and Hearing Association
10801 Rockville Pike
Rockville, Maryland 20852
(301) 897-5700

Consumer Reports Magazine
101 Truman Avenue
Yonkers, New York 10703-1057

Consumer Reports Buying Guide
256 Washington Street
Mount Vernon, N.Y. 10553

National Association of the Deaf
814 Thayer Avenue
Silver Spring, MD 20910
(301) 587-1788 (Voice)

Self-Help for Hard of Hearing People, Inc.
7910 Woodmont Avenue, Suite 1200
Bethesda, MD 20814
(301) 657-2248 (Voice) or (301) 657-2249(TT)

References

Abrahamson, J. 1991. Teaching coping strategies: A client education approach to aural rehabilitation. *Journal of the Academy of Rehabilitative Audiology* 24:43–53.

Alpiner, J. G., and B. Baker. 1981. Communication assessment procedures in the aural rehabilitation process. *Seminars in Speech-Language-Hearing* 2(3):189–294.

Andersson, Y. 1995. Personal communication. Gallaudet University, Washington, D.C.

Baker, C., and D. Cokely. 1980. *American sign language: A teacher's resource text on grammar and culture.* Silver Spring, Md.: T.J. Publishers, Inc.

Bally, S. J. 1987. *Communication Strategies Continuum.* Washington, D.C.: Gallaudet University, Department of Audiology and Speech-Language Pathology.

Bally, S. J., ed. 1991, 1995. *Communication science: A guide for deaf and hard of hearing consumers.* Washington, D.C.: Gallaudet University, Department of Audiology and Speech-Language Pathology.

Bally, S. J., and H. Kaplan. 1988. The Gallaudet University Elderhostels. *Journal of the Academy of Rehabilitative Audiology* 21:99–112.

Bally, S. J., and J. L. Pray. 1990. Problem solving approaches and communication strategies. Paper presented at the Fifth International SHHH Convention, Little Rock, Arkansas.

Bally, S. J., and S. Trychin. 1989. *A newcomer's guide to an old problem: Hearing loss.* Washington, D.C.: SHHH Publications.

Bally, S. J., and M. H. Hilley. 1992. *Repair strategies hierarchy for communication partners.* Washington, D.C.: Gallaudet University, Department of Audiology and Speech-Language Pathology.

Bally, S. J., M. P. Wilson, and J. Bergan. 1984. Effective communication strategies: A guide for the hearing impaired. Unpublished manuscript, Gallaudet University, Washington, D.C.

Bally, S. J., R. Goffen, and S. M. Scott. 1995. *Familiarization with unfamiliar vocabulary as an anticipatory strategy.* Study in progress, Gallaudet University, Washington, D.C.

Becker, G. 1987. Lifelong socialization and adaptive behavior of deaf people. In *Understanding deafness socially*, ed. P. C. Higgins and J. E. Nash. Springfield, Ill.: Charles C. Thomas.

Bias, J. 1995. Personal communication.

Castle, D. 1980. *Telephone training for the deaf.* Rochester, N.Y.: National Technical Institute for the Deaf.

Castle, D. L. 1988. *Telephone strategies: A technical and practical guide for hard-of-hearing people.* Washington, D.C.: Alexander Graham Bell Association for the Deaf.

Clark, H., and E. Clark. 1977. *Psychology and language.* New York: Harcourt, Brace & Jovanovich.

Cornett, O. R. 1972. Effects of cued speech upon speechreading. In *International symposium on speech communication and profound deafness*, ed. G. Fant. Washington, D.C.: Alexander Graham Bell Association for the Deaf.

DeFilippo, C. 1988. Tracking for speechreading training. *Volta Review* 90(5):215–239.

DeFilippo, C., and B. L. Scott. 1978. A method for training and evaluating the reception of ongoing speech. *Journal of the Acoustical Society of America* 63:1186–1192.

Demorest, M. E., and S. A. Erdman. 1986. Scale composition and item analysis of the Communication Profile for the Hearing Impaired. *Journal of Speech and Hearing Disorders* 29:515–535.

Demorest, M. E., and S. A. Erdman. 1987. Development of the communication profile for the hearing impaired. *Journal of Speech and Hearing Disorders* 52(4):129–143.

Deyo, D. 1984a. *Speechreading in context: Functional activities for student practice.* Washington, D.C.: Gallaudet University, Pre-College Programs.

———. 1984b. *Ring/Flash.* Washington, D.C.: Gallaudet University, Pre-College Programs.

Deyo, D., and M. Hallau. 1984. *Communicate with me: Communication strategies for deaf students.* Washington, D.C.: Gallaudet University, Pre-College Programs.

Elfenbein, J. 1992. Coping with communication breakdown: A program of strategy development for children who have hearing losses. *American Journal of Audiology: A Journal of Clinical Practice* 1:25–29.

Erber, N. P. 1982. *Auditory training*. Washington, D.C.: Alexander Graham Bell Association for the Deaf.

―――. 1985a. *Telephone communication and hearing impairment*. San Diego, Calif.: College Hill Press.

―――. 1985b. *QUEST?AR (Questions for Aural Rehabilitation)*. Victoria, Australia: Helographics.

―――. 1985c. *ASQUE (Answers/Statements/Questions)*. Victoria, Australia: Helographics.

―――. 1988. *Communication therapy for hearing-impaired adults*. Abbotsford, Victoria, Australia: Clavis Publishing.

―――. 1993. *Communication and adult hearing loss*. Melbourne, Australia: Clavis Publishing.

Erber, N. P., and C. W. Greer. 1973. Communication strategies used by teachers at an oral school for the deaf. *Volta Review* 75:480–485.

Erdman, S. A. 1993. Counseling hearing impaired adults. In *Rehabilitative audiology: Children and Adults*, 2d ed., ed. J. G. Alpiner and P. A. McCarthy. Baltimore: Williams & Wilkins.

Forgotch, M., and S. Trychin. 1988a. *Getting along*. Bethesda, Md.: SHHH Publications.

―――. *Getting along* (videotape). Bethesda, Md.: SHHH Publications.

For hearing people only: How do deaf people get each other's attention if they can't yell? *Deaf Life* 7:3.

Gagne, J-P., and K. M. Wyllie. 1989. Relative effectiveness of three repair strategies on the visual identification of misperceived words. *Ear and Hearing* 10:368–374.

Gagne, J-P., P. Stelacovich, and W. Yovetich. 1991. Reactions to requests for clarification used by hearing-impaired individuals. *Volta Review* 93(3):129–143.

Garretson, C. J., and S. C. Jordon. 1982. *Communication processes and the hearing impaired*. Washington, D.C.: Gallaudet University, Department of Communication Arts.

Garstecki, D., and J. Alpiner. 1982. In *Introduction to aural rehabilitation*, 2d ed., ed. R. L. Schow and M. A. Nerbonne. Austin, Tex.: Pro-Ed.

Hallberg, L. R. M., and S. G. Carlsson. 1991. A qualitative study of strategies for managing a hearing impairment. *British Journal of Audiology* 25(2):201–211.

Hilley, M., and S. J. Bally. 1990. Repair Strategies Hierarchy. Washington, D.C.: Gallaudet University, Department of Audiology and Speech-Language Pathology.

Horn, R., J. Mahshie, H. Kaplan, S. Bally, and M. P. Wilson. 1984. Assessing communication skills of hearing impaired adolescents and adults: A comprehensive approach. *ASHA* 26:10.

Kaplan, H. 1982. Facilitating adjustment. In *Rehabilitative audiology*, ed. R. H. Hull. New York: Grune & Stratton.

Kaplan, H., S. J. Bally, and C. Garretson. 1987. *Speechreading: A way to improve understanding,* 2d ed. Washington, D.C.: Gallaudet University Press.

Kaplan, H., S. J. Bally, and F. B. Brandt. 1991. Communication Self-Assessment Scale for Deaf Adults. *Journal of the American Academy of Audiology* 2(3):164–182.

Kaplan, H., S. J. Bally, F. Brandt, D. A. Busacco, and J. L. Pray. 1994. Effects of the Gallaudet University Elderhostel Programs on the lives of older adults with hearing loss. Presentation to the American Academy of Audiology Summer Institute, Salt Lake City, Utah.

Kemp, G. 1989. *It's a silent world.* Washington, D.C.: 4th International SHHH Convention.

Kipila, E., and B. Williams-Scott. 1990. Cued Speech: A response to "Controversy within sign language." In *Communication issues among Deaf people: A Deaf American monograph,* ed. M. D. Garretson. Silver Spring, Md.: National Association of the Deaf.

Kretschmer, R. R., and L. W. Kretschmer. 1978. *Language development and intervention with the hearing impaired.* Baltimore: University Park Press.

Marcus, I. S. 1985. *Your eyes hear for you: A self-help course in speechreading.* Bethesda, Md.: SHHH Publications.

Mayo, P., and P. Waldo. 1986. *Scripting.* Eau Claire, Wis.: Thinking Publications.

McCall, R. 1984. *Speechreading and listening tactics.* London, England: Robert Hale Limited.

Mezei, F., and S. Smith. 1993. *Lipreading naturally.* Mississauga, Ontario, Canada: The Canadian Hearing Society.

New York League for the Hard of Hearing. 1990. *I see what you're saying* (videotape, vol. 1 and 2). New York: New York League for the Hard of Hearing.

Nitchie, E. B. 1912. *Lipreading: Principles and practice.* New York: Frederick A. Stokes Co.

Owens, E., and C. C. Telleen. 1981. Tracking as an aural rehabilitative process. *Journal of the Academy of Rehabilitative Audiology* 14:259–273.

Owens, E., and M. Raggio. 1987. The UCSF tracking procedure for evaluation and training of speech reception by hearing-impaired adults. *Journal of Speech and Hearing Disorders* 52:120–128.

Palmer, L., L. Bement, and J. Kelly. 1990. Implications of deafness and cultural diversity on communication instruction: Strategies for intervention. *Journal of the Academy of Rehabilitative Audiology* 23:43–52.

Rezen, S. V., and C. Hausman. 1985. *Coping with hearing loss: A guide for adults and their families.* New York: Dembner Books.

Rohland, P. A., and B. Meath-Lang. 1984. Perceptions of deaf adults regarding audiologists and audiological services. *Journal of the Academy of Rehabilitative Audiology* 17:130–150.

Rosenthal, R. 1975. *The hearing loss handbook.* New York: Schocken Books.

Sanders, D. 1971. *Aural rehabilitation.* Englewood Cliffs, N.J.: Prentice-Hall.

Schow, R. L., and M. A. Nerbonne. 1977. Assessment of hearing handicap by nursing home residents and staff. *Journal of the Academy of Rehabilitative Audiology* 10:2–12.

———. 1982. *Introduction to aural rehabilitation,* 2d ed. Austin, Tex.: Pro-Ed.

Shimon, D. A. 1992. *Coping with hearing loss and hearing aids.* San Diego, Calif.: Singular Publishing Group, Inc.

Shroyer, E. H. 1982. *Signs of the times.* Washington, D.C.: Gallaudet University Press.

Sims, D., J. VonFeldt, F. Dowaliby, K. Hutchinson, and T. Meyers. 1979. A pilot experiment in computer assisted speechreading instruction utilizing the data analysis video interactive device (DAVID). *American Annals of the Deaf* 124:618–623.

Sternberg, M. L. A. 1994. *American sign language dictionary.* New York: Harper Perennial.

Trychin, S. 1987a. *Communication rules for hard of hearing people,* Bethesda, Md.: SHHH Publications.

———. 1987b. *Did I do that?* Bethesda, Md.: SHHH Publications.

———. 1987c. *Did I do that?* (videotape). Bethesda, Md.: SHHH Publications.

———. 1987d. *Relaxation training for hard of hearing people* (videotapes). Bethesda, Md.: SHHH Publications.

———. 1987e. *Relaxation training for hard of hearing people,* trainee's manual. Bethesda, Md.: SHHH Publications.

———. 1987f. *Relaxation training for hard of hearing people,* practitioner's manual. Bethesda, Md.: SHHH Publications.

———. 1987g. *Stress management* (information series 203), Bethesda, Md.: SHHH Publications.

———. 1988a. *Is that what you think?* Bethesda, Md.: SHHH Publications.

———. 1988b. *So that's the problem!* Bethesda, Md.: SHHH Publications.

———. 1990. *Living with hearing loss: training manual for group facilitators.* Washington, D.C.: Gallaudet University.

Tye-Murray, N. 1991. Repair strategy usage by hearing-impaired adults and changes following communication therapy. *Journal of Speech and Hearing Research* 34: 921–928.

———. 1992a. Communication therapy. In *Children with cochlear implants: A handbook for parents, teachers and speech and hearing professionals,* ed. N. Tye-Murray. Washington, D.C.: Alexander Graham Bell Association for the Deaf.

———. 1992b. Laser videodisc applications in the aural rehabilitation setting: Good news for the severely and profoundly hearing-impaired client. *The American Journal of Audiology: A Journal of Clinical Practice* 1:33–36.

————. 1992c. Preparing for communication interactions: The value of anticipatory strategies for adults with hearing impairment. *Journal of Speech and Hearing Research* 35:430–435.

————. 1994a. Communication strategies training. *Journal of the Academy of Rehabilitative Audiology Monograph Supplement* 27:193–207.

————. 1994b. *Let's converse.* Washington, D.C.: Alexander Graham Bell Association for the Deaf.

Tye-Murray, N., and L. Schum. 1994. Conversation training for frequent communication partners. *Journal of the Academy of Rehabilitative Audiology Monograph Supplement* 27:209–236.

Tye-Murray, N., S. C. Purdy, and G. Woodworth. 1992. The reported use of communication strategies by members of SHHH and its relationship to client, talker, and situational variables. *Journal of Speech and Hearing Research* 35:708–717.

Tye-Murray, N., R. S. Tyler, B. Bong, and T. Nares. 1988. Using laser videodisc technology to train speechreading and assertive listening skills. *Journal of the Academy of Rehabilitative Audiology* 21:143–152.

Tye-Murray, N., S. C. Purdy, G. C. Woodworth, and R. S. Tyler. 1990. Effects of repair strategies on visual identification of sentences. *Journal of Speech and Hearing Disorders* 55:621–627.

Tye-Murray, N., S. Witt, L. Schum, and C. Sobaski. 1994. Communication breakdowns: partner contingencies and partner reactions. *Journal of the Academy of Rehabilitative Audiologists* 27:107–133.

Ventry, I., and B. Weinstein. 1982. The Hearing Handicap Inventory for the Elderly: A new tool. *Ear and Hearing* 3:128–134.

Watzlawick, P., J. B. Bavelas, and D. D. Jackson. 1967. *Pragmatics of human communication.* New York: Norton.

Williams-Scott, B. 1994. *Cued speech news.* Washington, D.C.: Gallaudet University.

Zarnoch, J. M., and J. G. Alpiner. 1977. The Denver Scale of Communication Function for Seniors Living in Retirement Centers. Unpublished manuscript, University of Denver.

Zimmerman, G. I., J. L. Owen, and D. R. Seibert. 1977. *Speech communication: A contemporary introduction.* St. Paul, Minn.: West Publishing Co.

4

Informational and Adjustment Counseling

Harriet Kaplan

■ ■ ■ ■

Many deaf and hard of hearing people experience difficulty using spoken language to interact and communicate with hearing people. Messages tend to be misinterpreted because crucial words and nuances of meaning conveyed by inflections, pauses, and stress patterns are missed. Resultant difficulties involve spouses, children, employers, and friends as well as the deaf or hard of hearing person. Both clients and significant others often need help to meet the challenge of accepting the hearing loss, complying with recommended rehabilitation measures such as the use of amplification, and finding ways to manage difficult communication problems. Assertiveness training, use of communication strategies, help with acceptance of amplification, and the development of problem-solving skills for difficult communication situations should be considered for inclusion in group and individual rehabilitation programs, as needed.

The relatively small group of individuals who consider themselves culturally Deaf do not experience the same kind of adjustment problems as the much larger group of hard of hearing or deafened adults. Culturally Deaf adults are those who choose to use sign language as their primary means of communication and associate primarily with others who do likewise. Such individuals find a vast array of social and cultural support systems in the signing Deaf community (Kannapell and Adams 1984). However, many culturally Deaf adults need to communicate with nonsigning people in some aspects of their lives, perhaps in the vocational arena or with hearing relatives. Counseling is often needed along with skill development to facilitate communication by bridging gaps between Deaf and hearing cultures. In addition, not all profoundly deaf people who incurred loss of hearing before the development of spoken language are culturally Deaf. Some wish to be part of the "hearing world" and experience difficulty accepting themselves as deaf people.

The Integrated Therapy Model described in chapter 2 of this book involves remediation of five skill areas, represented by spokes radiating from a central core. Connecting all the skill areas are several concentric circles, one of which is counseling. The significance of this pictorial representation of the therapy model is that informational and adjustment counseling form part of all communication therapy. For example, successful use of amplification requires informational counseling in the use and care of the hearing aid and adjustment counseling in developing reasonable expectations of its benefits. Successful development of speechreading and communication strategies skills requires that the client understand these processes and be willing to acknowledge the presence of hearing loss to communication partners. Some form of informational and adjustment counseling is needed in communication therapy programs for most clients with hearing loss.

Definition of Informational and Adjustment Counseling

Counseling in aural rehabilitation may be thought of as the facilitative process used by clinicians to help clients accept hearing loss when necessary and resolve communication problems secondary to hearing loss. It often focuses on helping the individual handle specific situational communication problems and increase the effectiveness of interpersonal communication. Counseling involves "empathetic listening, which acknowledges and validates another's feelings; problem solving, which helps one examine choices and possible outcomes; and cognitive approaches, which examine how beliefs and thinking patterns shape behavior" (Stone and Olswang 1989, 28). Sanders (1975, 1980, 1988) discusses two types of counseling: personal adjustment counseling, which deals with feelings and attitudes, and informational counseling, which deals with dissemination or sharing of information. Although the two types of counseling may be discussed separately, the dichotomy is artificial. Affective and cognitive aspects of counseling are usually intertwined in the rehabilitation program because dissemination of information is an essential part of the problem-solving approach used to help clients find solutions to their difficulties.

Giolas (Schow and Nerbonne 1982) presents an outline of an eight-week adult aural rehabilitation group program for people with hearing loss and their significant others that combines personal adjustment and informational counseling. This program typifies a problem-solving approach. The goals of the program are "to analyze auditory failures and develop concrete behaviors which result in improved communication" (577). The group leader's function is to facilitate discussion by raising pertinent questions, by being a good listener, and by showing respect for all opinions. The aural rehabilitationist also serves as the expert on hearing and hearing disorders. Group activities involve mutual support, exchange of information, and exploration of communication problems for the purpose of finding solutions. At the end of each session, clients receive a homework assignment involving analysis and management of difficult communication situations: for example, identification of communication variables such as talker, environmental conditions, purpose of conversation, reasons for difficulty, and how problems were managed.

During each session, the following activities occur:

1. Discussion of homework assignment

2. Formal presentation on informational counseling

3. Discussion of formal presentation

4. Social break

5. Communication strategy activity

Personal Adjustment Counseling

This section of the chapter describes the nature of personal adjustment counseling and how it relates to other aspects of communication therapy. Discussion of how to recognize when it is appropriate to refer a client to a mental health professional is also included.

Nature of Personal Adjustment Counseling

In recent years, some audiologists have emphasized a counseling-oriented approach to help clients cope with communication situations and reduce anxiety (Alpiner 1982; Alpiner and McCarthy 1987; Fleming et al. 1973) as opposed to traditional speechreading and auditory training. The aural rehabilitationist functions as a facilitator to help clients modify negative attitudes about themselves as persons who are deaf or hard of hearing and adopt a problem-solving approach to resolve communication and psychosocial difficulties. (Psychosocial aspects of hearing loss are discussed in detail in chapter 5 of this book.)

Group sessions are effective vehicles for facilitating adjustment and communication improvement (Alpiner and Garstecki 1989). Clients become aware that others experience similar problems as a result of hearing loss and become more willing to discuss their difficulties openly. The stress and frustration caused by hearing loss can be ventilated. Group dynamics facilitate the problem-solving process because group members can share their successful coping strategies. The role of the aural rehabilitationist is to function as group leader to stimulate positive discussion. Although the benefits of counseling are more apparent in a group format, some of the same processes (e.g., ventilation and problem solving) are possible in individual therapy.

It is helpful to involve significant others in either individual or group counseling programs because communication problems occur in family, vocational, and social situations. The client may feel that family members do not make sufficient effort to help with communication whereas family members may consider the client unreasonably demanding. The client may withdraw from social contacts because communication has become too difficult, impacting the social lives of family members.

Acceptance of Amplification The clinician must not assume that because a client has come to the clinic for hearing aid evaluation, she has accepted the hearing loss. Some clients are simply appeasing family or are ambivalent about the need for amplification. If a client is not ready to accept amplification, it is better to encourage enrollment in a counseling-based aural rehabilitation program before fitting a hearing aid. The clinician should emphasize that participation in the program is not contingent on purchase of a hearing aid but that the audiologist is ready to assist with amplification if and when the client is ready.

Hearing aid orientation is considered to be a major part of aural rehabilitation for first-time hearing aid users and other clients with hearing aid related problems. In most cases, instruction in the technical aspects of hearing aid management is insufficient for acceptance and satisfactory use of hearing aids. Pre- and postfitting counseling must occur to create realistic understanding of the nature of the hearing loss, its effect on communication, and the benefits and limitations of hearing aid use. The client needs to be ready to accept amplification in order to use it well. Hearing aid orientation combines informational and personal adjustment counseling.

Attributes of a Facilitator Kodman (1967) discusses the attributes of a good facilitator. He speaks of *accurate empathy*, which refers to understanding by the counselor of the true feelings that underlie a client's statements. The counselor responds in such a way that the client's feelings are reflected back and then are viewed objectively. For example, a client might say, "If people would speak better, I wouldn't have any problems." The counselor might respond, "It must be terribly frustrating not to understand people. Let's talk about some of your experiences." A second attribute is *unconditional positive regard*, which involves acceptance of clients as they are, despite hostility, anger, or lack of cooperation. *Perspective taking,* the ability to take another's point of view (Erdman 1993), is a combination of accurate empathy and unconditional positive regard. A rehabilitationist can work with a client far better if he or she can see things from the client's viewpoint.

A third attribute is *genuineness,* which involves having a relaxed, friendly attitude toward the client, respect for the client's suggestions, the ability to accept criticism, and the ability to communicate in a manner the client can understand easily. A genuine clinician does not use professional jargon or inform a client that his or her opinion is wrong. An excellent discussion of issues involved in counseling adults with hearing loss can be found in Erdman (1993).

A communication therapist can be an effective facilitator if he or she brings the attributes discussed in the previous section to the counseling situation. In addition to these attributes, clinicians must make sure that their facial expressions, eye contact, gestures, and body language communicate empathy, genuineness, and unconditional positive regard. Typically, audiologists and speech-language pathologists receive little training in development of effective client-clinician relationships. However, they can develop successful interactional skills by practicing attentive listening and restating the client's content in a way that reflects the feelings underlying the client's statements. These counseling skills can be modeled, practiced through role playing, and evaluated by peers and supervisors (Erdman 1993). If the client is receptive, sessions can be videotaped for later analysis.

These attributes are particularly important when working with culturally Deaf clients, whose language (ASL) must be understood and respected. Clinicians who use ASL, even if not fluent in the language, are generally respected by culturally Deaf clients. The attempt to use ASL is often considered an indication of the genuineness of the relationship. Furthermore, it is important for the hearing clinician to respect the decisions of culturally Deaf clients not to mainstream into hearing culture. Some clients come to therapy because they wish to maximize their communicative independence in specific situations where use of English speech or writing is important. They still identify themselves as Deaf people, however, and communicate with sign language in social situations. Successful work with culturally Deaf clients requires the aural rehabilitationist to recognize that they tend to approach aural rehabilitation from a different perspective than hard of hearing clients. With such clients, the counseling focus tends to be on informational counseling and on helping the client facilitate communication with hearing people. A situation specific problem-solving approach described later in this chapter often works well.

Referring to a Mental Health Professional Many aural rehabilitationists are uncomfortable about their counseling roles partly because they are unclear as to when they need to refer to a mental health professional. Stone and Olswang (1989) discuss boundaries that define appropriate limits for the audiologist or speech language pathologist in the counseling process (see table 4.1). The counselor must establish a relationship with a client in which both clearly understand

Table 4.1   Boundaries for Aural Rehabilitation Counseling

Within the Boundaries	Outside the Boundaries
Rehabilitative Counseling	Psychotherapy
Deals with current feelings related to communication.	Changes unconscious patterns. Change basic ways of relating.
Focus or Content of Therapy	
Feelings, attitudes related to communication.	Feelings, attitudes not related to communication.
Dynamics of Client-Clinician Relationship	
Mutual respect between client and clinician.	Client overly dependent. Client and clinician emotionally involved.
Client active and empowered.	Client becomes unstable. Clinician becomes uncomfortable.

Source: Stone and Olswang 1989.

the boundaries. These boundaries may vary depending on the skills and experience of the professional and the constraints of the treatment setting (e.g., access to other professionals who may provide counseling service).

The first boundary discussed by Stone and Olswang (1989) involves the difference between psychotherapy and the type of supportive counseling performed during aural rehabilitation. Rehabilitation counseling strives to help the client deal with current feelings related to communication problems and make use of personal and societal resources to resolve those problems. Such counseling involves empathetic listening, and problem solving, and should take a cognitive approach. In contrast, psychotherapy attempts to change a client's unconscious patterns and a client's or family's basic way of relating. When a counseling relationship enters the realm of psychotherapy, the client needs to be referred to a mental health professional.

Stone and Olswang (1989) discuss two specific types of boundaries that the counselor needs to consider. One involves the focus or content of material discussed in therapy. Material within this boundary includes feelings, attitudes, or problems directly related to communication needs. Topics beyond the boundary are not related to communication (e.g., domestic violence, substance abuse, etc.)

and require referral. Sometimes it is not clear whether content is outside or challenging the boundaries (e.g., marital difficulties related to hearing loss). The counselor must then decide whether to redirect the client within the counseling situation or refer him elsewhere.

The second type of boundary concerns the dynamics of the client-counselor relationship. Relationships within the boundaries are mutually respectful; the client is active and empowered. Relationships are beyond the boundaries if the client becomes overly dependent, if the client and the counselor become emotionally involved with each other, or if the client's emotional and behavioral stability fluctuates repeatedly. Another indicator of a relationship outside the boundaries is persistent uncomfortable feelings on the part of the rehabilitationist. These are signs that the client's emotional problems have gone beyond the capabilities of the audiologist or speech-language pathologist and need to be addressed by a mental health professional.

When it becomes clear that a referral to a mental health professional is needed, the counselor should help the client enter into a relationship with that professional. The counselor can facilitate the client's acceptance of the need for referral, help set up the first appointment, or even accompany the client to the first appointment. In some cases, the counselor may continue working with the client on communication-based problems at the same time that the client is working with the mental health professional.

Informational Counseling

Informational or educational counseling involves dissemination of information about communication, hearing loss, and problem-solving strategies to help cope with communication difficulties. Such information is presented in the form of discussion and is integrated with other aural rehabilitation activities.

Included are topics such as:

1. The nature of the auditory system and hearing loss, including interpretation of the audiogram;

2. The effects of hearing loss on communication, the contributions of vowels and consonants to intelligibility, and the impact of background noise;

3. The importance of visual input, audiovisual integration, environmental conditions, and attending behavior;

4. The impact of talker differences and social conditions on communication;

5. The benefits and limitations of speechreading;

6. The benefits and limitations of hearing aids and assistive devices;

7. The use of anticipatory and repair strategies to facilitate communication;

8. The use of community resources such as self-help groups.

Informational counseling is integrated into all aspects of skill development. For example, speechreading training includes discussion of benefits and limitations of speechreading. Understanding the contribution of vowels and consonants to intelligibility facilitates articulation training. Informational counseling facilitates adjustment counseling. For example, successful use of anticipatory and repair strategies increases communicative confidence. Participation in self-help groups builds self-esteem and facilitates acceptance of the hearing loss.

Counseling Approaches

A number of counseling approaches have been found to be useful with deaf and hard of hearing clients. Many counselors have developed eclectic approaches by combining aspects of several programs. Below is a brief review of several systems, followed by a description of an approach found by this author to be useful with deaf and hard of hearing adults.

Rational Emotive Therapy Rational Emotive Therapy (RET) is an example of a cognitive approach to therapy that encourages expressions of emotions and beliefs accompanying hearing loss. It is founded on the premise that a relationship exists between thought, emotion, and behavior. The clinician assumes a supportive but directive role in helping the client identify and change inappropriate perceptions, beliefs, and attitudes about life circumstances (Ellis and Grieger 1977; Kelly 1992).

Client-Centered Therapy Affective or humanistic approaches focus on expression of emotion or feelings to facilitate adjustment rather than to direct change of behavior or thought processes. Carl Rogers's client-centered therapy is a well-known example of such an approach. The clinician assumes a nondirective role and helps the client to redirect his or her life through self-exploration (Rogers 1951; Erdman 1993). The qualities of accurate empathy and unconditional positive regard are considered essential to the successful use of this approach.

Bibliotherapy Bibliotherapy is being used by some aural rehabilitationists as an adjunct to audiologic counseling (Bryant and Roberts 1992). Clients are given reading material followed by guided discussion to facilitate positive growth. In addition to providing information, bibliotherapy is used to help the client understand that the communication problem is shared by others, to demonstrate that it is possible to develop a positive outlook, and to increase adjustment and communication options by illustrating problem-solving strategies not previously considered. Readings must be selected carefully with the needs of the client and significant others in mind.

Problem Solving The problem-solving approach has been found by this author to be well suited to individual and group aural rehabilitation counseling. Typically, the process starts by asking the client(s) to identify and prioritize difficult communication situations. One situation is selected for analysis in order to identify sources of difficulty. The following areas are included in the analysis:

1. Environmental conditions such as noise or visual barriers

2. The nature or purpose of the conversation

3. The client's typical reaction to the communication difficulty

4. The roles of client and communication partner in the conversation (e.g., patient and physician)

5. The communication partner's reaction to the communication problem

6. Passive, aggressive, or assertive behavior as used by client and communication partner

After problems have been identified, the client(s) brainstorm alternative solutions and write appropriate dialogues. Role playing is performed to try out these solutions in the safety of the class or individual session. After tentative solutions have been selected, homework is assigned to test these solutions in real-life situations. Erdman (1993) and Hull (1992) discuss this approach in greater detail.

A problem-solving approach can be effective in teaching assertive behavior, described in detail in chapter 3. Client and clinician select a problem situation, describe passive, aggressive, and assertive ways of handling that situation, and discuss advantages and disadvantages of each approach. Role playing can be incorporated to give clients the opportunity to define and practice appropriate behaviors. Successful role playing can be followed by homework assignments to use assertive behavior in specific situations. The homework is followed by discussions during subsequent aural rehabilitation sessions. Once clients are able to function assertively in difficult communication situations, they are ready to learn communication strategies. Detailed discussion of communication strategies and exercises for practice can be found in chapter 3 of this book: Kaplan, Bally, and Garretson (1988); Tye-Murray (1991, 1993); and Tye-Murray, Purdy, and Woodworth (1992).

Specific problems, goals, and counseling techniques vary from client to client. Many clients need to work on acceptance of hearing loss and development of effective communication ability. Some culturally Deaf people need to focus on ways to communicate more effectively with hearing people. An additional goal, acceptance of and adjustment to amplification, is important for those people who choose to use hearing aids or assistive listening devices.

Evaluation for Aural Rehabilitation Counseling

Assessment of overall communication function and adjustment difficulties is important in defining a client's strengths, weaknesses, and needs in the areas of interpersonal communication and adjustment to hearing loss. A starting point in such assessment is defining the client's attitudes toward communication, toward himself or herself as a deaf or hard of hearing person, and his or her perceptions of other people's attitudes toward hearing loss. Because a problem-solving approach focuses on specific communication situations, it is necessary to determine which communication situations create difficulty and how important each situation is to the client. The problem-solving approach evaluates alternative solutions to communicative difficulties, with an emphasis on communication strategies. Therefore, assessment procedures are needed to define both positive and negative strategies used by the client in order to know what should be reinforced and what should be unlearned. Because communication always involves at least two people, the perspectives, attitudes, communication strategies, and difficulties of frequent communication partners also need to be evaluated. This section of the chapter discusses various types of communication self-report scales developed for deaf and hard of hearing adults. Described in some detail is the Communication Self-Assessment Scale for Deaf Adults (CSDA), the only scale available for use with prelingually deaf adults.

Communication Self-Report Scales

Neither the audiogram, speech production tests, auditory or visual speech perception tests, nor language or pronunciation evaluation can provide information about difficult communication situations, communication strategies, or attitudes. Case history and anecdotal information obtained during interviews can be helpful, as can self-assessment inventories. These inventories include sections on problem communication situations, positive and negative communication strategies, use of amplification, clients' attitudes toward communication, and perceived attitudes of significant others. Some communication scales contain parallel forms for significant others. Information provided by these scales can form the basis for informational and adjustment counseling programming for individuals or groups. Those scales that have been evaluated psychometrically and have good reliability characteristics can be used to assess change as a function of intervention.

The following section describes the wide range of self-assessment communication scales available for hard of hearing and adventitiously deaf adults. These are listed in table 4.2. Some provide information designed to develop therapy goals, some are screening tools, and some have been designed specifically for elderly clients with hearing loss, some evaluate benefits of amplification. None of these scales, however, are suitable for most people who became deaf before the

Table 4.2 Communication Self-Report Scales

Comprehensive Scales for Hard of Hearing and Late-Deafened Adults

Hearing Performance Inventory (HPI)
Lamb, Owens, and Schubert (1983)

Communication Profile for the Hearing Impaired (CPHI)
Demorest and Erdman (1986)

Performance Inventory for Severe to Profound Hearing Loss (PIPSL)
Owens and Raggio (1984)

Intermediate-Length Scales for Hard of Hearing Adults

Hearing Handicap Scale
High, Fairbanks, and Glorig (1964)

Hearing Measurement Scale
Noble and Atherley (1970)

Denver Scale of Communication Function
Alpiner et al. (1974)

Quantified Denver Scale
Schow and Nerbonne (1980)

McCarthy Alpiner Scale of Hearing Handicap
McCarthy and Alpiner (1983)

Scale for Deaf Adults

Communication Self-Assessment Scale for Deaf Adults (CSDA)
Kaplan, Bally, and Brandt (1991)

Scales for Elderly People

Hearing Handicap Inventory for the Elderly (HHIE)
Ventry and Weinstein (1982)

Hearing Handicap Inventory for the Elderly: Spouses (HHIE-SP)
Newman and Weinstein (1986)

Hearing Handicap Inventory for the Elderly: Screening Version (HHIE-S)
Ventry and Weinstein (1982, 1983)

Self-Assessment of Communication (SAC)
Schow and Nerbonne (1982)

Table 4.2 *Continued*

Self-Assessment of Communication: Significant Others (SOAC)
    Schow and Nerbonne (1982)

Denver Scale of Communication Function for Senior Citizens Living in
    Retirement Centers
    Zarnoch and Alpiner (1977)

Nursing Home Hearing Handicap Index (NHHHI)
    Schow and Nerbonne (1977)

Communication Assessment Procedure for Seniors (CAPS)
    Alpiner and Baker (1981)

Scales to Quantify Hearing Aid Benefit

Hearing Problem Inventory
    Hutton (1980)

Hearing Aid Performance Inventory (HAPI)
    Walden, Demorest, and Hepler (1984)

Hearing Handicap Inventory for the Elderly (HHIE)
    Newman and Weinstein (1988)

Hearing Handicap Inventory for Elderly: Screening Version (HHIE-S)
    Newman et al. (1991)

development of spoken language because they contain inappropriate items, inappropriate language, and omit important content such as the ability to communicate with nonsigning people. The Communication Self-Assessment Scale for Deaf Adults (CSDA) was developed specifically for this population and will be discussed in a later section of this chapter.

Scales for Adventitiously Deaf and Hard of Hearing Adults The longer, more comprehensive scales for hard of hearing adults, such as the Hearing Performance Inventory (HPI) (Giolas et al. 1979; Lamb, Owens, and Schubert 1983) and the Communication Profile for the Hearing Impaired (CPHI) (Demorest and Erdman 1986, 1987), can provide baseline data to define the extent and nature of hearing disability, outline counseling goals, and monitor counseling progress. These scales provide extensive information about specific difficulties, reactions to those difficulties, and coping strategies. They may be used for detailed planning and assessment of rehabilitative procedures. Owens and Raggio (1984) developed a modification of the HPI called the Performance Inventory for Severe to Profound Hearing Loss (PIPSL) for use with clients who have incurred severe to profound hearing losses as adults.

A number of intermediate length self-report scales are available. The Hearing Handicap Scale (High, Fairbanks, and Glorig 1964) and the Hearing Measurement Scale (Noble and Atherley 1970) evaluate difficult communication situations, but do not deal with coping strategies or psychosocial factors. The Denver Scale of Communication Function (Alpiner et al. 1974) and a modification, the Quantified Denver Scale (Schow and Nerbonne 1980) focus on communication attitudes. The McCarthy Alpiner Scale of Hearing Handicap (McCarthy and Alpiner 1983) not only assesses the psychological, social, and vocational effects of adult hearing loss on an individual, but also has a parallel form for family members. This scale has good reliability characteristics and can be used for pre- and post-therapy assessment.

Scales for the Elderly Several scales have been designed with the elderly client with hearing loss in mind, although scales for the younger adult are quite satisfactory for many older adults. Typically, scales for the elderly tend to use fewer items, omit vocational items, and offer fewer response choices per item. Face to face presentation is often an option, especially with a multiply disabled, institutionalized population.

The best known of the scales for the elderly is the Hearing Handicap Inventory for the Elderly (HHIE) (Ventry and Weinstein 1982). This twenty-five item scale quantifies the emotional and social/situational impact of hearing loss on noninstitutionalized elderly persons. It has been extensively researched and found to have excellent reliability and low standard error of measurement (Weinstein, Spitzer, and Ventry 1986). In a pre/postintervention comparison, a change of 18 percent can be considered clinically significant (Weinstein, Spitzer, and Ventry 1986). A parallel form, the HHIE-SP, has been developed for spouses (Newman and Weinstein 1986), and a ten-item screening version, the Hearing Handicap Inventory for the Elderly: Screening Version (HHIE-S), has also been developed (Ventry and Weinstein 1982, 1983) to be used in conjunction with screening audiometry to determine which clients in an institutional setting should receive priority for rehabilitation (Jupiter 1989). Of course, staff and self-referral take precedence in determining rehabilitation priority.

Several other scales are available for the elderly population. The Self-Assessment of Communication (SAC), developed by Schow and Nerbonne in 1982, is an alternative screening tool to the HHIE-S and has a parallel form for significant others (SOAC). Both scales were recommended by the proposed ASHA Guidelines as tools for screening hearing loss in the elderly population. The Denver Scale of Communication Function for Senior Citizens Living in Retirement Centers (Zarnoch and Alpiner 1977) is an interview procedure that attempts to define problem areas related to family, other persons, home, general communication, self-concept, and group situations. The Nursing Home Hearing Handicap Index (NHHHI) was designed by Schow and Nerbonne (1977) for the same population. It has a parallel form for staff members that can be useful in planning in-service training. Alpiner and Baker (1981) developed the Communication Assessment Procedure for Seniors (CAPS), an interview type scale that attempts to evaluate specific difficult communication situations and the communication attitudes of people living in extended care facilities.

Scales to Quantify Hearing Aid Benefit Self-report scales can be used to quantify hearing aid benefit. The Hearing Problem Inventory (Hutton 1980) evaluates clients' perceptions of their communication problems with and without their hearing aids. The Hearing Aid Performance Inventory (HAPI) (Walden, Demorest, and Hepler 1984) evaluates benefits of amplification in noisy situations, in quiet situations with speaker close to the listener, in situations with reduced signal redundancy, and in situations with nonspeech stimuli. This scale has excellent internal consistency reliability. Both the HHIE (Newman and Weinstein 1988; Malinoff and Weinstein 1989) and the HHIE-S (Newman et al. 1991) have been used to assess perceived benefits of hearing aids.

Communication Self-Assessment Scale for Deaf Adults The Communication Self-Assessment Scale for Deaf Adults (CSDA) (Kaplan, Bally, and Brandt 1991) is a comprehensive diagnostic scale modeled after the Communication Profile for the Hearing Impaired (Demorest and Erdman 1986, 1987) and the Hearing Performance Inventory (Giolas et al. 1979) and was developed to facilitate management of communication problems of prelingually deaf adults because all of the other scales in current use were developed for people with adventitiously acquired hearing loss.

The CSDA consists of 125 items divided into four scales, dealing with difficult communication situations, their importance to the individual, communication strategies, and attitudes related to communication. The Communication Importance and Difficult Communication Situations Scales must be used together because they are based on the same items. The Communication Strategies and Communication Attitudes Scales, however, may be used independently of each other and of the Communication Importance and Difficult Communication Situations Scales. Each scale contains subscales.

Each item describes a situation, management strategy, or attitude in simple active declarative sentences (see appendix 4A). For three of the scales, the client indicates whether the item is considered to be true: (1) almost always, (2) sometimes, (3) almost never. For the Communication Importance Scale the three response choices are: (1) very important, (2) important, (3) not important (see appendix 2B). After all items have been scored (see appendix 2C), a profile of subscale scores can be plotted (see appendix 4D). A high score on the total scale or on any of the subscales indicates that the client has a high degree of difficulty in communicating.

Extensive developmental procedures—including item analysis, factor analysis, internal consistency, and test-retest reliability studies—have been performed on the scales. Description of these procedures can be found in Kaplan, Bally, and Brandt (1991). Internal consistency and test-retest reliability coefficients of .80 or higher have been obtained for all scales and subscales. The CSDA has been found useful in the planning of rehabilitative procedures as well as in counseling clients.

Sample Case The following discussion illustrates how the results of the CSDA may be used to help develop an integrated rehabilitation program for a prelingually deaf adult and indicates areas in which counseling could be useful.

AG is a prelingually deaf college senior who has requested communication therapy because she wishes to improve her communication skills with hearing people. She had participated in an off-campus internship in which no one used sign language and found that she could communicate with her coworkers only by writing. She had not used hearing aids or her voice for four years and expressed ambivalence about their use even when communicating with hearing people. Her social contacts, however, were exclusively within the signing Deaf community, and she did not want to change that aspect of her life.

An evaluation of her communication skills revealed:

1. Severe to profound bilateral sensorineural hearing loss with poor word recognition ability

2. Good audiovisual speechreading ability when using amplification

3. Poor speech intelligibility attributable to voice and articulation problems

4. Acceptable written English language skills.

AG's scores on the various subtests of the CSDA appear in figures 4.1 and 4.2. Analysis of the scores suggests the following:

1. As can be seen in figure 4.1, AG is experiencing significant difficulty hearing environmental sounds (sound awareness subscale), understanding speech (speech reception subscale), and being understood by others (speech intelligibility subscale). Scores on the Importance Scale, however, reveal that she considers her sound awareness difficulties of moderate importance. Her problems understanding speech and being understood are important in work-oriented but not social situations. This pattern of responses suggests that communication therapy needs to focus on work-oriented communication. Specific problem situations might be identified by inspection of individual items.

2. Scores on the Strategies Scale in figure 4.1 reveal that AG reports difficulty with both receptive and expressive repair strategies and a large number of maladaptive strategies; inspection of items in the Maladaptive Strategies Scale reveals a great deal of passive behavior. She seems to have less difficulty with anticipatory/environmental strategies. These results suggest that receptive and expressive repair strategies related to the workplace need to be incorporated into therapy, and maladaptive strategies need to be identified and unlearned.

COMMUNICATION SELF-ASSESSMENT SCALE FOR DEAF ADULTS
Profile Form
High Score = Increased Difficulty

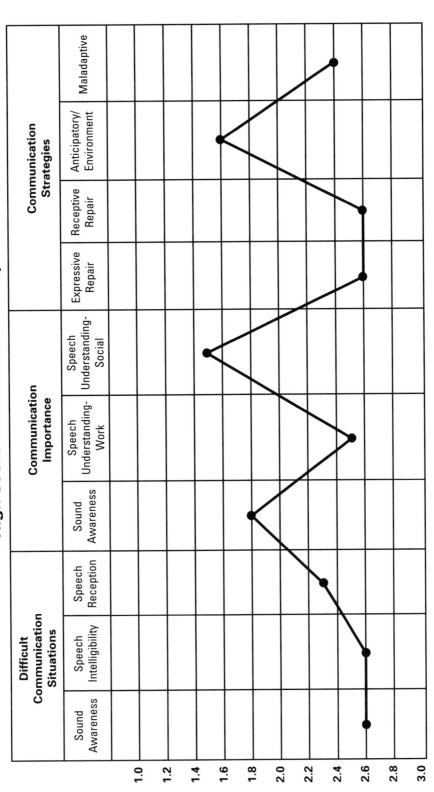

Figure 4.1. Client scores for the subscales of the Difficult Communications, Communication Importance, and Communication Strategies Scales of the CSDA

Source: Kaplan, Bally, and Brandt 1991.

COMMUNICATION SELF-ASSESSMENT SCALE FOR DEAF ADULTS
Profile Form
High Score = Increased Difficulty

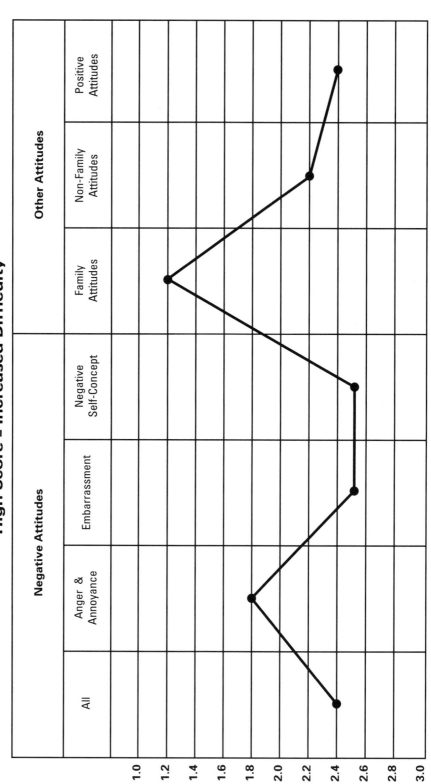

Figure 4.2. Client scores for the subscales of the Attitudes Scale of the CSDA

Source: Kaplan, Bally, and Brandt 1991.

3. Figure 4.2 reveals a high score in negative attitudes, specifically embarrassment and negative self-concept. AG also shows a high score on the Positive Attitudes Subscale, indicating limited positive attitudes toward communication with hearing people. The low score on the Family Attitudes Subscale suggests little difficulty with perceived attitudes of family members toward her deafness, but the high score on the Nonfamily Attitudes Subscale suggests a problem in that area. AG's scores on the Attitudes Subscales suggest the need for adjustment counseling to improve her communicative self-confidence and her attitudes toward communicating with nonfamily members.

The information obtained from AG's CSDA scores indicates that a problem-solving counseling approach focused on work-oriented situations might be useful. Because difficulty in receptive communication is evident, hearing aids and/or assistive devices evaluation and speechreading or auditory training might be attempted. However, counseling on the use of technology, if only in the workplace, is necessary. Expressive communication difficulties suggest the need for voice and articulation training, but counseling is necessary to develop willingness to use voice when communicating with hearing people. Improvement of receptive and expressive repair strategies and reduction of inappropriate communication strategies are also indicated, as is counseling to emphasize positive attitudes and perceptions about communication. AG is likely to be motivated to participate in this therapy program if it focuses on the work environment and respects her desire to communicate with sign language in social situations.

The CSDA profile of subscale scores, as shown in figures 4.1 and 4.2, has been found to be useful in explaining to clients their self-reported communication strengths and weaknesses. The graphs have helped in the negotiation process with AG to develop the type of rehabilitation program discussed in the previous section. The CSDA, however, is only one tool for use in the development of a counseling and rehabilitation program. Results of the scale provide a pattern of overall communication strengths, weaknesses, and needs as reported by the client. This information needs to be used with the results of communication skills evaluation, interview data, and especially negotiation and discussion with the client.

Summary

Integrated personal adjustment and informational counseling is a basic part of adult aural rehabilitation. An empathetic client-clinician relationship and a problem-solving approach to communication difficulties are essential in facilitating adjustment to hearing loss and resolving communication problems. Evaluative procedures such as interviews or communication scales are necessary to define the areas of rehabilitative focus. Many such scales are available for various purposes and different populations.

Appendix 4A
Communication Scale for Deaf Adults: Instructions and Items

We want to find out how your hearing loss affects your daily life. The following questions are about different communication situations, ways of managing situations, and attitudes about different situations.

Some of the items ask you whether you understand conversation. The word "understand" means knowing enough of what is said or signed to be able to answer appropriately. Always assume you are interested in what is being said.

We know that some people are easier to understand than others. Please answer the questions according to the way most people talk to you. We know that sounds and speakers vary. Please answer the questions as best you can.

If you wear a hearing aid, answer the questions as though you were wearing your aid.

SECTION I — DIFFICULT COMMUNICATIONS SITUATIONS

Please read each situation. Decide if the situation is true: 1) Almost always, 2) Sometimes, or 3) Almost never. If you have not experienced this situation DO NOT answer the question. GO on to the next question.

Then indicate if the situation is:
1) Very Important to you, 2) Important to you, 3) Not important to you.

Question # 1.
You are in class. The teacher is easy to lipread but is not signing. You understand.

Question # 2.
You meet a stranger on the street and ask for directions. He does not sign. You understand him.

Question # 3.
You are at work. It is quiet. Your supervisor gives you an order. She is not signing but her face is clearly visible. You understand her.

Question # 4.
You are at work. It is noisy. A hearing co-worker asks you to eat lunch with her. She does not sign but you can see her face. You understand her.

Question # 5.
You are visiting a friend. His hard-of-hearing child speaks to you about his school. The child does not sign. You understand.

Question # 6.
You are at a meeting. A hearing person speaks but does not sign. You know the subject. You understand.

Question # 7.
You are in class. A hearing person speaks but does not sign. You know the subject. You understand.

Question # 8.
You are at the dinner table at home. All your relatives are hearing. Your grandmother is talking. She does not sign. You do not know the topic. You understand her.

Question # 9.
You are introduced to a hearing person. You sign and speak at the same time. He understands you.

Question # 10.
You are at a meeting with five hearing people. No one signs but everyone's face can be seen. One person talks at a time. You understand the conversation.

Question # 11.
You are watching a movie on television. There is no captioning. It is quiet in the room. You understand.

Question # 12.
You are talking to the doctor. It is quiet. She does not sign. You can see her face clearly. You understand her.

Question # 13.
You are ordering lunch at McDonald's. You speak to the person behind the counter. She understands you.

Question # 14.
You are talking to one person at a noisy party. The person does not sign. You understand.

Question # 15.
You are talking to a family member on the telephone. It is quiet in the room. You understand.

Question # 16.
You are reading in a quiet room. Someone calls you from the next room. You hear the person's voice.

Question # 17.
You are sitting in a car next to the driver. The driver is talking. He is not signing. You understand him.

Question # 18.
You must give directions to hearing people at work. They understand your speech.

Question # 19.
I have trouble hearing fire alarms in buildings when other people can hear them.

Question # 20.
I have trouble hearing fire engines and ambulances when other people can hear them.

Question # 21.
I have trouble hearing cars or buses when other people can hear them.

Question # 22.
I have trouble hearing the telephone ring when I am in the same room.

Question # 23.
I have trouble hearing the telephone ring when I am in the next room.

Question # 24.
I have trouble hearing the doorbell when other people can hear it.

Question # 25.
I have trouble hearing a knock on the door when other people can hear it.

Question # 26.
I have trouble hearing music when it is loud enough for other people.

Question # 27.
I have trouble hearing a person's voice when he is talking in the same room.

Question # 28.
You explain a new project to a family member. He understands your speech.

Question # 29.
You tell a hearing friend about a new TV show. She understands your speech.

Question # 30.
You call your parents on the telephone. They understand your speech.

Question # 31.
You call your Doctor's office for an appointment. They understand your speech.

SECTION II — COMMUNICATION STRATEGIES

Please read each situation. Decide if the situation is true: 1) Almost always, 2) Sometimes, or 3) Almost never. If you have not experienced this situation DO NOT answer the question. GO on to the next question.

Question # 32.
You are talking with someone you do not know well. You do not understand. You ask her to repeat.

Question # 33.
You are talking with two people. You are not understanding. You change the topic so that you can control the conversation.

Question # 34.
You ask a stranger for directions. You understand part of what he says. You tell him the part you understand and ask him to repeat the rest.

Question # 35.
You answer a question but the other person doesn't understand. You repeat the answer.

Question # 36.
You are at work. Your boss gives you instructions. You do not understand. You ask him to say the instructions in a different way.

Question # 37.
A friend introduces you to a new person. You do not understand the person's name. You ask the person to spell her name.

Question # 38.

A person asks you for your name. He does not understand your speech. You spell your name.

Question # 39.

A stranger spells his name for you. You miss the first two letters. You ask him to say each letter and a word starting with each letter. (A as in Apple, B as in Boy.)

Question # 40.

A person tells you his address. You do not understand. You ask him to repeat the street number, one number at a time.

Question # 41.

You are talking with one person but are not understanding. You interrupt the person before he finishes to say what you think.

Question # 42.

You are telling a friend a story. Another friend arrives. You stop the story to tell the new friend what the conversation is about.

Question # 43.

You tell a bank teller your account number. She does not understand your speech. You repeat it, one number at a time.

Question # 44.

You are telling a friend about a math test. He doesn't understand your speech. You tell him again using easier words.

Question # 45.

A small child in your family is playing with matches. You tell him to stop but he does not understand your speech. You shake your finger and your head to tell him to stop.

Question # 46.

Your friend asks you to buy seven hamburgers. You do not understand how many he wants. You ask him to start counting from zero and stop at the correct number.

Question # 47.

You are in a restaurant. The waitress does not understand what you want. You point to the item on the menu.

Question # 48.

You are in class. The teacher says something you do not understand. You pretend to understand and hope to get the information from the book later.

Question # 49.

You are at the dinner table with your family. Someone does not understand you. You say the same thing a different way.

Question # 50.

Someone who does not sign asks you for your phone number. You say each number and show the correct number of fingers as you speak.

Question # 51.

Two people are talking. You do not understand the conversation. You ask them to tell you the topic.

Question # 52.

You are talking with one person in a restaurant. His face is in the shadows. You know you could understand better if you changed seats with him. You ask to change seats.

Question # 53.

You are at the airport. You want to buy a ticket for a flight home. The clerk does not understand you. You write the information.

Question # 54.

You are visiting the doctor. He tells you what to do for your sickness. You do not understand his speech. You ask him to write.

Question # 55.

You are at a meeting. The speaker does not look at you when he talks. You feel angry but do nothing about it.

Question # 56.

You meet a deaf friend who is with another person. The other person talks to you but does not sign. You ask her to sign.

Question # 57.

You are at a meeting. You realize you are too far from the speaker to understand. There are empty seats in the front of the room. You change your seat.

Question # 58.

You are at a meeting at work. You are the only deaf person. You are afraid that you will not understand but you do not ask for help. You do the best you can.

Question # 59.

You are talking to the dentist. He speaks very fast. You cannot lipread him. You ask him to slow down.

Question # 60.

You are in class. The teacher talks while she writes on the board. You talk to her after class. You explain that you need to see her face in order to speechread.

Question # 61.

Your teacher likes to move around the room while she teaches. You have problems reading her signs. You ask her after class to lecture from one place so you can understand her signing.

Question # 62.

You are going to a series of meetings or lectures. The speaker does not sign. You ask the speaker to use the slides, pictures, or the overhead projector whenever possible.

Question # 63.

You are going to a series of meetings or lectures. The speaker does not sign. You ask him to find a person to take notes for you.

Question # 64.

You are going to a series of meetings or lectures. The speaker does not sign. You ask for an interpreter.

Question # 65.

You are going to a series of meetings or lectures. The speaker does not sign. You ask for an outline or a reading list.

Question # 66.

You are going to a play. It will not be signed. You read the play or reviews of the play before you see it.

Question # 67.

You are going to a job interview. You act out the situation in advance with a friend to prepare yourself for the experience.

Question # 68.

You are talking with a clerk at the bank. A fire truck goes by. You ask him to stop talking until the noise stops.

Question # 69.

You ask a person to repeat because you don't understand. He seems annoyed. You stop asking and pretend to understand.

Question # 70.

You ask a stranger for directions to a place. You really want to understand his speech. You ask very specific questions like: "Is this place north or south of here? Do I turn left or right at the corner?"

Question # 71.

You need to ask directions. You avoid asking a stranger because you think you will have trouble understanding him.

Question # 72.

You must make a phone call to a hearing person. The person does not have a TDD. You ask a hearing friend to make the call and interpret for you.

Question # 73.

You are at a store. You have trouble hearing the clerk because his voice is soft. You explain you are hearing impaired and ask him to talk louder.

Question # 74.

You are at home. You ask your family to get your attention before they speak to you.

Question # 75.

You are with five or six friends. No one is signing. You miss something important. You ask the person next to you what was said.

Question # 76.

You have trouble understanding a man who is chewing gum. You explain that you need to speechread. You politely ask him to remove the gum when he talks.

Question # 77.

You try to avoid people when you know you will have trouble hearing them.

Question # 78.

You hate to bother other people with your hearing problem. So, you pretend to understand.

Question # 79.
You avoid wearing your hearing aid because it makes you feel different.

SECTION III — ATTITUDES

Please read each situation. Decide if the situation is true: 1) Almost always, 2) Sometimes, or 3) Almost never. If you have not experienced this situation DO NOT answer the question. GO on to the next question.

Question # 80.
I feel embarrassed when I don't understand someone.

Question # 81.
I get upset when I can't follow a conversation.

Question # 82.
I become angry when people do not speak clearly enough for me to understand.

Question # 83.
I feel stupid when I misunderstand what a person is saying.

Question # 84.
It's hard for me to ask someone to repeat things. I feel embarrassed.

Question # 85.
Most people think I could understand better if I paid more attention.

Question # 86.
I get angry when people speak too softly or too fast.

Question # 87.
Sometimes I can't follow conversations at home. I still feel part of family life.

Question # 88.
I feel frustrated when I try to communicate with hearing people.

Question # 89.
Most hearing people do not understand what it is like to be deaf. This makes me angry.

Question # 90.
I am ashamed of being hearing impaired.

Question # 91.
I get angry when someone speaks with his mouth covered or with his back to me.

Question # 92.
I prefer to be alone most of the time.

Question # 93.
I am uncomfortable with people who communicate differently than I do.

Question # 94.
My hearing loss makes me nervous.

Question # 95.
My hearing loss makes me feel depressed.

Question # 96.
My family does not understand my hearing loss.

Question # 97.
I get annoyed when people shout at me because I have a hearing loss.

Question # 98.
People treat me like a stupid person when I don't understand their speech.

Question # 99.
People treat me like a stupid person when they don't understand me.

Question # 100.
Deaf people and hearing people often have difficulty communicating. It is only the responsiblility of the hearing person to improve communication.

Question # 101.
Deaf people and hearing people often have difficulty communicating. It is only the responsibility of the deaf person to improve communication.

Question # 102.
Members of my family get annoyed when I have trouble understanding them.

Question # 103.
People who know I have a hearing loss think I can hear when I want to.

Question # 104.
Members of my family don't leave me out of conversations.

Question # 105.
Hearing aids don't always help people understand speech but they can help in other ways.

Question # 106.
I feel speechreading (lipreading) is helpful to me.

Question # 107.
I feel the only useful communication system for a deaf person is sign language.

Question # 108.
Even though people know I have a hearing loss, they don't help me by speaking clearly or repeating.

Question # 109.
My family is willing to make telephone calls for me.

Question # 110.
My family is willing to repeat as often as necessary when I don't understand them.

Question # 111.
Hearing people get frustrated when I don't understand what they say.

Question # 112.
Hearing people get embarrassed when they don't understand my speech.

Question # 113.
Hearing people pretend to understand me when they really don't.

Question # 114.
I feel the only useful communications system for a deaf person is speech and lipreading.

Question # 115.
I feel embarrassed when hearing people don't understand my speech.

Question # 116.
I do not mind repeating when people have trouble understanding my speech.

Question # 117.
I prefer to write when I communicate with hearing people because I am ashamed of my speech.

Question # 118.
I feel that most hearing people try to understand my speech.

Question # 119.
I feel that my family tries to understand my speech.

Question # 120.
I feel that strangers try to understand my speech.

Question # 121.
Members of my family make it is easy for me to speechread them.

Question # 122.
Strangers make it easy for me to speechread them.

Question # 123.
I am embarrassed to use my voice in public.

Question # 124.
I would like to improve my speech.

Question # 125.
I would like to improve my speechreading ability.

IDENTIFYING INFORMATION

Name _____

                Last   First   Middle Initial

Social Security # _____

                         (Gallaudet Student use ID Number)

Current Location (Check One)

    ( ) Gallaudet University
    ( ) NTID
    ( ) Other (Please Specify) _____

Age _____   Sex ( ) Male   ( ) Female

When did you become deaf?
      (   ) Between Birth–2 years of age
      (   ) Between Age 2–6 years of age
      (   ) Between Age 6–12 years of age
      (   ) Between Age 12–18 years of age
      (   ) After age 18

Current Education Status:

      (   ) In High School
      (   ) In undergraduate college program
      (   ) In graduate college program
      (   ) Not in School

Highest Educational Level Completed:

      (   ) High School
      (   ) Associate or Technical Degree
      (   ) Undergraduate Degree
      (   ) Graduate Degree

Did you take most of your important classes (English, Math, Social Studies, Science) through high school in:

      (   ) Deaf Classes
      (   ) Mainstreamed Classes
      (   ) Combination of Both

How long did you attend each of the following programs after High School:
(Enter 0 if you did not attend and .5 if you attended less than a full year.)

      Gallaudet University, NTID, or other program   _____ year(s) _____ mo.
      for Deaf people

      Hearing College or program   _____ year(s) _____ mo.

How do you communicate most of the time:

At Home:	( ) Sign Language	( ) Speech & Speechreading	( ) Both
At School:	( ) Sign Language	( ) Speech & Speechreading	( ) Both
At Work:	( ) Sign Language	( ) Speech & Speechreading	( ) Both
In your home community:	( ) Sign Language	( ) Speech & Speechreading	( ) Both

Do you own a hearing aid(s) now?   (   ) Yes
                                     (   ) No

How often do you use a hearing aid now?

      (   ) Not at all
      (   ) Sometimes
      (   ) Most of the time

Do you wear an aid in:
      (   ) One ear
      (   ) Both ears

Type of aid currently in use: (Check all that you use)

( ) Behind-the-ear aid
( ) In-the-ear aid
( ) Body-worn or eyeglass aid
( ) Vibrotactile aid
( ) Cochlear Implant

Source: Kaplan, Bally, and Brandt 1991.

Appendix 4B
Communication Scales

ANSWER SHEET

Name _____

Social Security # _____

SECTION I
DIFFICULT COMMUNICATION SITUATIONS

Response Scale for Communication

   1) Almost Always True
   2) Sometimes True
   3) Almost Never True

Response Scale for Importance

   1) Very Important
   2) Important
   3) Not Important

1)	1 2 3	1 2 3	17) 1 2 3	1 2 3
2)	1 2 3	1 2 3	18) 1 2 3	1 2 3
3)	1 2 3	1 2 3	19) 1 2 3	1 2 3
4)	1 2 3	1 2 3	20) 1 2 3	1 2 3
5)	1 2 3	1 2 3	21) 1 2 3	1 2 3
6)	1 2 3	1 2 3	22) 1 2 3	1 2 3
7)	1 2 3	1 2 3	23) 1 2 3	1 2 3
8)	1 2 3	1 2 3	24) 1 2 3	1 2 3
9)	1 2 3	1 2 3	25) 1 2 3	1 2 3
10)	1 2 3	1 2 3	26) 1 2 3	1 2 3
11)	1 2 3	1 2 3	27) 1 2 3	1 2 3
12)	1 2 3	1 2 3	28) 1 2 3	1 2 3
13)	1 2 3	1 2 3	29) 1 2 3	1 2 3
14)	1 2 3	1 2 3	30) 1 2 3	1 2 3
15)	1 2 3	1 2 3	31) 1 2 3	1 2 3
16)	1 2 3	1 2 3		

Name _____

Social Security # _____

SECTION II
COMMUNICATION STRATEGIES

1) Almost Always True
2) Sometimes True
3) Almost Never True

32)	1	2	3	56)	1	2	3
33)	1	2	3	57)	1	2	3
34)	1	2	3	58)	1	2	3
35)	1	2	3	59)	1	2	3
36)	1	2	3	60)	1	2	3
37)	1	2	3	61)	1	2	3
38)	1	2	3	62)	1	2	3
39)	1	2	3	63)	1	2	3
40)	1	2	3	64)	1	2	3
41)	1	2	3	65)	1	2	3
42)	1	2	3	66)	1	2	3
43)	1	2	3	67)	1	2	3
44)	1	2	3	68)	1	2	3
45)	1	2	3	69)	1	2	3
46)	1	2	3	70)	1	2	3
47)	1	2	3	71)	1	2	3
48)	1	2	3	72)	1	2	3
49)	1	2	3	73)	1	2	3
50)	1	2	3	74)	1	2	3
51)	1	2	3	75)	1	2	3
52)	1	2	3	76)	1	2	3
53)	1	2	3	77)	1	2	3
54)	1	2	3	78)	1	2	3
55)	1	2	3	79)	1	2	3

Name _____

Social Security # _____

SECTION III
COMMUNICATION ATTITUDES

1) Almost Always True
2) Sometimes True
3) Almost Never True

80)	1	2	3		103)	1	2	3
81)	1	2	3		104)	1	2	3
82)	1	2	3		105)	1	2	3
83)	1	2	3		106)	1	2	3
84)	1	2	3		107)	1	2	3
85)	1	2	3		108)	1	2	3
86)	1	2	3		109)	1	2	3
87)	1	2	3		110)	1	2	3
88)	1	2	3		111)	1	2	3
89)	1	2	3		112)	1	2	3
90)	1	2	3		113)	1	2	3
91)	1	2	3		114)	1	2	3
92)	1	2	3		115)	1	2	3
93)	1	2	3		116)	1	2	3
94)	1	2	3		117)	1	2	3
95)	1	2	3		118)	1	2	3
96)	1	2	3		119)	1	2	3
97)	1	2	3		120)	1	2	3
98)	1	2	3		121)	1	2	3
99)	1	2	3		122)	1	2	3
100)	1	2	3		123)	1	2	3
101)	1	2	3		124)	1	2	3
102)	1	2	3		125)	1	2	3

Source: Kaplan, Bally, and Brandt 1991.

Appendix 4C
Scoring Form for the CSDA

Difficult Communication Situations

Sound Awareness*

Item #	19	20	21	22	23	24	25	26	27	Average
Answer (1–3)										

* This is a reversed scored scale. For this subscale, record every number 1 response as a 3 and every number 3 response as a 1.

Speech Reception

Item #	1	2	3	4	5	6	7	8	
Answer (1–3)									
Item #	10	11	12	14	15	16	17		Average
Answer (1–3)									

Speech Intelligibility

Item #	9	13	18	28	29	30	31				Average
Answer (1–3)											

Sound Awareness Importance

Item #	16	19	20	21	22	23	24	25	26	27	Average
Answer (1–3)											

Work Communication Importance

Item #	1	3	4	6	7	10	18				Average
Answer (1–3)											

Social Importance

Item #	2	5	8	9	11	12	13				
Answer (1–3)											
Item #	14	15	17	28	29	30	31				Average
Answer (1–3)											

COMMUNICATION SCALE
SCORING FORM

Communication Strategies
Version 3

Expressive Repair

Item #	35	38	42	43	44	45	47	49	50	53	Average
Answer (1–3)											

Receptive Repair

Item #	32	34	36	37	39	40	46	51			
Answer (1–3)											
Item #	54	56	59	68	70	72	73	75			Average
Answer (1–3)											

Anticipatory/Environmental

Item #	52	57	60	61	62	63	64				
Answer (1–3)											
Item #	65	66	67	72	74	76					Average
Answer (1–3)											

Maladaptive Strategies*

Item #	33	41	48	55	58	69	71	77	78	79	Average
Answer (1–3)											

*This is a reversed scored scale. For this subscale, record every number 1 response as a 3 and every number 3 response as a 1.

COMMUNICATION SCALE
SCORING FORM

Communication Attitudes
Version 3

Negative Attitudes—All*

Item #	80	81	82	83	84	86	88			
Answer (1–3)										
Item #	89	90	91	92	93	94	95			
Answer (1–3)										
Item #	97	100	101	107	114	115	117	123		Average
Answer (1–3)										

*This is a reversed scored scale. For this subscale, record every number 1 response as a 3 and every number 3 response as a 1.

Negative Attitudes—Anger & Annoyance*

Item #	82	86	89	91	97		Average
Average (1–3)							

* This is a reversed scored scale. For this subscale, record every number 1 response as a 3 and every number 3 response as a 1.

Negative Attitudes—Embarrassment*

Item #	80	84	90	115	117	123		Average
Average (1–3)								

* This is a reversed scored scale. For this subscale, record every number 1 response as a 3 and every number 3 response as a 1.

Negative Attitudes—Negative Self Concept*

Item #	81	83	88	92	93	94	95		Average
Average (1–3)									

* This is a reversed scored scale. For this subscale, record every number 1 response as a 3 and every number 3 response as a 1.

References

Alpiner, J. G. 1982. Evaluation of communication function. In *Handbook of adult rehabilitative audiology,* ed. J. G. Alpiner. Baltimore: Williams & Wilkins.

Alpiner, J. G., and B. Baker. 1981. Communication assessment procedures in the aural rehabilitation process. *Seminars Speech, Language, Hearing* 2:189–204.

Alpiner, J. G., and P. McCarthy, eds. 1987. *Rehabilitative audiology: Children and adults.* Baltimore: Williams & Wilkins.

Alpiner, J. G., and D.C. Garstecki. 1989. Aural rehabilitation for adults. In *Introduction to aural rehabilitation,* 2d ed., ed. R. L. Schow and M. A. Nerbonne. Austin, Tex.: Pro-Ed.

Alpiner, J. G., W. Chevrette, C. Glascoe, M. Metz, and B. Olsen. 1974. The Denver Scale of Communication Function. Unpublished study, University of Denver.

Bryant, J. D., and S. D. Roberts. 1992. Bibliotherapy: An adjunct to audiologic counseling. *Journal of the Academy of Rehabilitative Audiology* 24:51–68.

Demorest, M. E., and S. A. Erdman. 1986. Scale composition and item analysis of the communication profile for the hearing impaired. *Journal of Speech and Hearing Research* 29:515–535.

———. 1987. Development of the Communication Profile for the Hearing Impaired. *Journal of Speech and Hearing Disorders* 52:129–142.

Ellis, A., and R. Grieger. 1977. *Handbook of rational-emotive therapy*. New York: Springer.

Erdman, S. A. 1993. Counseling hearing-impaired adults. In *Rehabilitative audiology: Children and adults,* 2d ed., ed. J. G. Alpiner and P. A. McCarthy. Baltimore: Williams & Wilkins.

Fleming, M., L. Birkle, I. Kolman, G. Miltenberger, and R. Israel. 1973. Development of workable aural rehabilitation programs. *Journal of the Academy of Rehabilitative Audiology* 6:35–36.

Giolas, T. A. 1989. Sample eight-week adult aural rehabilitation group outline. In *Introduction to aural rehabilitation,* 2d ed., ed. R. L. Schow and M. A. Nerbonne. Austin, Tex.: Pro-Ed., 577.

Giolas, T. A., E. Owens, S. H. Lamb, and E. D. Schubert. 1979. Hearing Performance Inventory. *Journal of Speech and Hearing Disorders* 44:169–195.

High, W. S., G. Fairbanks, and A. Glorig. 1964. Scale for Self-Assessment of Hearing Handicap. *Journal of Speech and Hearing Disorders* 29:215–230.

Hull, R. H. 1992. Techniques of aural rehabilitation treatment for older adults. In *Aural Rehabilitation,* 2d ed., ed. R. H. Hull. San Diego, Calif.: Singular Publishing Group.

Hutton, C. L. 1980. Responses to a hearing problem inventory. *Journal of the Academy of Rehabilitative Audiology* 13:133–154.

Jupiter, T. 1989. A community hearing screening program for the elderly. *Hearing Journal* 42(1):14–17.

Kannapell, B., and R. Adams. 1984. *An orientation to deafness: A handbook and resource guide*. Washington, D.C.: Gallaudet University.

Kaplan, H., S. J. Bally, and C. Garretson. 1987. *Speechreading: A way to improve understanding*. 2d ed. Washington, D.C.: Gallaudet University Press.

Kaplan, H., S. J. Bally, and F. Brandt. 1991. Communication Self-Assessment Scale Inventory for Deaf Adults. *Journal of the American Academy of Audiology* 2(3):164–182.

Kelly, L. J. 1992. Rational-emotive therapy and aural rehabilitation. *Journal of the Academy of Rehabilitative Audiology* 24:43–50.

Kodman, F. 1967. Techniques for counseling the hearing aid client. *Maico audiolog-*

ical library series, vol. 8, reports 23–25. Minneapolis, Minn.: Maico Hearing Instruments.

Lamb, S. H., E. Owens, and E. D. Schubert. 1983. The revised form of the Hearing Performance Inventory. *Ear and Hearing* 4:152–159.

Malinoff, R. L., and B. E. Weinstein. 1989. Changes in self-assessment of hearing handicap over the first year of hearing aid use by older adults. *Journal of the Academy of Rehabilitative Audiology* 22:54–60.

McCarthy, P. A., and J. G. Alpiner. 1983. An assessment scale of hearing handicap for use in family counseling. *Journal of the Academy of Rehabilitative Audiology* 16:256-270.

Newman, C. W., and B. E. Weinstein. 1986. Judgments of perceived hearing handicap by hearing-impaired elderly men and their spouses. *Journal of the Academy of Rehabilitative Audiology* 19:109–115.

Newman, C. W., and B. E. Weinstein. 1988. The Hearing Handicap Inventory for the Elderly as a measure of hearing aid benefit. *Ear and Hearing* 9(2):81–85.

Newman, C. W., G. P. Jacobson, G. A. Hug, B. E. Weinstein, and R. L. Malinoff. 1991. Practical method for quantifying hearing aid benefit in older adults. *Journal of the American Academy of Audiology* 2:70–75.

Noble, W. G., and G. R. C. Atherley. 1970. The Hearing Measurement Scale: A questionnaire for the assessment of auditory disability. *Journal of Auditory Research* 10:229-250.

Owens, E., and M. W. Raggio. 1984. *Hearing Performance Inventory for Severe to Profound Hearing Loss.* San Francisco: University of California Press.

Rogers, C. R. 1951. *Client-centered therapy.* Boston: Houghton Mifflin.

Sanders, D. A. 1975. Hearing aid orientation and counseling. In *Amplification for the Hearing Impaired,* ed. M. C. Pollack. New York: Grune & Stratton.

————. 1980. Hearing aid orientation and counseling. In *Amplification for the Hearing Impaired,* ed. M. C. Pollack. New York: Grune & Stratton.

————, D.A. 1988. Hearing aid orientation and counseling. In *Amplification for the Hearing Impaired,* ed. M. C. Pollack. New York: Grune & Stratton.

Schow, R. L., and M. A. Nerbonne. 1977. Assessment of hearing handicap by nursing home residents and staff. *Journal of the Academy of Rehabilitative Audiology* 10:10–12.

————. 1980. *Introduction to aural rehabilitation.* Baltimore: University Park Press.

————. 1982. Communication screening profile: Use with elderly clients. *Ear and Hearing* 3:135–147.

Stone, J. R., and L. B. Olswang. 1989. The hidden challenge in counseling. *ASHA* 31:27–31.

Tye-Murray, N. 1991. Repair strategy usage by hearing-impaired adults and changes following communication therapy. *Journal of Speech and Hearing Research* 34:921–928.

————. 1993. Aural rehabilitation and patient management. In *Cochlear implants: Audiological foundations*, ed. R. S. Tyler. San Diego, Calif.: Singular Publishing Group.

Tye-Murray, N., S. C. Purdy, and G. G. Woodworth. 1992. Reported use of communication strategies by SHHH members: Client, talker, and situational variables. *Journal of Speech and Hearing Research* 35:708–717.

Ventry, I., and B. Weinstein. 1982. The Hearing Handicap Inventory for the Elderly: A new tool. *Ear and Hearing* 3:128–134.

————. 1983. Identification of elderly people with hearing problems. *ASHA* 25:37–42.

Walden, B. E., M. E. Demorest, and E. H. Hepler. 1984. Self-report approach to assessing benefit derived from amplification. *Journal of Speech and Hearing Research* 9:91–109.

Weinstein, B., J. Spitzer, and I. Ventry. 1986. Test-retest reliability of the Hearing Handicap for the Elderly. *Ear and Hearing* 7:295–299.

Zarnoch, J. M., and J. C. Alpiner. 1977. The Denver Scale of Communication Function for Senior Citizens Living in Retirement Centers. Unpublished study, Denver, Colorado.

5

Psychosocial Aspects of Adult Aural Rehabilitation

Janet L. Pray

■ ■ ■ ■

Clinicians in the rehabilitation field have long known that the effects of a disability and successful adaptation to a disability are not determined solely by the severity of the particular condition (Asch 1984; Goffman 1963; Ladieu, Adler, and Dembo 1948; Pray 1992; Roth 1983; Schultz and Decker 1985; Wright 1983). Despite significant physical limitations imposed by amyotrophic lateral sclerosis (a severe and progressive neurological disease), the brilliant scientist Stephen Hawking continues to make major contributions to his field. A young man in the Navy, I. King Jordan, became profoundly deaf as the result of a motorcycle accident, yet went on to become the president of Gallaudet University. Unlike Hawking and Jordan, however, other individuals may experience major difficulties adapting to similar conditions or even to those conditions that the clinician might consider insignificant.

What accounts for such differences? Whether an individual is deaf, hard of hearing, or has some other condition or disability that sets him or her apart from what is considered to be the norm in society, adaptation is influenced by a complex interplay of biological, psychological, and social factors. This chapter examines the "biopsychosocial dynamics" that contribute to the subjective experience of being deaf, Deaf,[1] or hard of hearing and considers the implications of these dynamics for students and professionals in the field of adult aural rehabilitation.

---

[1] For the significance of the capitalized "D," see Kinsella-Meier's discussion of Deaf culture in chapter 1.

The experience of this author and of colleagues with whom she has been engaged in interdisciplinary work is that understanding the unique biopsychosocial factors related to the phenomenon of being Deaf, deaf, or hard of hearing contributes to effective rehabilitative efforts.

The Biopsychosocial Perspective

The biopsychosocial perspective considers that the effects of hearing loss and adjustment to hearing loss are determined by a number of factors within the biological, psychological, and social realms. The terms "biopsychosocial" and "biopsychosocial dynamics" suggest that these factors do not occur in isolation; rather, they are engaged in a process of dynamic interaction with one another. Because of these dynamics, the audiologist, speech-language pathologist, and other members of the aural rehabilitation network can expect clients to present diverse reactions to the hearing loss, to assessment of the hearing loss, and to recommendations for hearing aids, assistive listening devices, speechreading classes, and the like. Examination of hearing loss within a biopsychosocial context provides a framework for understanding the diversity of reactions to hearing loss and for developing strategies that will maximize the effectiveness of interventions by audiologists, speech-language pathologists, and other professionals.

Biological/Physiological Factors

The *nature and severity of the hearing loss* are likely to be the first factors considered by the clinician: for example, the type of loss—sensorineural, conductive, or mixed; the degree and configuration of loss; discrimination ability; age at onset; sudden or gradual onset; cause of the loss; and progression of the loss. Other aspects to be considered include whether the person has *other physical conditions or disabilities* because the energy required to manage other physical conditions is likely to affect the emotional resources available for coping with the hearing loss. Such conditions include those that may be related to the hearing loss, including tinnitus or balance problems. The presence of other physical or health conditions is one of many reasons it is important for the clinician to recognize that frequently a linear relationship does not exist between the nature and severity of hearing loss and its effects on the individual or on the individual's receptivity to professional recommendations.

Mrs. M. illustrates the role that other physical disabilities have in adaptation to hearing loss. Mrs. M. is a seventy-one-year-old woman with a mild sensorineural hearing loss. She enrolled in an aural rehabilitation program reluctantly, pressured by her husband, who expressed frustration with her refusal to wear her hearing aid, her withdrawal from family and friends, and her pattern of crying whenever her hearing loss was mentioned. An interview with the client revealed that she also had diabetes, a heart condition, and a vascular disorder. Whereas her husband's perspective was that the hearing loss was insignificant compared to her other conditions, she experienced the hearing loss as "the straw that broke the camel's back"—one further indication of aging and its attendant losses. This recognition led to the decision to have the social worker on the aural rehabilitation team counsel the couple concerning their differing perspectives on the impact of the hearing loss.

The social work plan was to provide emotional support to Mrs. M. as she struggled to cope with the combined effects of her multiple physical conditions, to acknowledge Mr. M.'s perspective, to explore how the hearing loss affected his life, and to encourage Mr. M. to express understanding of his wife's feelings and support her in participating in aural rehabilitation at a pace comfortable for her. Close collaboration among audiologist, speech-language pathologist, and social worker helped to ensure that the introductions of ALDs and emphasis on developing effective communication strategies parallelled Mrs. M.'s psychological readiness.

This approach conveyed to Mrs. M. that her feelings were regarded as important. Thus, she was gradually able to become more actively involved in the aural rehabilitation program that focused on better understanding of the hearing loss; on selection and use of hearing aids, ALDs, and communication strategies; and on psychosocial adjustment.

The case of Mrs. M. illustrates the importance of assessing clients' health and other conditions that may affect adaptation to hearing loss. It also demonstrates the value of understanding the family context and of utilizing an interdisciplinary approach.

Psychological/Emotional Factors

People vary greatly in their psychological makeup and in the ways in which they respond to events in their lives. The following aspects of psychological and emotional functioning are of particular relevance in understanding the deaf or hard of hearing person and for planning appropriate professional interventions.

Personality and Patterns of Coping with Stress The personality of the individual and patterns of coping with stress are important indicators of how that person will adapt to the hearing loss. Persons who have a history of coping effectively with other stresses in their lives are likely to bring those effective coping resources to bear on the effects of their hearing loss. Conversely, persons who do not manage stress well or who have had difficulty adapting to illness or disability are likely to have difficulty adapting to hearing loss.

For some individuals, the stress of the onset (as in the case of sudden onset of deafness), diagnosis, or confirmation of hearing loss may precipitate a crisis. According to crisis theory, when customary approaches to coping are not adequate to deal successfully with a stressful situation, a state of crisis characterized by disequilibrium and diminished capacity to function may result (Aguilera 1994). Clients in the midst of a crisis may be functioning at less than their usual or optimum level and are likely to require additional time and support for processing information and for following through with recommendations. Clients may exhibit a host of different and sometimes conflicting feelings and behaviors, some of which may be directed at the clinician. These include anxiety, anger, frustration, irritability, helplessness, loss of confidence, insecurity, reduced self-esteem, depression, withdrawal, and dependence, among others (Martin, Krall, and O'Neal 1990; Orlans and Meadow-Orlans 1985; Pray 1992).

Although the clinician may be concerned about the intensity of feeling displayed and the extent of disorganization, working with clients during an active crisis has advantages because people in crisis feel vulnerable and, having exhausted internal resources, are inclined to be open to professional intervention. Crises are known to resolve within six to twelve weeks, with or without professional intervention (Aguilera 1994). The individual may remain at a diminished level of functioning, may return to the level of functioning prior to the onset of the crisis, or may attain a higher, more effective level of functioning because of successful resolution of the crisis and the achievement of new strengths and coping capacities. The clinician's involvement with clients in a state of crisis not only will assist them in managing their hearing loss more effectively, but also may facilitate the process of restoration or even enhancement of prior levels of functioning that extend to areas beyond coping with the hearing loss.

The clinician should also consider the presence of other stresses or problems. He or she needs to know if clients are attempting to cope with other problems and stresses in addition to those presented by the hearing loss because, inevitably, such problems will affect the personal resources available to deal with the hearing loss. In some instances, these stresses or problems are within the individual and may include personal adjustment problems and psychological disorders. In other situations, stresses or problems may be more interactional or transactional in nature, deriving from roles, expectations, and relationships involving family, friends, and others in the person's social system. These situations are discussed below in the section on interpersonal and social factors, although in actual clinical practice personal and interpersonal factors should be considered together.

The Grieving Process A preponderance of the clinical and research literature makes note of the strong emotional reactions experienced by those who develop hearing loss as adolescents or adults (Glass 1985; Meadow-Orlans 1985; Pray 1992; Schlesinger 1985; Thomas 1984). Many in the field of disability have noted a grief and mourning process experienced by those who have lost functional capacities as the result of spinal cord injuries, by those who have had limbs amputated, by women who have had mastectomies, etc. This process has most often been described as having parallels with stages in the grieving process identified originally by Kubler-Ross in her pioneering work with dying patients (Kubler-

Ross 1969). Grief and mourning has also been described as a phenomenon oc-curring among those who experience adult-onset hearing loss (Clark and Martin 1994; Luterman 1991; Pray 1990; Scheuerle 1992; Tanner 1980). In a qualitative study of older persons with late-onset hearing loss, Pray (1992) found a grieving process among many of the participants with hearing loss as well as among the spouses and significant others in their lives.

The literature cited above shows that many persons experiencing hearing loss in adulthood must also experience a process of coming to terms on an emo-tional level with the reality of having lost the ease of communication they had previously. Many of the characteristics described by Kubler-Ross are commonly found in this process, particularly denial, anger, depression, and ultimately ac-ceptance. Note, however, that this author finds the term *adaptation* preferable to Kubler-Ross's term *acceptance*. *Acceptance* implies passivity and resignation, which is probably appropriate as a phase or stage in the dying process. The con-cept of *adaptation* is more consistent with the assertiveness essential for coping effectively with hearing loss.

Spouses, families, and friends often express the view that they recognized the hearing loss long before the individual with the loss, and the assumption is made that the deaf or hard of hearing person's delayed recognition represents *denial*. This view is reinforced when a significant period of time elapses between first suspicion of hearing loss by family or friends and the initial clinical assess-ment. In a qualitative study of twenty-eight persons age sixty and older, Pray (1992) found the period of time from first suspicion to initial assessment ranged from several months to six or seven years or, in one instance, fifteen years. The results of the same study suggest that some people experience a prolonged period of denial even when the hearing loss is evident to virtually everyone else.

Pray also noted that because the onset of hearing loss may be slow and in-sidious, it is likely that some individuals are not denying their hearing loss; they are simply unaware of it or unaware that the difficulties they are experiencing are caused by hearing loss. Considered within this context, a client who complains that people have begun to "mumble" may respond well to a careful explanation about the nature of sensorineural hearing loss.

Persons who refuse to be evaluated or clients who challenge the results of the audiological assessment are the individuals who are more likely to be denying their hearing loss. Those who refuse an evaluation may not reach the clinician's office, or they may come only because they are pressured to do so by a spouse or other family members. Clients who do not accept the results of the assessment or the recommendations are unlikely to respond favorably if they are pressed with further information or if they are confronted with their denial. Such clients may be more receptive if asked to discuss with the clinician their feelings about the results of the assessment. This approach may not result in relinquishment of the denial, but it conveys to the client that the clinician recognizes his or her feelings as important and legitimate and lays the groundwork for a clinician-client rapport that may make it possible for the client to return at a later time.

Appropriate timing is important when conveying the results of the audiologic assessment. Pacing the informational counseling to the readiness of the client to hear and accept professional advice is a key factor in success with any client, especially with one who has not been able to accept the hearing loss. To the extent possible within the constraints of busy clinics and offices, it is important to build in time for the client to think about the information and recommendations and to be able to return to have questions answered and for further counseling before making a commitment to any further course of action.

Anger is a significant component in the grieving process, and because anger is a powerful emotion, it can be a difficult one with which to deal. It is useful to recognize that when clients direct anger at the clinician, usually this is a displacement from the real source of the anger. Consistent with the Kubler-Ross model, clients may be angry about the effects that hearing loss has on their lives. The most important guideline for responding to the angry client is to avoid taking the anger personally, even if the client is provoking a response by challenging credentials, competence, or fees. The best approach to angry clients is to acknowledge that they are angry and to engage them in a discussion of how they are feeling. This is not to suggest that the clinician assume the role of psychotherapist. An acknowledgment of the client's feelings and an opportunity to express them conveys to the client the clinician's capacity for empathy, which may be sufficient for the client to focus appropriately on the purpose for the visit to the office or clinic. As Kaplan notes in chapter 4, when the client's anger extends beyond what the clinician feels comfortable or competent to deal with, that is an indication for making a referral to another professional, such as a social worker, psychologist, or counselor. Specific issues to be considered in making such referrals are included in the discussion concerning deafened adults.

Although *depression* is part of a normal grieving process, one cannot assume that when clients talk about being depressed, they are, in fact, clinically depressed. An individual may be feeling very sad without being depressed, and if the clinician is concerned about whether the client needs to be referred for counseling or therapy, it will be important to explore the client's feelings. Indications for referral include disturbances in patterns of eating or sleeping over an extended period of time, complaints of always feeling tired or exhausted, loss of satisfaction with life, or thoughts of suicide.

Most people know Kubler-Ross's theory as a stage theory, and stage theories seem to suggest an orderly progression from one stage to another. A careful study of stage theories, including Kubler-Ross's, indicates that rarely does the theorist suggest that an individual simply completes the tasks of one stage, closes the door on that stage, and moves on to the next (Erikson 1959, 1968; Kubler-Ross 1969). Most of these theories make provision for progression and regression between stages in recognition of the multiple factors that influence development through life. Thus, it is not to be expected that an individual will arrive at the final stage of adaptation, never again to contend with the issues, conflicts, and tasks associated with earlier stages. Kubler-Ross cautioned that a person who at one moment might be in the stage of acceptance, at another moment might be found in the stage of denial.

The implication for the clinician is that it is important to assess and reassess the feelings of the client and respond according to what the client is feeling at each point of contact. For example, if it were assumed that once having achieved good adaptation a client would never again experience feelings of depression, the clinician may overlook or dismiss signs of a recurrence of feelings that could respond best to early intervention.

Meaning of Hearing Loss to the Individual A critical factor in assessing the effects of the hearing loss on the adolescent, adult, and older adult client is understanding the meaning of hearing loss to the individual. In chapter 1 Kinsella-Meier discussed the population that considers itself culturally Deaf, a cultural and linguistic minority distinct from those who view deafness as a medical/pathological condition. Those who take pride in their culture and in their language (American Sign Language) consider being Deaf a difference—not a deficit and not a "loss."

Most Deaf and deaf individuals have heard throughout their lives that they must develop skills required for functioning in the "hearing world." It could be argued that this is an ethnocentric view, inconsistent with the emphasis in the 1980s and 1990s on multiculturalism in this country. Just as the "melting pot" philosophy that subordinated minority cultures to the majority culture in the United States gave way to a philosophy of appreciating cultural diversity, the hearing majority may need to develop greater appreciation and respect for the strengths in Deaf culture and for those who identify themselves as part of that culture.

Wilson and Scott indicate in chapter 2 that culturally Deaf persons often seek aural rehabilitation services to enhance their ability to function independently in situations such as the workplace. Because most aural rehabilitation professionals are hearing, they are in a unique position to help bridge the gap between hearing society and Deaf society, which comprise our multicultural world.[2] Basic to most types of counseling are the related concepts of acceptance, best described by Carl Rogers as "unconditional positive regard" (Rogers 1979), and respect for clients' values. Genuineness in accepting Deaf clients' desires to preserve their culture while enhancing their ability to communicate effectively with hearing society is a critical aspect of working effectively with this population. Failure of the clinician to value the client's personal identity will usually result in resistance to aural rehabilitation services proffered to enhance competence in communicating with the hearing majority.

Adjustment Issues for Adolescents and Young Adults Hearing loss in adolescents and young adults of high school and college age presents particular challenges to those age groups and to the professionals providing services to those populations.

[2] The term "multicultural world" is a more appropriate designation than "hearing world," conveying inclusiveness rather than exclusiveness.

Superimposed upon the usual stresses associated with this stage of life are those created by the hearing loss. At a time when acceptance by peers assumes primary importance, differences imposed by having a hearing loss, and perhaps by having to wear a hearing aid, may become intolerable. Young adults who are deaf and communicate most comfortably in sign language may deal with the need for peer group acceptance by identifying totally with the Deaf community and Deaf culture. For some, this process involves the rejection of hearing aids and the decision not to use their voices, especially if their speech draws attention to their deafness and is the object of ridicule by hearing peers.

Considered within the context of the normal tasks of adolescence and young adulthood for identity development and for achieving independence from parents or other adults in authority positions, the foregoing adaptation is not difficult to understand (Erikson 1959, 1968). The clinician working with this population has the greatest potential for success if he or she accepts the client's choice of a Deaf identity as appropriate, but at the same time introduces or reinforces the concept of developing skills for functioning successfully in the society of hearing people as well as in the society of Deaf people. Such an approach avoids the pitfall inherent in attempting to persuade (even by implication) adolescents and young adults that they should choose membership in the majority culture at a time when they feel alienated from hearing persons.

Adjustment Process for Deafened Adults Deafened adults face a unique set of circumstances because they have a well-established identity as hearing persons and suddenly find themselves isolated and alienated from persons who are hearing as well as from those who are culturally Deaf and who communicate using American Sign Language. The ability to communicate with ease, typically taken for granted, suddenly has become seriously impaired, and some obstacles initially may seem insurmountable. They may wonder how they will sustain relationships with family and friends, function in the workplace, participate in social activities, and retain their humanity. According to Oyer and Oyer (1976), "One of the most humanizing elements in the adjustment of mankind is the ability to communicate" (ix–x). Typically, deafened adults initially find their ability to communicate severely compromised. These questions and concerns contribute to their vulnerability to crisis and to the likelihood of their experiencing a grief and mourning process as discussed earlier in this chapter.

It is common for a deafened adult to experience each of the discrete stages described by Kubler-Ross. A person suddenly becoming deaf after surgery for removal of a tumor on the auditory nerve, after an acute episode of Meniere's, after an illness, or after a serious accident is likely to experience *shock and denial* initially: "This cannot be happening to me!" When the onset of deafness is sudden, the quality of the response to it is likely to be more intense and dramatic than it is for a gradual-onset hearing loss.

In the phase of shock and denial, the deafened individual may question the permanence of the deafness and seek additional professional opinions in hopes of obtaining a more favorable prognosis. It is important for professionals not to interpret this need to secure other opinions as a challenge to their competence or credentials. What usually underlies the search for multiple opinions is the client's inability to come to terms with the psychological pain of having become deaf. The clinician can be helpful in moving the adjustment process forward by expressing understanding of the client's struggle with what happened and by articulating empathy for the wish to find someone who offers hope for restoration of hearing. It is not helpful to confront clients with the belief that they must face the reality of the irreversability of the deafness. As Kubler-Ross has stressed, people should not have hope stripped away even in the case of terminal illness. Clients can be encouraged to utilize appropriate services even while they seek a cure that the clinician knows will not be forthcoming.

When the shock passes and denial gives way to recognition of the reality of deafness, the client may wonder, "Why me?" The individual in this phase may experience *guilt* because of the feeling that becoming deaf must be a punishment or retribution for some misdeed. In a process similar to that associated with adjustment to other disabilities, some people who have become deaf will indicate that as they searched for answers, they concluded that they must have done something wrong to "deserve" their particular situation.

The belief that the fault is in the individual is replaced by some with the belief that the fault is elsewhere, and they may direct anger at the health care system—at the physician or surgeon, or even at the members of the aural rehabilitation team. Anger may not always appear logical, but it can be understood as part of the individual's effort to explain what has happened, to fix responsibility for what has happened, and to cope with other real and perceived losses attributable to the deafness. Sometimes expressions of anger directed to the clinician or other professionals are actually projections of the client's own feelings of guilt stemming from the perception that the hearing loss is punishment for some real or imagined misdeed. Projecting blame or responsibility elsewhere represents an effort—usually an unconscious one—to reduce feelings of personal responsibility and guilt.

Anger may also be a straightforward expression of feeling about the enormity of the impact of the hearing loss on the person's life and of the adjustments required. Although the feelings may be straightforward, frequently they are directed in a seemingly random fashion, conveying the impression to the observer that the deafened person is "angry at the world." This observation may be entirely accurate if the person is observed to express anger indiscriminately towards family, friends, and professionals. What may not be so apparent is that the person is sometimes angry at himself or herself, reflecting a diminished self-esteem and a rejection of the involuntary identity as a deaf person.

Bargaining (Kubler-Ross 1969) is an effort to negotiate one's way out of the unacceptable situation, usually by promising more desirable behavior in return. Bargaining might take the following form: "If I could just get my hearing back, I would never again complain about minor aches and pains." With a client who is communicating in bargaining language, it is more likely to be effective for the clinician to express awareness of how badly the person feels about becoming deaf than to confront the client for having unrealistic expectations. If clients believe that their feelings are understood and are legitimate, they are more likely to co-operate with professional recommendations than they will if they feel that the appropriateness of their feelings is being questioned or challenged.

Deafened adults may experience a period of *depression* as part of the process of dealing with the complex changes and additional losses that accompany the loss of hearing. If withdrawal from significant relationships and social situations occurs, it may be difficult to assess whether this behavior is related primarily to the reality of frustrating attempts to communicate or whether it is symptomatic of depression. In addition to the indications for suspecting depression mentioned earlier in the chapter, a sense of helplessness and hopelessness and an inability to participate meaningfully in problem-solving efforts with the clinician may be in-dications of depression and/or significant difficulties adjusting to being deaf. If any of these indicators are identified, a referral to a social worker, psychologist, or counselor should be considered, preferably someone who has experience in counseling persons with significant hearing loss.

One of the practical difficulties involved in making referrals to counseling professionals is that only a limited number has knowledge of the effects of hearing loss. Thus, the clinician is often in the position of having to take responsibility for identifying counseling professionals who have this knowledge and who un-derstand the process of successful adaptation. The most desirable situation is one in which the social worker, psychologist, or counselor is familiar with a model of integrated therapy such as that described in chapter 2 and functions as part of an interdisciplinary team. The counseling or psychotherapy can then be provided in a more holistic fashion as part of an integrated program of aural rehabilitation.

Most counseling professionals begin their work by assessing the factors that precipitated the request for service. In situations where collaborative teamwork is not possible, this assessment process can be facilitated if the clinician secures the client's permission to send a report. The report should include the usual clini-cal assessment as well as the specific reasons for recommending counseling. The counseling professional then will have a clear context within which to assess the client's needs, a situation far more beneficial to clients than a simple recommen-dation that they seek professional counseling. The most effective referrals are those in which there is communication between the professionals.

Successful *adjustment or adaptation* is, of course, the desired outcome for the deafened adult. The knowledge, skills, and technology available to the audiologist and speech-language pathologist are critically important to successful adaptation, but a key element is client readiness and receptivity to that expertise. Effective-ness in aural rehabilitation will be enhanced if assessment includes (1) identifying where the client is emotionally in the process of dealing with having become deaf and (2) developing a plan that takes into consideration the emotional aspects of adjustment.

Progress toward successful adaptation is most likely to occur when recommendations and therapy take into account client readiness. As discussed earlier in the chapter, appropriate timing is essential. The clinician may be inclined to develop an aggressive aural rehabilitation program for a newly deafened individual because it is logical that such a program is essential for the most effective functioning possible. This will be the appropriate approach for a person whose pattern of coping with problems is to obtain as much information as possible and to pursue solutions aggressively. For an individual who is devastated by the deafness and is depressed at the time of the initial assessment, a more appropriate approach will be to acknowledge the extent of her emotional response to the deafness, to provide information about the range of resources available (which should include resources to help manage the emotional response), and to assure the client that the pace of intervention will respect her feelings and readiness. In such situations, the clinician may encourage clients to try a particular recommendation, such as participating in a speechreading class or joining a self-help group, but should also carefully assess the client's reactions. When the client is clearly uncomfortable or resistant to the recommendation, a positive clinician-client relationship can be maintained if the clinician expresses understanding of the client's feelings and simply suggests that the recommendation be kept in mind for the future. When the timing is right for clients, they have the information and can act on it without feeling pressured into something for which they were not ready earlier.

When clients appear to be coping poorly because of depression or other emotional adjustment difficulties, clinicians have to determine the limits of their expertise in those areas and their comfort level in dealing with feelings. The issue of whether audiologists and speech-language pathologists should limit their role to informational counseling or whether the role appropriately includes personal adjustment counseling has been discussed and studied by numerous writers in those fields (Clark 1994; Erber 1988; Flahive and White 1982; Luterman 1991; Scheuerle 1992), but is not the focus of this chapter. Whichever stance the clinician takes, however, personal adjustment should not be ignored; the clinician should either deal with it or make a referral to a social worker, counselor, or psychologist who has expertise in this area. If clinicians do not heed personal adjustment issues, the consequence to some clients will be less effective coping with their hearing loss. Such an outcome would be particularly regrettable at a time when there is emphasis on holistic approaches in the health care delivery system and in the education of health care professionals.

Interpersonal and Social Factors

Because hearing loss effects communication, it is apparent that spouse, family, friends, coworkers, and anyone in a communication exchange with the deaf or hard of hearing individual are affected to some degree by the hearing loss and the related communication problems. It is important to recognize that each person involved is both affected by and has an effect on the adaptation of the person with hearing loss. Clearly, the closer the relationship (as with family members relationships), the more power there is in the relationship (as in employer-employee), and the more frequent the contact, the more significant the mutual effects are likely to be and the greater their impact. The concept that persons within the communication network of people with hearing loss are affected by the hearing loss and its consequences has important implications for aural rehabilitation and is elaborated below.

Support System Members of the support system are often looked to for the role they can have in the adjustment process for persons with a disability. Before expecting family and friends to offer support in coping with hearing loss or any disability, it is important to consider first how they are affected. Substantial evidence in the reports of clinicians, researchers, family members, and persons with hearing loss shows that hearing loss has significant effects on the support system (Ashley 1985; Beck 1991; Harvey 1989; Kyle and Wood 1983; McKnight 1981; Pray 1992; Sonnenschein 1987; Trychin 1990). Effects described by members of the support system frequently parallel the effects described by the individuals with hearing loss and include loss of intimacy, strain on the relationship, decrease in quantity and quality of communication, change in social activities, helplessness, frustration, bewilderment, and role reversal.

Spouses experience diverse reactions to the hearing loss, and these reactions can have a major effect on the individual's adjustment. Many spouses have great empathy and concern, whereas others feel imposed upon and resent how the hearing loss has affected their lives. Some are disappointed about changes in their social lives and struggle with whether to pressure the spouse with hearing loss to socialize more, to relinquish social situations stressful for the spouse with hearing loss, or to participate in some or all social activities alone. Many find the nature of communication in the relationship changing; communication is reduced to only what is essential. Some spouses feel that their problems are not understood or considered significant. Some spouses become protective and "take over" in communication situations, and others find their roles have changed. A number of spouses feel guilty for their reactions, and some indicate they have experienced or are in the midst of a grieving process themselves (Pray 1992).

The extent to which the hearing loss affects the spouse and family suggests that plans for managing the effects on the individual with hearing loss should focus on ways in which spouse and family members can be assisted as well. To look only at how the support system can assist the person with hearing loss fails to address spouse and family member needs and may also fail to secure their involvement. Ways in which significant others can be involved include having them participate in meetings at which the clinician interprets results of the audiological assessment and makes recommendations; inviting them to participate in the aural rehabilitation program, including speechreading classes with the person with hearing loss; and focusing joint counseling sessions on how each can be sensitive to the needs of the other and how to seek balance in the relationship in view of the difficulties stemming from the hearing loss.

Another dimension of the relationship with spouse and family is that the problems observed in the relationship may not be related primarily to the hearing loss. There may have been problems in marital or family relationships prior to the onset of the hearing loss, and these problems may have become more acute because of the additional stress. Such a situation is more difficult to deal with, and referral for counseling is often advisable.

Social Interaction A number of studies have found social isolation and loneliness among persons with hearing loss and that feelings of loneliness and isolation increase with increased severity of hearing loss (Christian, Dluhy, and O'Neill 1989; Thomas and Gilhome-Herbst 1980; Weinstein 1980; Weinstein and Ventry 1982). Other studies, however, have not found an association between hearing loss and loneliness or social isolation (Downs 1979; Manzella 1982; Norris and Cunningham 1981; Powers and Powers 1978). These inconsistent findings suggest that the clinician cannot make assumptions about how the hearing loss will affect the extent of social interaction, but if a client was experiencing isolation prior to the hearing loss, it would be reasonable to consider the possibility that the hearing loss may be an additional barrier to social interaction. Furthermore, because many studies and the experience of clinicians have shown that many people do experience difficulty maintaining the same quality of social relationships, this is an area warranting attention.

The ability to maintain satisfying interpersonal relationships clearly presents a challenge when communication is difficult because of hearing loss. Many years of clinical experience with persons with hearing loss has led the author to conclude that in situations involving a deaf or hard of hearing person and a hearing person, a number of reactions or responses are triggered in each when attempts at communication are unsuccessful. The reactions in both individuals are frequently quite similar in nature, escalate in intensity, and have a predictable outcome if the communication impasse is not resolved with the use of appropriate and effective strategies by one or both of the participants in the situation. The common progression of feelings and behavior in such situations is presented in table 5.1, a chart developed by the author for use in workshops with individuals with hearing loss and with their families.

The chart represents an effort to demonstrate a process characterized by increasing discomfort on the part of the person with hearing loss and the hearing person, a process that leads to withdrawal by both. Experience using this chart in workshops has shown that not every person will experience every reaction, but the general pattern is a common one. The chart draws attention to the progression of feelings when communication is unsuccessful and to the reasons for the feelings. Both the person with hearing loss and the person with normal hearing are experiencing isolation in this process—isolation with respect to the content of communication and to the source of their feelings. Not only is withdrawal from

Table 5.1 Parallel Reactions to Unsuccessful Communication

Person with Hearing Loss (PHL)	Person with Normal Hearing (PNH)
Frustration: can't understand	Frustration: can't make self understood
Anxiety, discomfort: fear of appearing stupid	Anxiety, discomfort: feeling awkward, not knowing what to do
Impatience: with PNH for not speaking clearly and slowly, etc.	Impatience: with PHL for not understanding, wondering if this is worth the effort
Anger: at PNH for not trying harder	Anger: at PHL for complaining, making demands, and getting angry
Feeling of loss of competence and self-esteem: another failure in efforts to communicate; reinforcement of loss of ability to communicate easily and effectively	Feelings of incompetence: inability to deal with communication barrier; lacks skills to cope with the situation; may view PHL as not competent
Self-pity: "poor me"; "it's not worth trying"	Self-pity, pity: "poor me"; pity for PHL
Guilt: for making demands, for being a burden	Guilt: for not knowing what to do, for being impatient and angry
Withdrawal: too uncomfortable to remain in the situation	Withdrawal: too uncomfortable to remain in the situation

the situation the unfortunate outcome, but there is also the potential for misunderstanding by the person with hearing loss and by the person with normal hearing about why the other has withdrawn.

Although it may be clear to both parties that there was frustration and anger, it may not be clear at all to both that each of them was experiencing feelings of incompetence. Neither individual may know that the other person was feeling guilty about the failed communication or feeling guilty about his or her frustration, impatience, and anger. What is likely is that each is more aware of her or his own frustration and sense of failure and of a desire to avoid similar situations in the future.

Insight into these parallel reactions has important implications for aural rehabilitation. Work with individuals with hearing loss as well as with those in their support system or in their employment environment can be enhanced by emphasizing a problem-solving approach that begins with both groups not only identifying their own feelings but also developing an appreciation for how the others feel. Often, persons with hearing loss are surprised to learn that those with normal hearing experience some of the same frustrations about the communication problems and that the feelings they express are not motivated by rejection and lack of interest or concern. Such insights foster greater understanding and can help motivate people—both those with hearing loss and those with normal hearing—to learn more effective communication strategies.

Communication strategies that will enhance communication and resolve communication problems require the ability to be assertive (see Bally, chapter 3). For many persons with hearing loss, becoming assertive poses a significant challenge. Many older people note that they were raised during a time when asserting their needs or rights was considered aggressive and unacceptable. Many people of all ages feel stigmatized by their hearing loss and do not want to draw further attention to it by making their communication needs known. The fact that so many people have difficulty being assertive suggests that when teaching communication strategies, the clinician should consider the personality of the client and assess his or her level of comfort with being assertive.

In a study of the coping patterns of twenty-eight older persons, their spouses, and significant others, Pray (1992) found that the majority of persons with hearing loss were either very passive in dealing with the loss or dependent upon a spouse or family member to take responsibility for dealing with problems in communication. Many of the spouses were very protective and "took over" for the person with hearing loss. It was not clear from the data if the deaf or hard of hearing person's passive approach to coping precipitated such behavior in the spouse, the spouse's personality produced the response, or it was some combination of these factors. Although the population studied was very small, the findings do suggest that it could be important to focus aural rehabilitation efforts on the spouses and significant others as well as on the person with hearing loss. A small number of such participants in the study indicated that they wished they had been included in reports of the results of the audiological assessment as well as in follow-up services that had been provided.

Invaluable support for people coping with hearing loss and for their families can be provided by self-help organizations such as Self-Help for Hard of Hearing People, Inc. (SHHH) and the Association of Late-Deafened Adults (ALDA).[3] Both of these organizations have chapters in many states that typically meet monthly

[3] SHHH, 7910 Woodmont Avenue, Suite 1200, Bethesda, MD 20814.
ALDA, 1027 Oakton, Evanston, IL 60202.

for mutual support, education, advocacy, and socialization. SHHH publishes a journal for consumers, and ALDA publishes a newsletter. Because of numerous benefits available, it is advisable to include a recommendation for membership in a self-help group as part of any aural rehabilitation plan.

Employment Situation If the client is employed, the nature of the employment situation and the amount and nature of communication required will play a role in the effects of the hearing loss. For a deafened client, major adaptations may be required and in some situations may involve a change of employment. The Americans with Disabilities Act requires employers to make reasonable accommodations for persons with hearing loss. Provisions of TDDs and interpreters for clients who communicate in sign language facilitate successful functioning in the workplace. Clients with mild to moderate hearing loss may find communication on the job stressful but manageable, especially if they have developed effective communication strategies and if employers provide amplified telephones where use of the telephone is required on the job.

Some clients are reluctant to acknowledge their hearing loss because they are fearful that to do so will result in their being viewed as less competent and thus denied opportunities for advancement. For older persons, the development of a hearing loss may influence the timing of retirement if they find communication stressful. These are situations in which the clinician may assist the client in developing specific job-related strategies and, if need be, in proposing to an employer ways a job might be restructured to make it possible for the employee to continue to be productive on the job.

Other Losses or Changes Any loss or change requires adaptation, and multiple changes or losses increase the demands on an individual's resources for coping. Thus, when people experience hearing loss, it is important to determine the extent of other demands on their coping resources. The stress created by another disability or health problem has already been discussed. Among other areas to be explored are change of job or loss of job, responsibility for care of a spouse or parent, a recent move, or any other major change requiring adjustment. Particularly in the case of older persons, factors to be considered are recent widowhood, death of friends, recent move of adult children or close friends, adjustment to retirement, or change of financial circumstances.

Understanding that these other life stresses may come into play enables the clinician to place the hearing loss within the context of the client's whole life experience. An assessment of these factors helps determine the extent of emotional resources the client has available for aural rehabilitation as well as the priority he or she places on adjustment to the hearing loss, thus contributing to the development of a realistic aural rehabilitation program.

Nature of Activities How people spend their time will have an impact upon the extent to which hearing loss affects their lives and the kinds of adaptations they need to make. Persons who will experience significant difficulty are those who lead very active social lives that include interaction with people in large groups, a great deal of entertaining, or attending the theater and concerts regularly. Persons with families with young children or grandchildren frequently express sadness and frustration at not being able to understand young children's voices at family gatherings.

When an individual develops a hearing loss, often his or her first inclination is to withdraw from social situations that cause frustration because of difficulty hearing or understanding. One of the contributions of the clinician can be to help the client think through acceptable alternatives to particularly stressful activities. For example, a client who has always led an active social life can be encouraged to consider smaller gatherings as a substitute for large parties rather than give up entertaining completely. A client who enjoys taking courses or attending lectures can be encouraged to become assertive about identifying lecturers whose style is conducive to good communication, about locating and obtaining seating that will maximize ability to understand, and about requesting the use of assistive technology such as FM and infrared systems.

Societal Attitudes toward Hearing Loss Watson and Maxwell (1977) assert that social criteria rather than physical criteria define disability. Calhoun and Lipman (1984), citing the work of Erving Goffman (1963), suggest that true disability is not related to the physical condition but to the "spoiled identity" resulting from stigma and alienation from interaction with others. Older persons experience devalued status (Rosow 1974) and "ageism" (Butler and Lewis 1973) and are in "double jeopardy" if they also have hearing loss because they have an additional kind of devalued status or stigma (Wax 1982). A typical example of "double jeopardy" is Ms. J., a retired businesswoman who is reluctant to use a hearing aid. Ms. J. believes that as an older retired person she no longer enjoys the respect she had as a business executive. She worries that wearing a hearing aid will further stigmatize her as a person with a disability.

One intriguing social context in which deafness was not defined as a disability occurred on Martha's Vineyard between the late 1600s and the early 1900s, during which time there was an unusually high prevalence of hereditary deafness. Because hearing people on the island communicated in sign language, deaf people were not considered to be disabled (Groce 1985).

A situation that occurred several years ago underscores indelibly the existence of stigma with respect to deafness. While boarding a flight to a national conference on deafness and deaf people, the writer observed that the flight attendants were distressed by the large number of deaf people using sign language as they boarded the plane. When they noticed a young woman both signing and speaking, they appeared relieved and asked, "Are you their leader?" Puzzled, the young woman asked what they meant. One of the flight attendants replied, "Well, do they know how to fly?"

The previous example is only one among many that demonstrate considerable evidence for the existence of stigma associated with hearing loss. One of the factors in clients' reluctance to purchase a hearing aid, in their greater preference for the smallest possible hearing aid, and in their reluctance to acknowledge having a hearing loss is concern about stigma. Although vanity is sometimes considered a factor in clients' unwillingness to acknowledge hearing loss or to use a hearing aid, it may be worth reevaluating that assumption, in view of the substantial evidence that hearing loss is a stigmatizing condition, and instead more clearly identifying stigma as one of the factors to be dealt with in the process of adapting to hearing loss.

Summary

The focus of this chapter has been on the interaction of the biological, psychological, and social aspects of hearing loss and how those aspects affect adjustment. The biopsychosocial perspective can be utilized as a guide to understanding the diverse feelings and behaviors that clients may exhibit during the aural rehabilitation process. The chapter suggests approaches that may be taken to address difficulties the client may experience in the psychosocial aspects of his life and emphasizes the importance of the clinician's responses to the client's feelings and of the timing of interventions to fit various phases of adjustment. Also emphasized is how the various meanings of being Deaf, deaf, deafened, or hard of hearing affect approaches to assessment and intervention.

References

Aguilera, D. C. 1994. *Crisis intervention: Theory and methodology.* St. Louis: C. V. Mosby.

Asch, A. 1984. The experience of disability: A challenge for psychology. *American Psychologist* 39:529–536.

Ashley, P. 1985. Deafness and the family. In *Adjustment to adult hearing loss,* ed. H. Orlans. San Diego, Calif.: College-Hill Press.

Beck, R. L. 1991. The forgotten family. *SHHH Journal* 12(1):7–9.

Butler, R. N., and M. I. Lewis. 1973. *Aging and mental health: Positive psychosocial approaches.* St. Louis: C. V. Mosby.

Calhoun, D. W., and A. Lipman. 1984. The disabled. In *Handbook on the aged in the United States,* ed. E. B. Palmore. Westport, Conn.: Greenwood Press.

Christian, E., N. Dluhy, and R. O'Neill. 1989. Sounds of silence: Coping with hearing loss and loneliness. *Journal of Gerontological Nursing* 15(11):4–9.

Clark, J. G. 1994. Audiologists' counseling purview. In *Effective counseling in audiology: Perspectives and practice,* ed. J. G. Clark and F. N. Martin. Englewood Cliffs, N.J.: Prentice Hall.

Clark, J. G., and F. N. Martin, eds. 1994. *Effective counseling in audiology: Perspectives and practice.* Englewood Cliffs, N.J.: Prentice Hall.

Downs, M. B. 1979. *The influence of mild to moderate hearing impairment and decreased social interaction on the verbal communication behavior of elderly women.* Unpublished doctoral dissertation. University of Maryland, Baltimore.

Erber, N. P. 1988. *Communication therapy for hearing-impaired adults.* Abbotsford, Victoria, Australia: Clavis Publishing.

Erikson, E. H. 1959. *Identity and the life cycle.* New York: International Universities Press.

———. 1968. *Identity, youth, and crisis.* New York: Norton.

Flahive, M., and S. White. 1982. Audiologists and counseling. *Journal of the Academy of Rehabilitative Audiology* 10:275–287.

Glass, L. E. 1985. Psychosocial aspects of hearing loss in adulthood. In *Adjustment to adult hearing loss,* ed. H. Orlans. San Diego, Calif.: College-Hill Press.

Goffman, E. 1963. *Stigma: Notes on the management of spoiled identity.* Englewood Cliffs, N.J.: Prentice-Hall.

Groce, N. E. 1985. *Everyone here spoke sign language; Hereditary deafness on Martha's Vineyard.* Cambridge: Harvard University Press.

Harvey, M. J. 1989. *Psychotherapy with deaf and hard of hearing persons.* Hillsdale, N.J.: Lawrence Erlbaum Associates.

Hunt, P. 1969. *Stigma: The experience of disability.* London: Chapman and Hall.

Kubler-Ross, E. 1969. *On death and dying.* New York: Macmillan.

Kyle, J. G., and P. Wood. 1983. *Social and vocational aspects of acquired hearing loss.* Final Report to MSC, School of Education, Bristol, England.

Ladieu, G., D. L. Adler, and T. Dembo. 1948. Studies in adjustment to visible injuries: Social acceptance of the injured. *Journal of Social Issues* 4(4):55–61.

Luterman, D. M. 1991. *Counseling the communicatively disordered and their families.* Austin, Tex.: Pro-Ed.

Manzella, D. S. 1982. *Activity patterns of hearing impaired older women.* Unpublished doctoral dissertation. University of California, Los Angeles.

Martin, F. N., L. Krall, and J. O'Neal. 1990. Diagnosis: Hearing loss! A study of adult patients' impressions. *SHHH Journal* 11(4):21–23.

McKnight, J. 1981. Professionalized service and disabling help. In *Handicap in a social world,* eds. A. Brechin, P. Liddiard, and J. Swain. London: Hodder & Stoughton.

Meadow-Orlans, K. P. 1985. Social and psychological effects of hearing loss in adulthood:

A literature review. In *Adjustment of adult hearing loss,* ed. H. Orlans. San Diego, Calif.: College-Hill Press.

Norris, M. L., and D. R. Cunningham. 1981. Social impact of hearing loss in the aged. *Journal of Gerontology* 36:727–729.

Orlans, H., and K. P. Meadow-Orlans. 1985. Responses to hearing loss: Effects on social life, leisure, and work. *SHHH Journal* 6(1):4–7.

Oyer, J. J., and E. J. Oyer. 1976. Preface. *Aging and communication.* Baltimore: University Park Press.

Powers, J. K., and E. A. Powers. 1978. Hearing problems of elderly persons: Social consequences and prevalence. *ASHA* 20: 79–83.

Pray, J. L. 1990. Aging and hearing loss: Mental health implications. *Gallaudet Today* 20(3):36–39.

————. 1992. *Aging and hearing loss: Patterns of coping with the effects of late-onset hearing loss among persons age sixty and older and their spouses/significant others.* Unpublished doctoral dissertation, The Union Institute, Cincinnati, Ohio.

Rogers, C. R. 1979. Foundations of the person-centered approach. *Education* (100)2: 98–107.

Rosow, I. 1974. *Socialization to old age.* Berkeley, Calif.: University of California Press.

Roth, W. 1983. Handicap as a social construct. *Society* March-April:55–61.

Scheuerle, J. 1992. *Counseling in speech-language pathology and audiology.* New York: Macmillan.

Schlesinger, H. S. 1985. The psychology of hearing loss. In *Adjustment to adult hearing loss,* ed. H. Orlans. San Diego, Calif.: College-Hill Press.

Schultz, R., and S. Decker. 1985. Long-term adjustment to physical disability: The role of social support, perceived control, and self-blame. *Journal of Personality and Social Psychology* 48:1162–1172.

Sonnenschein, M. A. 1987. How does my hearing loss affect my spouse? *SHHH Journal* 8(5): 27–28.

Tanner, D. C. 1980. Loss and grief: Implications for the speech-language pathologist and audiologist. *ASHA* 22:916–922.

Thomas, A. J. 1984. *Acquired hearing loss: Psychological and psychosocial implications.* Orlando, Fla.: Academic Press.

Thomas, A. J., and K. Gilhome-Herbst. 1980. Social and psychological implications of acquired deafness in adults of employment age. *British Journal of Audiology* 14: 76–85.

Trychin, S. 1990. You . . . me . . . and hearing loss makes three. *SHHH Journal* 11(1):7–11.

Watson, W. H., and R. J. Maxwell. 1977. *Human aging and dying: A study in sociocultural gerontology.* New York: St. Martin's Press.

Wax, T. 1982. The hearing-impaired aged: Double jeopardy or double challenge? *Gallaudet Today* 12(2):3–7.

Weinstein, B. E. 1980. *Hearing impairment and social isolation.* Unpublished doctoral dissertation. Columbia University, New York.

Weinstein, B. E., and I. M. Ventry. 1982. Hearing impairment and social isolation in the elderly. *Journal of Speech and Hearing Research* 25:593–595.

Wright, B. A. 1983. *Physical disability: A psychosocial approach.* New York: Harper and Row.

6

Technology for Aural Rehabilitation

Harriet Kaplan

■ ■ ■ ■

Basic to any aural rehabilitation program is the consideration and selection of appropriate amplification systems such as hearing aids, assistive listening systems, and cochlear implants. Equally important are telecommunication systems—auditory, visual, and vibrotactile alerting devices, as well as tactile aids. Technology is an integral part of the integrated therapy model described in chapter 2 of this book. It is depicted in the model as one of the concentric circles, indicating that it is an important consideration for all aspects of communication therapy. For example, auditory training is predicated on the use of hearing aids, cochlear implants, or assistive listening systems. Training of auditory skills is of little value if the client is unable to hear sound. Therefore, a client needs to be evaluated and fitted with appropriate amplification early in the rehabilitation process. If the client does not wish to use amplification, then aspects of rehabilitation other than auditory training can be explored.

Telephone training requires use of telephone amplifiers, TTYs, or both. Telephone technology appropriate to the client needs to be selected early in therapy. Speech production and speechreading training are facilitated when technology can be used to provide some auditory or tactile input. For these reasons, the client's ability to benefit from technology is usually considered early in communication therapy.

The purpose of this chapter is to provide an overview of four general technologies that facilitate receptive communication: hearing aids, assistive devices, cochlear implants, and tactile aids. In-depth discussions can be found in other texts, which are referenced in appropriate sections of the chapter. Aids to expressive communication and rehabilitation techniques are discussed in other chapters of this book.

The hearing aid section describes types of hearing aids and earmolds, and discusses candidacy and selection issues. The assistive technology section focuses on listening, telecommunication, and alerting systems, including their benefits and limitations. The sections on cochlear implants and tactile aids also consist of description, candidacy issues, and benefits and limitations. Because of the adult focus of this book, issues relating specifically to children will not be included.

Hearing Aids

All types of hearing aids share the same basic components: a microphone, an amplifier, a receiver, and a battery to power the instrument. Figure 6.1 shows a schematic of the basic configuration of a hearing aid.

Transducers

Microphones and receivers are the transducers used in all hearing aids to convert one form of energy to another. The microphone changes acoustic energy to electrical energy for the purpose of amplification whereas the receiver changes amplified electrical energy back to its acoustic analog so that it may be delivered to the ear.

The Microphone Virtually all microphones today have the capability of responding to a wide range of frequencies with minimal distortion, low internal noise, and low sensitivity to mechanical vibration and temperature change. A more complete description of microphone technology can be found in Olsen 1986, 22–24; Killion and Carlson 1974; and Killion 1993a.

Many behind-the-ear hearing aids (and assistive listening devices) provide the option of a directional microphone which is designed to reduce amplification of sound (particularly low frequencies) from the rear of the listener. Because speech signals originate from the front of the listener and noise from the rear, listening in noise is enhanced. Studies by Mueller (1981), Mueller, Grimes, and Erdman (1983), Madison and Hawkins (1983), Hawkins and Yacullo (1984), and Mueller, Hawkins, and Sedge (1984) indicate that listeners consider directional microphones superior or equal to omnidirectional microphones in noisy situations. Mueller and Grimes (1987) recommend the selection of a directional microphone for all hearing aid fittings.

The Telecoil Although not a transducer because it does not change one form of energy to another, the hearing aid telecoil is an alternative to a microphone as a way of transmitting sound information to the amplifier. It is activated by moving a switch on the hearing aid from microphone (M) to telecoil (T). The telecoil is a

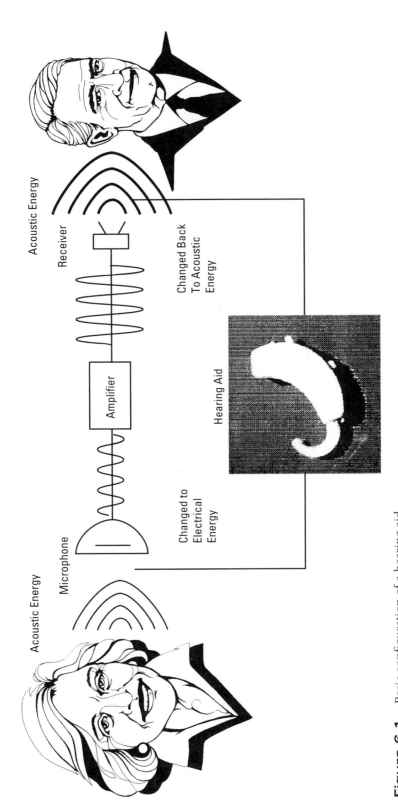

Figure 6.1. Basic configuration of a hearing aid

Source: Brandt 1995.

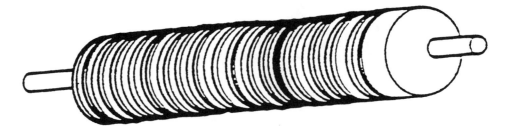

Figure 6.2. Hearing aid telecoil
Source: Electronic Industries Association 1993.

small metal rod surrounded by coils of wire that are attached to the amplifier (see figure 6.2). It picks up electromagnetic signals emanating from the sound source (e.g., telephone) and sends them to the amplifier. Because the microphone is turned off, background noise is not picked up. It is possible to order a hearing aid that allows both microphone and telecoil to function simultaneously (an MT position), allowing the listener to monitor his or her voice, to hear environmental sounds such a door bell, and to hear comments of talkers in the environment. Telecoils are important for use with assistive listening devices that use induction loop amplification. Such systems are discussed in the assistive devices section of this chapter.

Telecoils come in a variety of sizes, and some are more powerful than others. All behind-the-ear aids can be ordered with telecoils if they are not already standard equipment. Behind the-ear aids generally have stronger telecoils than in-the-ear aids, but there is considerable variation. Although most in-the-ear hearing aids can be equipped with telecoils, they are not standard equipment. It is often necessary to special order a strengthened telecoil, particularly for in-the-ear aids (Compton 1991a).

There are no standards concerning the position or orientation of the telecoil within the hearing aid. If the hearing aid is to be used with induction loop assistive listening systems, the telecoil should be mounted vertically within the hearing aid. A horizontal orientation is optimal for telephone use. If, however, the telecoil is to be used both for telephone and induction loop systems, a vertical orientation is preferable. The user must then angle the telephone receiver for best reception. Because telecoils may be placed in different positions in different hearing aids, the user must search for the location of the telecoil by moving the telephone receiver around the hearing aid case until the telephone signal is loudest and clearest; the telephone receiver must be maintained in that position for the duration of the conversation. In addition, the listener usually needs to increase the hearing aid volume when the telephone switch is turned to "T" position. If there is need to hear both electromagnetic signals from a loop system or telephone and environmental sounds simultaneously, the "MT" switching option on the hearing aid should be activated. When both input systems are used, it is desirable for the hearing aid to provide a slight increase in telecoil gain relative to microphone gain.

The Receiver The function of the receiver (sometimes called the earphone) is to convert (transduce) the amplified electrical signal back to sound so that it can be delivered to the ear. A small number of hearing-impaired individuals cannot benefit from air-conducted sound because of atresia of the ear canal or some medical condition that requires the ear canal to remain unoccluded. In such situations, a bone conduction vibrator may be used. The vibrator is placed on the mastoid process of the amplified ear, where it transduces the electrical signal from the amplifier into mechanical vibrations that are transmitted to the cochlea by way of the temporal bone. Bone conduction vibrators are inefficient transducers because of limited output, restricted frequency response, and high battery consumption. They are usually considered only if there is no other amplification alternative.

The Amplifier

The amplifier determines the gain, frequency response, and maximum power output (SSPL-90) of the hearing aid. Maximum power output can be set in two ways. With peak clipping, the peaks of sound that exceed the maximum power output are electronically clipped, with some resultant distortion. With signal compression, the level of the entire signal is automatically reduced when a sound exceeds a predetermined level. Compression technology is used for several purposes. Compression limiting or high-level compression is used to compress high-level signals to prevent distortion. Dynamic-range compression (also called wide-range compression, syllabic compression, or log-linear compression) compresses most of the dynamic range of speech so that the listener is able to hear the speech within his or her range of residual hearing. Automatic volume control or automatic gain control systems automatically control the gain as a function of the level of the input signal. Compression technology is present in almost all programmable hearing aids and many nonprogrammable instruments. A hearing aid may be designed to compress the entire signal, or the signal may first be divided into frequency bands, and each band processed independently. Further discussion of compression technology can be found in Fabry (1993), Letowski (1993), Fabry (1991), Braida et al. (1979), Stypulkowski (1993), Killion and Fikret-Pasa (1993), Johnson (1993), and Hickson (1994).

Specific gain, frequency response, maximum power output, and compression parameters are selected based on the client's audiogram, usually by using a prescription formula. Further information on prescriptive procedures can be found in Humes (1991), Bratt and Sammeth (1991), and Byrne, Parkinson, and Newall (1991). Changes in output and frequency response may be made manually using switches or screwdriver adjustments. With digital hearing aids the adjustments are programmed into the amplifier with a computer.

Most hearing aids are equipped with volume controls that allow users to select the amount of amplification for their needs in various situations. In most cases, the volume control is located on the hearing aid, but some of the smaller instruments use a remote control device similar to that used for television. Remote controls can be useful to clients who cannot manipulate very small controls. However, they can be misplaced; this becomes extremely problematic if the hearing aid cannot function without the remote control.

Digital Programmable Hearing Aids

All present hearing aid amplifiers use traditional (analog) circuitry. However, increasing numbers of hearing aids have digital controls. Some digitally controlled aids are programmed at the factory and cannot be reprogrammed by the audiologist. Others allow the audiologist to program adjustments using computers, computerlike systems, or handheld programmers. These adjustments are stored in memory on the small microchip in the hearing aid. Once the amplifier adjustments are made, the signal is sent to the receiver and the ear in the same manner as a totally analog hearing aid.

Some programmable aids have multiple memories and allow the audiologist to program several different frequency responses into the hearing aid to correspond to the requirements of different listening situations. The hearing aid contains a switch that allows the user to shift between programs as needed.

Types of adjustments are similar with digital and analog technology, but digital control permits more precise settings better customized to the needs of the individual. Programmable hearing aids allow the audiologist to reprogram the aid if the person's hearing changes over time. Multiple memories, not possible in analog aids, allow differential programming for different listening situations.

Programmable hearing aids vary in their features. Mueller (1994) divides programmable (digitally controlled) hearing aids into Tier I (single-channel) and Tier II (multichannel). Both Tier I and Tier II hearing aids use some form of adjustable compression.

According to Mueller (1994), as many as 80 percent of all hearing aid clients are candidates for programmable hearing aids. Some clients, however, are not good candidates. Although the situation may change, most programmable instruments do not provide sufficient gain and output for severe to profound hearing losses. Wireless CROS or BICROS fittings are not available in programmable instruments. Some programmable hearing aids, particularly the Tier II systems, are significantly more expensive than traditional analog instruments. Aural rehabilitationists can refer clients who are interested in trying programmable hearing aids to certified audiologists with knowledge and experience in this area. A trial with a refund option needs to be included in the evaluation, however.

Additional information on digital programmable hearing aids can be found in Compton, Van Middlesworth, and Di Pietro (1992); Fabry (1991); Bentler (1991); Mueller (1994); and Berkey et al. (1992).

Noise Reduction Circuitry

Hearing aids with automatic noise reduction circuitry are called adaptive frequency response (AFR), level-dependent frequency response (LDFR), automatic signal processing (ASP), and automatic noise reduction (ANR) instruments. Noise reduction circuity is available in both analog and digital hearing aids. One type of noise reduction circuitry attempts to filter out background noise, usually low frequencies. They are activated by the overall level of background sound or by sound levels in specific frequency bands. These instruments sometimes reduce the number of low-frequency speech cues as well. Research data on such noise reduction hearing aids do not indicate improved speech intelligibility when the noise is competing with speech (Fabry and Van Tasell 1990; Hochberg et al. 1992). Because some clients report improvement with noise reduction circuitry, a trial/experience period needs to be provided when noise reduction hearing aids are considered.

Other types of noise reduction circuits, such as the K-Amp, reduce high-frequency gain in response to high-intensity sound (Killion 1990). Using compression technology, maximum gain is provided for low-level input and minimal gain for high-intensity signals. This type of processing is combined with a low-distortion Class D amplifier and wide bandwidth. Research has shown that this type of technology does improve listening in noise, not by eliminating noise but by increasing available speech cues (Killion 1993; Killion and Villchur 1993). Killion (1993) cautions, however, that K-Amp fittings may be problematic with clients who have moderate to severe flat losses or near-normal low-frequency hearing.

More information on noise reduction circuits can be found in Fabry (1991) and Bentler (1991).

Batteries

Batteries provide the power source for all hearing aids and come in various sizes for different hearing aids. Hearing aid batteries generally are made of mercury, silver oxide, or zinc-air. Because the zinc-air battery is activated only by exposure to air when a protective covering is removed, it has a long shelf life. The actual life of a hearing aid battery depends on the power of the hearing aid, the volume control setting used by the listener, and the number of hours per day the hearing aid is used. All batteries maintain relatively constant voltage until used up, allowing stable hearing aid performance. A few hearing aids can use nickel cadmium (nicad) rechargeable batteries, but nicad batteries are much more common in assistive-listening devices.

Direct Audio Input

A hearing aid containing direct audio input is equipped with a special electrical connection at the bottom or the side of the hearing aid (see figure 6.5, p. 165).

This allows an external microphone or assistive-listening device to plug directly into the hearing aid amplifier via an audio shoe. By bypassing the hearing aid microphone, environmental noise and microphone distortion are eliminated. Many behind-the-ear hearing aids provide direct audio input as standard equipment; it can be special-ordered for other behind-the-ear and some in-the-ear hearing aids. Presently, canal aids do not provide this feature. Hearing aids can be used with both direct audio input and environmental microphone activated. Even though hearing aid manufacturers are moving toward universally compatible direct audio input systems, present technology requires that each hearing aid must be used with its own audio shoe and cord.

Types of Hearing Aids

Today there are four types of hearing aids on the market (see figure 6.3): (1) in-the-ear (ITE), including in-the-canal (ITC), (2) behind-the-ear (BTE), (3) eyeglass, and (4) body-worn.

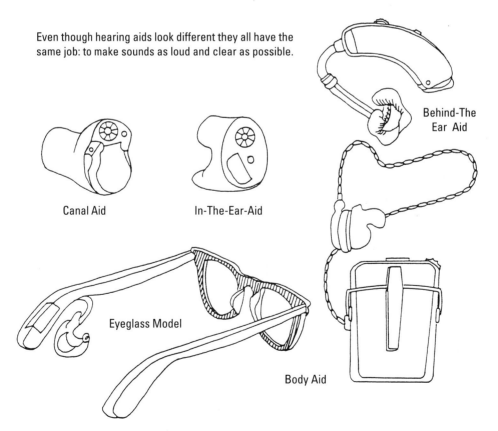

Even though hearing aids look different they all have the same job: to make sounds as loud and clear as possible.

Behind-The Ear Aid

Canal Aid

In-The-Ear-Aid

Eyeglass Model

Body Aid

Figure 6.3. The five types of hearing aids
Source: National Information Center on Deafness 1988.

In-the-Ear (ITE) and In-the-Canal (ITC) Hearing Aids

ITE and ITC hearing aids are the most popular type of instruments sold today. An in-the-ear hearing aid consists of a shell that is custom-fitted to the listener's ear from the same type of ear impression used to make an earmold for a behind-the-ear instrument. This shell contains the microphone, amplifier, receiver, user controls, battery compartment and, if space permits, other hearing aid components such as a telecoil. The custom, full in-the-ear aid fills the concha completely. Smaller versions include the low-profile and half-concha, which fill part of the concha. The in-the-canal (ITC) hearing aid fits primarily into the ear canal.

In today's market, the in-the-ear instrument is the hearing aid of choice for most adults with mild to moderately severe (sometimes severe) hearing losses. Custom, full in-the-ear instruments can generally fit most hearing losses unless the needed amount of gain exceeds the capability of the aid. Although strong, properly oriented telecoils and direct audio input capability are easier to obtain in behind-the-ear aids, these features are possible in ITEs if the size and shape of the listener's ear allow sufficient space in the hearing aid.

The major advantage of the ITE and especially the ITC hearing aid is that users consider them more cosmetically acceptable. In addition, many people find them easier to manipulate, although some elderly people report difficulty handling the miniature batteries and with inserting and removing the aids from their ears. Neither the ITE nor the ITC provides the fitting flexibility of the behind-the-ear instrument with its gain, frequency response, and maximum power output trimpots.

Behind-the-Ear (BTE) Hearing Aids

The BTE hearing aid consists of a shell contoured to fit behind the ear (see figure 6.3). It contains all hearing aid components and can be powerful enough to fit a profound hearing loss. The amplified acoustic signal leaving the receiver travels through attached tubing that continues as the sound channel through the custom-fitted earmold. The BTE is the most flexible of all hearing aids because of the many available electroacoustic fitting adjustments and because of its ability to use earmold modifications to meet the client's specific needs. BTEs are used when high power is needed or when a client is a poor candidate for an ITE for other reasons.

Body-Worn and Eyeglass Hearing Aids

Body-worn hearing aids consist of a case that contains all hearing aid components except for an external receiver, which is connected to it with a cord. The button-type receiver snaps on to the earmold. The body-worn hearing aid is rarely used today because the BTE can provide sufficient power for the vast majority of hearing losses. Those few people who still use this style do so because they require more gain than the strongest BTE can provide without feedback and large visible controls to accomodate manual dexterity problems, or because the pinna cannot accomodate a BTE. Body-worn hearing aids can perform like a vibrotactile device with the bone conduction vibrator delivering the vibrotactile signal.

Eyeglass hearing aids are glasses that can accommodate hearing aid components in one or both temples. Functionally, they are similar to behind-the-ear aids. Eyeglass hearing aids have fallen into disuse because the need to accommodate visual and auditory needs in a single prosthesis causes fitting, adjustment, and repair problems that are greater than with other hearing aids.

Earmolds

Earmolds are part of the sound conducting mechanism of the hearing aid. With BTE and eyeglass aids, the earmold attaches to tubing, which in turn connects to the receiver. Earmolds of body-worn aids snap directly to the receiver button. The earmold is a vital part of the hearing aid fitting process because a variety of modifications are possible to achieve different acoustic goals. With ITE and ITC hearing aids, the hearing aid itself replaces the earmold. Some of the same acoustic modifications used with earmolds (primarily venting) can be incorporated into the ITE shell. The frequency response of a hearing aid can be modified by venting, damping, or horning the earmold, earhook, or tubing; these modifications are discussed below. Detailed information on earmold acoustics can be found in Hodgson (1986, 71–108).

Venting

An earmold vent is an opening separate from the sound channel that extends from the outside surface of the earmold to its tip in the ear canal. Most vents run parallel to the sound channel and are used primarily to attenuate low frequencies. Vents are also used to permit sound that does not require amplification (e.g., frequencies at which hearing is normal) to reach the ear and to reduce pressure buildup against the eardrum often present with closed earmolds. The larger the vent, the greater the reduction of low frequencies. The ultimate vent is a nonoccluding earmold, also referred to as a free field, CROS, IROS, or open mold. For relief of pressure, only a small vent is needed. When clinicians are uncertain about the optimal vent size, they usually order earmolds with a positive venting valve (PVV) or a select-a-vent (SAV) system. Each system provides a large vent and inserts of different diameters. Similar effects may be achieved with an ITE hearing aid by venting the hearing aid shell.

The major undesirable effect of venting is feedback, familiar as a high-pitched squeal. Feedback occurs when amplified sound delivered to the ear canal escapes around a loosely fitted earmold or hearing aid, through poorly fitted or cracked tubing, or through a vent, and then enters the hearing aid microphone to be reamplified. The risk of feedback increases with the power of the hearing aid and the proximity of the sound leak to the hearing aid microphone. If venting results in feedback, the vent must be plugged.

Damping

Damping is the result of inserting an occluding-type filter into the tubing of BTE hearing aids, usually at the tone hook. Damping smooths peaks in the frequency response created by the receiver-earmold system and reduces overall output, primarily in the midfrequency region. Dampers of different ohm values are available to affect differentially the frequency response of the hearing aid. By eliminating undesirable peaks in the frequency response, damping can improve sound quality, eliminate or reduce feedback that usually occurs at the frequency of the peak, and improve tolerance for amplified sound.

Horn Effects

Acoustic horns are used with wide-band receivers to increase acoustic energy in high-frequency regions. A horn is created in a BTE hearing aid when the tubing and sound channel of the earmold gradually increase in diameter to a typical maximum of 4mm at the tip of the earmold. Because most hearing losses are greater in the high rather than in the low frequencies, horns are used frequently. Horn-type plumbing is difficult to use with ITE hearing aids, however, because of space constraints and the small distance between the hearing aid receiver and the opening into the ear canal.

Binaural Amplification

There is considerable research evidence to indicate that most deaf and hard of hearing clients can benefit from binaural amplification (Hawkins and Yacullo 1984; Byrne 1981). Binaural amplification often:

1. improves localization in the horizontal plane (Dermody and Byrne 1975);

2. allows use of less gain than one hearing aid, reducing the possibility of exceeding uncomfortable listening level (binaural thresholds are approximately 3 dB better than monaural);

3. eliminates the head shadow effect by allowing the user to hear speech originating from either side of the head;

4. improves the ability to understand speech in the presence of noise.

Binaural amplification should be considered if a client has two aidable ears, even if ear symmetry is lacking (Causey and Bender 1980; Nabelek and Mason 1981). Those clients who function better with monaural amplification can be identified during hearing aid evaluation or during the thirty-day trial following purchase.

Candidacy Issues

According to the Vanderbilt/VA Hearing Aid Conference 1990 Consensus Statement, "Anyone who describes hearing difficulties in communicative situations should be considered a potential candidate for hearing aids or other assistive devices" (Hawkins et al. 1991, 37). Hearing aid candidacy cannot be determined by pure tone thresholds or word recognition scores alone.

Motivation

Many audiologists consider motivation the most important factor for predicting successful hearing aid use, particularly with elderly people who sometimes deny their communication difficulty or feel that a hearing aid will not make an appreciable difference. Sometimes, these feelings are reinforced by lack of understanding of the nature of the hearing loss, by poor advice from medical personnel, or by financial considerations. Younger people with hearing loss, in contrast, are often motivated to use amplification by workplace pressures. Older individuals who lead mentally, physically, and emotionally active lives are more likely to be successful hearing aid users than those who have withdrawn from society. Sometimes a period of aural rehabilitation is necessary to create motivation for amplification.

Culturally Deaf individuals may have different reasons for lack of interest in amplification. Some Deaf clients who seem to be good candidates for amplification, based on the audiogram, choose not to use oral communication; they rely on sign language and writing for communication. They feel no need to hear or understand speech, even if a hearing aid would make it possible.

Hearing aids can provide benefits other than speech understanding, such as:

1. Awareness and identification of alarms, sirens, car horns, babies crying, phones ringing, and other environmental sounds

2. Voice monitoring

3. Support for speechreading

4. Ability to hear music and awareness of dance rhythm

Some Deaf people feel that if speech understanding through audition is not possible, amplification is of no value. Demonstration of the above benefits, however, may motivate them to try amplification. It is clear that some profoundly deaf people are candidates for hearing aids. This issue is discussed in greater depth in the section on Hearing Aid Orientation in chapter 7 of this book.

Understanding and Acceptance of Loss

These factors are closely related to motivation. A client must accept the reality of the hearing loss and the limitation it imposes on life activities. Until denial ceases, the individual is not ready for the fitting and adjustment to a hearing aid. Denial is more common with people having mild hearing losses of gradual onset who tend to blame their communication difficulties on the communication setting or the communication partner. Assessing acceptance of loss, perhaps with one of the communication inventories discussed in chapter 4, helps to determine whether the client is ready for hearing aid use. Realistic expectations of the benefits of amplification are very important to successful use. Some people become disappointed that the hearing aid does not restore hearing to normal and may discard the instrument (the familiar "dresser drawer" syndrome). Others expect the hearing aid to be of little value, and never make the effort to adjust to the instrument. Counseling about benefits and limitations of amplification should start after completion of the basic hearing evaluation and continue as needed throughout the rehabilitation process.

Degree of Hearing Loss

Although degree of hearing loss does not determine hearing aid candidacy, many individuals with mild hearing losses are marginal candidates. This is particularly true of individuals with: (1) normal hearing through 2000 Hz and hearing loss of 30 dB or greater at higher frequencies, and (2) mild to moderate low-frequency loss with normal hearing in the high frequencies. Because such clients are difficult to fit, they are sometimes discouraged from using amplification even though they experience communication difficulty. Current technology can sometimes meet these needs, so amplification may be attempted if the individual is motivated to try hearing aids.

Other Problems

Other factors that affect success of hearing aid use, particularly with elderly clients, include manual dexterity and ability to care for oneself. A person who cannot manipulate and take care of a hearing aid will not be a successful hearing aid user unless a significant other is consistently present to assist.

Hearing Aid Evaluation

Following the selection of type of aid, electroacoustic characteristics, and ear/s to be fitted, some type of formal evaluation is performed. With an ITE fitting, the audiologist sends the client's audiogram, an earmold impression, and a list of desired special features to the manufacturer who then custom designs a hearing aid. Some audiologists select a specific frequency response from a target matrix book provided by the manufacturer. When the hearing aid arrives, it is fitted to the client, often using real ear procedures, which involve placing a small soft microphone in the ear canal along with the hearing aid to measure the frequency response of the aid in the ear canal. Probe microphone real ear procedures are used primarily for fitting verification and optimization. If the expected result of fitting is not seen on the screen of the real ear equipment, the audiologist may fine-tune the hearing aid, using the available hearing aid trimpots or return the instrument to the manufacturer for adjustment. If the aid is programmable, it will be reprogrammed by the audiologist.

The visual display of audibility targets can be used as a counseling tool to demonstrate to the client what is being accomplished. Most audiologists use real ear procedures to help determine the desired electroacoustic characteristics. The client's audiogram and other pertinent information (e.g., the client's unaided insertion gain) are entered into the equipment and one of the target formulas (e.g., NAL) is selected. The equipment will compute a target hearing aid response for the client. Detailed information about probe microphone real ear procedures can be found in the book on probe microphone measurements edited by Mueller, Hawkins, and Northern (1992). Additional information can be found in Cole (1993), Tecca (1993), and Pence, Cunningham, and Windmill (1993).

Other possible evaluation procedures include word recognition testing and/or functional gain measures. Functional gain involves comparing frequency-specific aided and unaided pure tone thresholds. Regardless of the specific procedures that are used, the client is always given the opportunity to comment on the quality and intelligibility of the hearing aid. If the fitting is not satisfactory, the hearing aid is returned to the manufacturer for adjustment.

Because BTE, eyeglass, and body-worn hearing aids do not have to be custom designed, the dispenser may perform comparative tests of different instruments in the clinic. The comparative evaluation may consist of real ear procedures, functional gain procedures, word recognition tests, subjective judgments of quality and intelligibility, or some combination of these procedures. At the end of the evaluation, a specific instrument is recommended or dispensed.

Regardless of the type of hearing aid or the specific hearing aid evaluation procedures, it is important for the client to have at least a thirty-day home trial with the instrument. During this trial period, the client receives any needed counseling and help with hearing aid adjustment. Sometimes, modifications to either the hearing aid or the earmold are made during this trial period. Proper preselection, hearing aid evaluation, and client counseling minimize returns and maximize successful hearing aid use.

Assistive Listening Devices

Although the personal hearing aid is the foundation of any auditory-based aural rehabilitation program, there are many communication situations in which its benefits are minimal. Hearing aids function poorly under conditions of noise, reverberation, distance listening, and multiple talkers. The problem is that the hearing aid microphone on the listener's head is equally distant from both noise and speech, making the hearing aid equally sensitive to both signals. Under the best of conditions, the person with sensorineural hearing loss has more difficulty separating speech from noise than the normal hearing person because of the "built-in" distortion that is part of the hearing problem (Ross 1982). Therefore, although hearing aids may be very effective for one-to-one communication in quiet, they do not separate signal from noise or compensate for distance listening at meetings, lectures, places of worship, theatres, or social situations.

Assistive listening devices (ALDs) can be very useful in these difficult communication situations. All ALDs use high-fidelity microphones held within 3 to 6 inches from the sound source (see figure 6.4). Once the speech enters the microphone, it is processed in such a way that it does not lose energy because of distance. Competing noise is generally located much farther away from the microphone than speech and reaches the listener at a significantly lower level. Some ALDs plug directly into the radio or television amplifier and deliver only the electronic signal to the listener's ear, thereby eliminating background noise.

Assistive listening systems may be used for large area amplification in auditoriums, meeting rooms, classrooms, or houses of worship. They may also be used for personal communication between individuals and for radio, television,

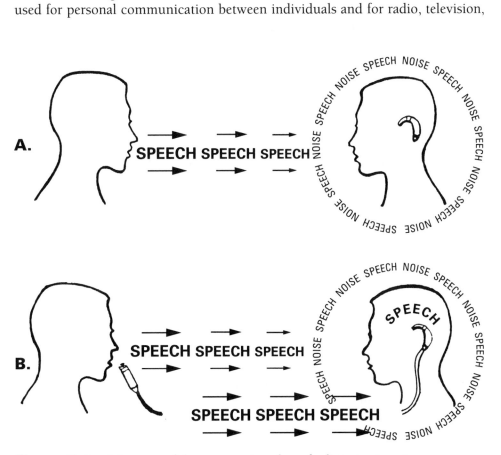

Figure 6.4. Advantage of the remote microphone for listening in noise
Source: Compton 1986.

stereo, or dictaphone listening. Hardwired and wireless technologies are available for these applications; the wireless technologies include FM, infrared, and induction loop systems.

At a lecture or meeting, the ALD user must be willing to ask the speaker to talk into the ALD microphone. During a party, family dinner, or small discussion group, the microphone needs to be passed from speaker to speaker or placed in the middle of a table if the group is small. In one-to-one communication situations, such as visits to physicians, lawyers, or religious counselors, the ALD user must ask the speaker to talk directly into the microphone. Some clients may not have the psychological strength to make such requests. They need assertiveness training and help with communication strategies to develop the ability to function well with assistive listening devices. ALDs must be considered part of a comprehensive aural rehabilitation program.

In one-to-one situations, even when noise is present, the strategy of "self-wiring" may be used as an alternative to passing a microphone. The listener attaches the ALD microphone to his or her own clothing and places himself or herself close to the speaker (Vaughn and Lightfoot 1992).

Assistive listening devices may be interfaced with personal hearing aids either by using direct audio input or a neckloop and the hearing aid telecoil (inductive coupling). The silhouette inductor is an alternative to the neckloop. It is a flat piece of plastic shaped like a behind-the-ear hearing aid and attached to a microphone or an ALD receiver; the silhouette, which contains an induction coil, is worn between the BTE hearing aid and the skull. Electromagnetic energy from the induction coil enters the telecoil of the hearing aid.

It is advantageous to use an ALD with a hearing aid because the hearing aid circuitry can optimize the frequency response of the ALD signal for the client. The hearing aid also prevents sound from exceeding the listener's uncomfortable listening level. In most cases, the hearing aid environmental microphone is available to the user when the ALD is used. It may be turned off to eliminate background noise or may be left on should the listener need to hear environmental sound as well as ALD-processed sound (e.g., comments of people other than the speaker). When the ALD and environmental microphones are functioning simultaneously, the ALD signal is generally somewhat stronger. ALDs may also be used with earphones. This makes them accessible to deaf or hard of hearing people who do not use hearing aids.

Hardwired Systems

A hardwired system (see figure 6.5) physically connects the listener to the sound source, restricting mobility to the area defined by the length of the cord. The system usually consists of a microphone, with or without an amplifier, attached to earphones by cord or to a hearing aid by direct audio input, telecoil, or silhouette inductor. When the sound source is electronic (e.g., radio or television), a plug/jack arrangement may substitute for the microphone. The plug/jack connector, however, turns off the loudspeaker unless the sound system is specially

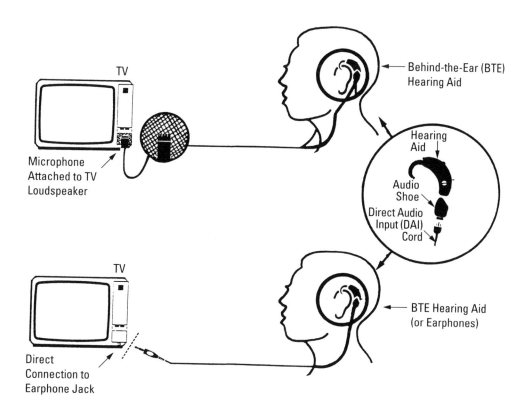

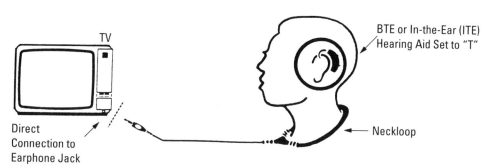

Figure 6.5. Use of remote microphone and direct connect hardwired systems with television
Source: Compton 1991.

adapted to allow the loudspeaker to remain on. Turning off the loudspeaker can be an advantage if the deaf or hard of hearing person wishes to watch television in privacy. If other people are watching, a microphone may be attached to the television loudspeaker so that others can also listen.

Hardwired systems used for personal amplification look like body-worn hearing aids with remote microphones. The microphone is connected by cord to an amplifier, which in turn is connected to an external receiver. Such systems are useful for one-to-one communication in situations where mobility is not an issue. Hardwired systems have been found useful by many hospitals, clinics, and emergency facilities for communication with people who do not use hearing aids. Many long-term care facilities have found that personal amplifiers with their large, easy-to-operate controls provide a practical alternative to the conventional hearing aid for elderly people who are physically or mentally incapable of operating hearing aids. They are self-contained, portable, and are designed with large, easily accessible controls, making them easy to use by people with visual or manual dexterity problems. The personal amplifier can also serve as a backup system to the hearing aid. Hardwired systems are inexpensive compared to personal hearing aids and other assistive listening systems.

FM Systems

Functionally, frequency modulation (FM) systems (see figure 6.6) are small radio stations. A microphone picks up the speech signal and delivers it to a transmitter via cord or radio frequency. The transmitter generates radio frequency carrier waves that transmit speech through the air to an FM receiver worn by a listener. The FM receiver removes the speech signal from the carrier wave, amplifies it,

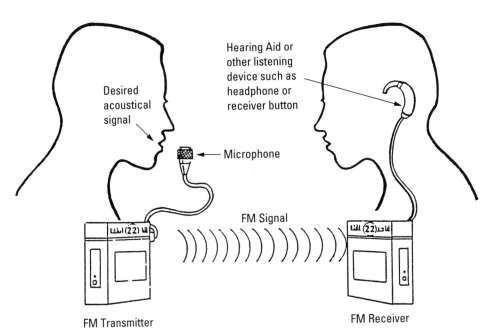

Figure 6.6. An FM system "booted" to the listener's hearing aid
Source: Compton and Brandt 1986.

and delivers it to an earphone or hearing aid. Both the transmitter and receiver are powered by batteries that may be rechargeable or disposable. The Federal Communications Commission (FCC) has allocated eight wideband and thirty-two narrowband FM channels between 72 and 76 Megahertz for communication purposes. The transmitter and receiver used for a specific communication situation must be set for the same channel.

FM systems are high-fidelity transmission systems and are very versatile in their applications. A single transmitter-receiver combination can be used by an individual for classes or other lectures (the speaker is asked to use the microphone transmitter); small group activities (the microphone is passed from speaker to speaker); one-to-one communication (using self-wiring); in the car (microphone is used by the speaker and receiver by the listener); and radio, television, or stereo listening (microphone is attached to the loudspeaker or a plug/jack arrangement is used). A special kind of FM device, called a TV Band Radio, is a portable radio that can pick up TV channels. The deaf or hard of hearing person tunes in the appropriate TV channel, uses controls on the radio to adjust the volume, and listens through attached earphones or personal hearing aid.

FM systems can be used for large area amplification by substituting a base station for the portable microphone transmitter. When used in this manner, the system usually interfaces with a public address system via a mixer. FM systems can be used indoors or outdoors. They transmit through walls, which may be desirable or undesirable, depending on the situation. Systems can be purchased with or without environmental microphones, with the capability of recording a lecture while listening to it, and with or without built-in personal amplification.

The major disadvantage of FM technology in comparison to other technologies is its cost. In addition, FM receivers are not universally compatible; they must be set to the same channel as the transmitter. Narrowband and wideband systems are not compatible. Therefore, an individual may not be able to use a personal FM receiver with a large area FM system in a local theatre unless the individual is able to tune the receiver from one channel to another. Another problem with FM is that the 72 to 76 Megahertz band is not restricted to use by deaf and hard of hearing people. Interference from other radio transmission systems, such as pagers or airport flight control systems, may occur.

Infrared Systems

Infrared technology (see figure 6.7) is similar to FM in concept but uses infrared light rays rather than radio frequencies as the carrier. The speech signal from the microphone or directly from the sound source amplifier is sent to an infrared transmitter/emitter that generates the infrared carrier. The listener wears an infrared receiver that accepts the airborne signal, removes the carrier, amplifies the speech, and delivers it to the ear via earphones, induction, or direct audio input. Infrared can be used for large area amplification, for small group situations, and for television listening at home; base stations and multiple emitters are used for

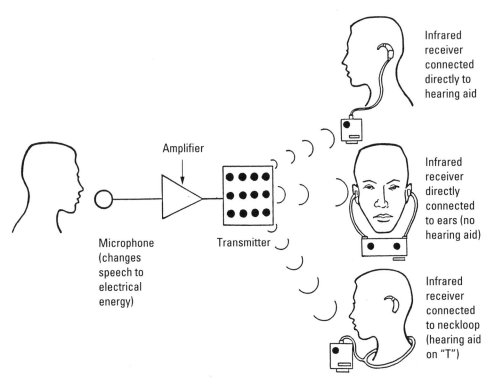

Figure 6.7. Infrared system and three ways it can input to a listener's ear
Source: Compton and Brandt 1986.

large area amplification. Receivers are portable and wearable, and may be used in most situations in which infrared transmission is available (most infrared systems transmit on a 95 KHz carrier frequency). However, unlike FM, infrared transmitters are not wearable because they must be powered by line current; therefore, infrared cannot be considered a personal amplification system.

Advantages of infrared include high-fidelity signal transmission (like FM), receivers that are not restricted to specific channels (unlike FM), and the ability to use the system with or without a hearing aid (like FM). Infrared signals will not travel through walls, thus allowing installation in adjacent rooms. Infrared is a good choice when security is an issue because speech from one room cannot be transmitted through the walls to another.

Limitations of infrared include: (1) less versatility than FM because transmitters are not wearable; (2) unsuitability for outside use because they are subject to interference from sunlight; (3) more limited signal strength than FM (therefore not suitable for profound hearing losses); (4) directional nature of infrared signals, requiring the user to face in the direction of the emitter to receive the signal clearly.

Schematic 1.

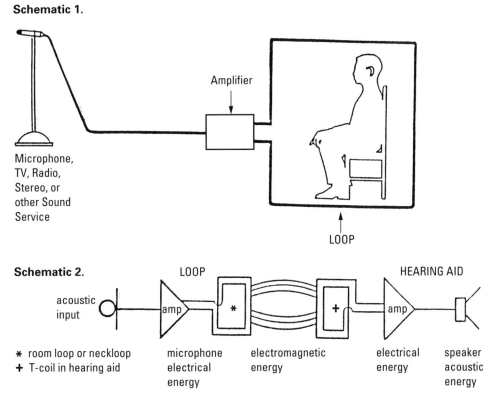

Figure 6.8. An induction loop system and how it interfaces with the telecoil of a hearing aid
Source: Compton and Brandt 1986.

Audio Loops

Amplified sound from a microphone, tape recorder, television, or other source is fed into a wire cable (loop) (see figure 6.8) encircling a room or smaller area. The amplified sound emanates from the loop in the form of electromagnetic energy. Any listener who is wearing a hearing aid containing a strong, properly function-ing telecoil and is within the loop or a specified distance outside the loop can pick up this energy. There are special pocket-size telecoil receivers and earphones for people who lack hearing aid telecoils. The neckloop described earlier in this chapter is a small version of the room loop.

The person who wishes to use a loop system must turn on the telecoil (t-switch) in the hearing aid and usually turn up the volume control, perhaps to full-on. The microphone of the hearing aid is thereby inactivated so that environ-mental noise will not be heard; only the signals entering the microphone of the loop system will be picked up by the telecoil. If it is important to be able to hear environmental sound as well as signals transmitted through the loop system, the hearing aid should be positioned on the MT setting. This activates both telecoil and microphone.

An audio loop is primarily a large area amplification system, although a small version can be used for television. It may be a permanent installation or an easy-to-install portable system. A major advantage of the induction loop for large area amplification is that it is considerably less expensive than FM or infrared. Another advantage is that special receivers are not necessary, provided listeners have hearing aid telecoils.

Spillover, a major problem with loop systems, occurs when signals from a looped area can be heard in vertically or horizontally adjacent areas by anyone listening through a hearing aid telecoil or hearing aid compatible phone. Therefore, it is not possible to loop adjacent areas in which different activities are occurring. In addition, with some loop installations, there is reduction of signal strength with distance from the loop and lack of uniformity of amplification within the loop. A new loop on the market, called the 3-D system and invented by Norman Lederman of Oval Window Audio, consists of three audio loops varying in amplitude and phase, embedded in a foam pad placed under a carpet. Testing has revealed dramatically reduced spillover effects and excellent uniformity of amplification (Gilmore 1992). The signal output from the 3-D system is maintained at a constant level within the confines of the loop (the foam pad) and attenuates rapidly outside of the loop. Measurements made at 3 feet from the 3-D loop edge revealed signal attenuation of 30 dB compared to 9 dB for a conventional induction loop. Vertical attenuation in a room directly below the 3-D system was 40 dB compared to 20 dB for a conventional loop system (Gilmore 1992).

Another problem with audio loops involves 60-cycle hum interference from fluorescent lights, transformers, and other magnetic systems. In addition, the use of loop systems in steel structures or in buildings with metal walls may result in poor transmission of signal; additional power may be required to overcome this problem.

Telecommunication Systems

Telecommunication systems include telephone amplifiers, text telephones (TTs, also called TDDs), dual party relay systems, facsimile machines, closed captioning, computer-assisted notetaking, and other computer-based systems.

Telephone Amplifiers

Telephone amplifiers are available as replacement handsets, in-line amplifiers, and portable amplifiers. In addition, two companies (Walker and Williams Sound) market telephones with amplifiers, adjustable gain controls, and low-frequency ringers built into the body of the phone. Williams Sound has two models, differing in power, that have adjustable frequency responses. The more powerful unit can connect to a personal hearing aid via direct audio input or induction.

Replacement handsets, containing built-in amplifiers and gain controls, substitute for regular handsets on modular phones. An amplified handset must be electronically matched to the telephone with which it is used to avoid distortion or loss of power. It can be used with or without a hearing aid on either the microphone or telecoil settings; it is best to use the handset with the telecoil because background noise is thereby eliminated. Some people with profound losses can use amplified handsets with hearing aid telecoils for telephone use, provided the handset is hearing aid compatible and the telecoil is strong and properly oriented.

The volume controls on some replacement handsets automatically return to zero upon completion of a call. This is a desirable feature if the telephone is also used by hearing people.

Some people with mild hearing loss may find use of the replacement handset with the hearing aid microphone (acoustic coupling) satisfactory, provided feedback is not a problem. A foam telepad or plastic coupler placed on the telephone earpiece can sometimes eliminate feedback caused by acoustic coupling. In-line amplifiers are inserted between the body and earpiece of modular telephones.

A variety of portable audio amplifiers on the market attach to the telephone earpiece. Most of these devices require hearing aid compatible phones because they function by picking up electromagnetic energy from the telephone, amplifying it, and changing it to acoustic energy. The Hearing Aid Compatibility Act of 1988 (Public Law 100-394) requires all telephones, corded and cordless, manufactured or imported for use in the United States to be hearing aid compatible. However, this legislation exempts private radio services, telephones used for security purposes, and telephones used with public mobile services; in addition, it does not require individuals to replace previously purchased noncompatible phones. Because noncompatible phones will not function with magnetically coupled amplifiers, acoustically coupled amplifiers must be used. Acoustically coupled amplifiers have built-in telecoils to add magnetic energy to the telephone signal. One such unit can be used only with a hearing aid telecoil; another—the AT&T Portable Amplifier—can be used with the naked ear or coupled to a hearing aid magnetically or acoustically. AT&T also markets an amplifier that is attached to the mouthpiece of the telephone to increase the volume of the talker's voice.

Telephone training is an important part of communication therapy. It includes selection of the optimal amplification system for use with the voice phone, listening training using telephone messages, speech production training focusing on increased speech intelligibility during telephone communication, and use of telephone strategies (e.g., spelling and code words for names). These issues will be discussed in much greater detail in chapter 12 of this book, "Telephone Communication Training."

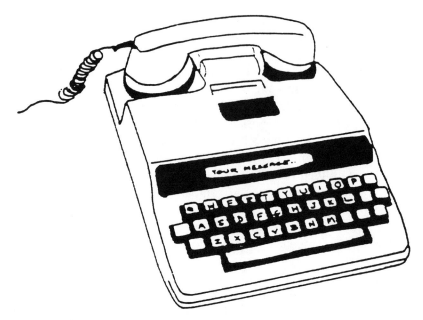

Figure 6.9. TDD with telephone receiver in the modem
Source: National Information Center on Deafness 1988.

Text Telephones (TTs), TTYs, or TDDs

Text telephones, also called telecommunication devices for the deaf (TDDs), are useful for deaf or hard of hearing people who cannot understand speech, even with a telephone amplifier. TTs can also be useful to people who cannot be understood because of speech problems.

Personal TTs are available for use in the home or office. Small portable units can be used for travel. TTs are available in most public places such as airports, train stations, and hospitals.

For TT communication, both parties must use small terminals containing keyboards and message display screens (see figure 6.9). Although most systems contain cradles (modems) in which the telephone handset is inserted, some systems attach the TT directly into the telephone line via a modular connector. After placing a call via voice telephone, the handset is placed in the modem, and the two parties communicate by typing messages to each other; these messages are transmitted over the telephone lines and appear on the message display screen.

TTs vary in complexity from simple portable versions to those containing printers, memory, large print, braille output for people who are blind, automatic redialing, answering machines, and computer compatibility. Some have speech synthesizers that announce for the benefit of hearing callers, "Hearing-impaired caller, use TDD." Prerecorded audiotapes are available for sending emergency messages via TT transmission. Costs increase with the number of features.

Dual-Party Relay Systems

Public dual-party relay systems are available in all states to facilitate communication between users of TTs and voice telephones. Title IV of the Americans with Disabilities Act (ADA) of 1990 required all telephone companies to provide intra- and interstate relay services by July 1993 (Strauss 1992). A relay system employs a specially trained operator to function as an intermediary, delivering a message received from a TT to a hearing person via voice phone and a voice message to a deaf person via TT. Most relay systems provide voice carryover, which allows a deaf person with intelligible speech to do his or her own talking.

Other visually based telephone technologies include facsimile (FAX) transmission and computers equipped with modems and software that allow transmission via telephone lines. FAX machines allow hard copy messages to be sent over telephone lines to other FAX machines, but are too slow for communication that requires turn-taking.

Real-Time Graphic Display

Closed Captioning. Closed captioning is a system that allows a person to see hidden subtitles on a television screen when the television is equipped with a special electronic decoder. The Television Decoder Circuitry Act requires decoder circuitry to be installed in all new televisions with screens thirteen inches or larger. For older televisions or those with smaller screens the viewer must purchase a special decoder that attaches to the television. Decoders are compatible with cable and allow captions to be recorded on VCRs. In addition to its use on television, captioning is used on large screens for meetings and public events such as graduations.

Computer-assisted notetaking and other systems. Computer-assisted notetaking is a simpler and less costly alternative to real-time captioning and is useful for meetings or lectures. The system requires the services of a typist who can type at least sixty words per minute accurately and can paraphrase the message as it occurs. As a speaker talks, the typist uses a standard word processing system to input the speech into the system via computer keyboard; the output is displayed on a projection screen and can be saved for later distribution as hard copy.

Other computer-based systems used primarily in business environments include electronic mail and bulletin boards. Further discussion of real-time graphic display can be found in Compton (1992), Harkins (1991), and Stuckless (1994).

Alerting Devices

Alerting and warning devices allow deaf and hard of hearing people to monitor important environmental sounds, usually in the home. These sounds include telephone ringers, doorbells, alarm clocks, smoke alarms, the voice of a person in another room, or even such sounds as kitchen timers and computer prompts.

Such systems are not limited to use by deaf people; many hard of hearing people are also unaware of important sounds when not wearing their hearing aids or when there is background noise.

Alerting devices monitor sounds with a microphone, direct electrical connection, or induction (for doorbell or telephone ringer). When the sound is picked up by the sensor, it is transmitted through line current or FM to a receiver that may be located at the sound source (e.g., alarm clock) or at some remote location. Types of alerting signals include loud and/or low-pitched sound (e.g., special telephone ringer), flashing lights, or vibrators (e.g., bed shakers or paging systems). It is also possible to use a strong fan as an alerting signal to meet special needs: for example, the need to avoid flashing lights because of seizure problems. If several sounds are monitored by a flashing light system, they can be differentiated by different flash patterns.

Portable vibratory pagers are available. Some transmit over short distances whereas others transmit over thousands of miles using telephone lines and satellite networks.

As another type of alerting "device," hearing dogs are professionally trained to alert their owners to important sounds in the home. When such sounds occur, the dog attracts the owner's attention and leads him or her to the sound. Almost all states have legislation giving hearing dogs equal status to Seeing Eye dogs. Fact sheets on hearing ear dogs can be obtained from the National Information Center on Deafness at Gallaudet University or the American Humane Association Center for Hearing Dog Information, Denver, Colorado.[1]

Selection of Appropriate Devices

Because there are many assistive devices on the market, it is important for the aural rehabilitationist to help clients select appropriate systems for their needs. Discussion of needs assessment can be found in chapter 7 of this book and in Vaughn and Lightfoot (1992); Compton (1991a); Beaulac, Pehringer, and Shough (1989); and Killingsworth (1989).

Cochlear Implants

A cochlear implant is an electronic device—part of which is worn on the body and part of which is surgically implanted in the ear—that sends electrical signals to auditory nerve fibers in the inner ear. A hearing aid, in contrast, stimulates the hair cells of the inner ear. The purpose of a cochlear implant is to provide sound

---

[1] Hearing Dog information:
American Humane Association, Center for Hearing Dog Information, 9725 East Hampden Avenue, Denver, Colorado 80231.
National Information Center on Deafness, Gallaudet University, 800 Florida Ave., N.E., Washington, D.C. 20002.

and speech information to individuals who are so profoundly deaf that they cannot benefit from hearing aids. This occurs when the hair cells are severely damaged but the auditory nerve fibers and their connections to the brain are intact. If there is a problem with the auditory nerve or its connections, the cochlear implant is of no value.

Research on single channel cochlear implants began during the 1960s with the House group in Los Angeles (House et al. 1976), Michelson at the University of California (Michelson 1971), and Simmons at Stanford (Simmons 1966). In the 1970s, research began in Europe, Asia, and Australia. Extensive discussion of the research in the United States and abroad can be found in House and Berliner (1991) and in Mecklenburg and Lehnhardt (1991).

The Nucleus 22-channel cochlear implant (Cochlear Corporation) is the system most widely used today with both children and adults in the United States. Six additional systems developed in Europe and Australia and used outside the United States are described by Mecklenburg and Lehnhardt (1991).

The most recent cochlear implant system, the Clarion, was developed at the University of California, San Francisco, and at the Research Triangle Institute of North Carolina. The Clarion has been granted Food and Drug Administration (FDA) investigational approval to undergo clinical trials at specified cochlear implant centers. Clinical research, demonstrating the safety and effectiveness of a system, is required by the FDA before the device can be approved for commercial sale. The Clarion is currently being tested with adults, eighteen years or older, who are profoundly deaf in both ears and lost their hearing after the development of speech. The unique feature of the Clarion is that it is capable of processing and coding speech in several different ways, allowing the coding system to be customized for the individual client. In contrast, all other cochlear implant speech processors permit only one type of speech coding. Further discussion of the Clarion cochlear implant can be found in Schindler and Kessler (1993) and Kessler and Schindler (1993).

The Auditory Brainstem Implant is a single channel system in which the electrode is positioned near the dorsal cochlear nucleus. It is undergoing clinical trials at the House Ear Institute and several other sites with adults who have bilateral eighth nerve problems because of tumor removal.

Description of the Cochlear Implant

Microphone Like the hearing aid, the cochlear implant uses a microphone to transduce acoustic information into electrical signals, which are then transmitted via cord to a speech processor worn somewhere on the body. The microphone is worn near the ear.

Speech Processor The speech processor looks like a body-worn hearing aid. It codes the incoming signal in such a way that frequency, intensity, and temporal information are maximally useful to the auditory nerve fibers. With most single channel implants, all the sound information is delivered to one electrode that stimulates only one site in the inner ear. Although single channel systems are not currently being implanted in the United States, many earlier-implanted children and adults are still using them.

Multichannel systems use one of two types of speech processing strategies: wideband or filterband and speech feature extraction. With both types of processing, intensity is coded as strength of current.

With wideband processing, the entire speech spectrum is presented. Filters are used to divide the incoming signal into frequency bands and sends these bands to different electrodes placed along the basilar membrane of the inner ear. The brain receives the entire signal and extracts speech features important for speech understanding.

The philosophy behind speech feature extraction is that the total speech signal is too complex for the cochlear implant to deliver effectively; better speech perception is possible when important speech features are extracted from the signal and coded explicitly by the implant. The most commonly used cochlear implant, Nucleus 22, now features a wideband processor, the Spectra 22 with the SPEAK coding strategy. Former versions of the Nucleus 22 processor used various feature-extraction processing strategies. However, recent research data (McKay et al. 1992; McKay and McDermott 1993) have shown speech perception superiority of wideband processing over feature extraction, particularly in noise. An excellent discussion of cochlear implant signal processing can be found in Wilson (1993).

The speech processor can be easily disconnected from the rest of the system, allowing a person to receive a new processor without additional surgery. The processor is powered by rechargeable or disposable batteries and has user controls (e.g., on-off switch, volume control).

Channels and Electrodes All cochlear implants must have at least one pair of electrodes because current must flow from an active electrode to a ground electrode. The word "channels" refers to the number of electrodes that can convey different stimulus information to different neurons. Although single electrode systems (one active electrode and one ground) are always single channel, with multielectrode systems it is not necessary to activate all the electrodes; therefore there may be fewer channels than electrodes. The Nucleus has twenty-two electrodes that allow for a maximum of twenty-one channels, but sometimes not all electrodes are activated because some may cause discomfort. Hochmair and Hochmair-Desoyer (1985) used a four-electrode single-channel device, selecting for each client the best available electrodes based on word recognition.

External Transmitter and Internal Receiver: Linkage The speech processor sends the coded signal to a small transmitter held against the mastoid process. The transmitter sends the signal to the internal receiver, surgically embedded beneath the scalp of the mastoid process. There are two methods of passing the stimulus from the external transmitter to the internal receiver: transcutaneous and percutaneous.

With a transcutaneous system such as the Nucleus 22, the transmitter and receiver are held in alignment by magnets in both components. The signal is transmitted across the scalp via electromagnetic induction; there is no physical connection. Signal transmission may be influenced by skin and hair thickness.

Percutaneous transmission involves a direct hard-wire plug/socket connection through the scalp. The connection can be capped to allow the user to bathe or swim. Advocates of this type of linkage feel that it allows for more flexibility in modifying processing schemes. There has been concern, however, about the susceptibility of the external plug to dirt, moisture, and mechanical damage and about the possibility of infection. At present, all cochlear implant systems use transcutaneous linkage.

Site of Stimulation Although there is continuing research with extracochlear implant systems, most currently implanted systems (e.g., Nucleus 22 and Clarion) are intracochlear. With extracochlear implants, the active electrode is usually located in the round window niche of the middle ear. The major advantage of extracochlear placement is that the electrode array does not invade the cochlea. However, intracochlear placement, in which electrodes are inserted into the cochlea through the round window, places the electrodes closer to the eighth nerve endings, allowing more effective stimulation of nerve fibers and requiring less current.

More extensive description of cochlear implant technology can be found in Patrick and Clark (1991), Eddington (1980), and Tyler and Tye-Murray (1991).

FDA Status There are two types of FDA approval: investigational and full. A new system first receives investigational status, which requires very rigid selection, evaluation, surgical, and postoperative follow-up protocols. Only approved medical teams and implant centers are permitted to perform the surgery and follow-up procedures. No marketing or commercialization of the implant is permitted.

When research has proven that the cochlear implant is safe and effective, it receives full FDA marketing approval. A system is considered effective if it does what it claims to do. The manufacturer must state its claims clearly and then demonstrate that those claims have been achieved. For example, a manufacturer may claim that the cochlear implant provides enhanced sound detection and improved audiovisual speech perception compared to hearing aids. Full FDA approval is granted if those claims are realized, even if open-set speech understanding through audition only (which has not been claimed) is not demonstrated. It is important that users of cochlear implants understand what the efficacy claims are based on.

When full FDA approval has been achieved, any qualified medical team can perform the surgery and follow-up. Less stringent candidate selection criteria, more relaxed training requirements for physicians and audiologists, and more marketing options are possible. When full FDA approval is granted, medicare and other third party payees may cover the procedure. In the United States, investigational and full market approval of systems have been granted at separate times for children and adults. At present, only the Nucleus 22 has received full market approval for both groups. The Clarion has been granted investigational approval for adults over eighteen years of age and may receive investigational approval for children shortly.

Candidacy Issues

In May 1988, a Consensus Development Conference was held at the National Institutes of Health in order to arrive at a consensus statement concerning candidate selection criteria and a number of other issues (NIH 1988). The following recommendations were made at that conference.

Audiological Criteria

1. A cochlear implant candidate should demonstrate a profound bilateral sensorineural hearing loss in excess of 95 dB in the better ear.

2. The client should receive no benefit from a hearing aid. Lack of benefit is defined as aided thresholds poorer than 60 dB, 0–4 percent on an open-set word recognition test, and no significant improvement in lipreading with a hearing aid.

   Although these criteria are generally accepted by most implant teams, research is exploring the effectiveness of the cochlear implant for people with less severe hearing losses. Some cochlear implant programs are investigating the use of implants with clients who score as high as 10 percent on the W-22 word lists. There is also research interest in combining the cochlear implant with a hearing aid in the nonimplanted ear. Clients may be considered for implants if they achieve as much as 25 percent open-set sentence identification in the better ear so long as the poorer ear has less than 10 percent word recognition (Luxford 1994). These areas of research were recommended by the 1988 Consensus Conference.

Medical Fitness

1. The cochlear implant candidate must demonstrate absence of physical or mental problems that would contraindicate surgery or interfere with ability to learn to use the device. People with developmental delay and/ or psychiatric disorders are usually not considered viable candidates. However, some clinical teams are exploring the efficacy of cochlear implants for multihandicapped individuals.

2. The potential candidate is sometimes evaluated to determine whether there is sufficient eighth nerve function for electrical stimulation to produce hearing sensations. Some groups perform a "promontory" test as the first procedure just prior to implantation. An electrode, inserted through the tympanic membrane, is placed either on the promontory or the round window niche of the middle ear; current is passed between

that electrode and a reference electrode placed somewhere outside the ear. Auditory sensations occur if neural elements are functioning. If there is no response, implantation is not continued. The promontory test, however, cannot determine the number of functioning neurons, and therefore cannot predict how well the candidate will perform with a cochlear implant. The use of the promontory test is not universal.

3. Some ear diseases, particularly meningitis, cause bony growth in the cochlea; insertion of an electrode array becomes difficult, if not impossible. Although some surgeons perform CAT scans or other radiological procedures to assess the condition of the cochlea, presence of bony growth does not always disqualify an otherwise acceptable candidate. Many surgeons have successfully implanted such individuals by drilling through the bone and inserting a shortened or sometimes complete electrode array. Further discussion of medical issues may be found in Cooper (1991), Abbas and Brown (1991), and Gray (1991).

Psychological Status In order to benefit from a cochlear implant, the client must be motivated to use it, be willing to commit to follow-up training and rehabilitation, have realistic expectations of what to expect from the implant, and be emotionally stable. Clients are generally evaluated prior to surgery, and both client and family are counselled regarding benefits and limitations of the device. Family counseling is particularly important when the implantee is a child or adolescent (defined as individuals from age two to eighteen). An older child or adolescent must be intrinsically motivated to use the device; parent motivation is not sufficient. The largest group of nonusers among individuals who have received cochlear implants are adolescents. Another factor that tends to facilitate successful use of implants is late onset of hearing loss, probably because the individual has memory for sound and considers it important. Prior successful use of amplification as occurs with progressive losses increases the probability of successful use of an implant.

Age of Implantation and Age of Onset of Deafness Much of the controversy surrounding cochlear implants relates to their use with children, which is beyond the scope of this book. The majority of cochlear implant recipients are postlingually deaf adults who have experienced normal hearing. Although prelingually deaf people have not been excluded as candidates, research has shown that they rarely achieve the open-set word recognition that some postlingually deaf adults achieve. (Berliner, Luxford, and House 1985). However, highly motivated and oral prelingually deaf adults have been implanted and have achieved improved speechreading, environmental sound identification, and in some cases, closed-set word recognition (Osberger 1990; Cohen, Hoffman, and Strosthein 1988). A second NIH Consensus Conference, held in May 1995, recommended extending cochlear implant candidacy to adults with severe hearing impairment and open-set sentence discrimination that is less than or equal to 30 percent in the best aided condition. (NIH 1995)

Training and Rehabilitation

Approximately four to six weeks after surgery, when sufficient healing has occurred, the speech processor is attached to the system, and the electrodes are programmed. Sensitivity and output at maximum comfortable level for each active electrode are determined based on client reports. These settings, called a MAP, are transferred from a large computer to the memory chip of the speech processor; the goal is to obtain low sensitivity thresholds and high comfort levels (large dynamic range) for each channel. Sometimes, not all electrodes are activated. Because threshold and comfort levels tend to vary in the first few months following initial programming, the client needs to be monitored and possibly "remapped"until the levels are stabilized.

Concurrent with or following development of the MAP, the client is started on a program of analytic and synthetic auditory training (see chapter 7 for details), audiovisual training, communication strategies, and speech and voice training if necessary. Some cochlear implant users can benefit from telephone training, including recognition of telephone signals and whatever degree of speech understanding is possible. Counseling regarding benefits and limitations of the implant should be started prior to surgery and continued as long as necessary. A number of training manuals have been developed to provide detailed guidelines and materials. *Commtram* was written by Geoffrey Plant (1984) in Sydney, Australia, to provide training for profoundly deafened adults, including those using hearing aids, cochlear implants, and tactile aids. Stout and Windle (1990) developed an auditory training curriculum for deaf and hard of hearing children called *Developmental Approach to Successful Listening (DASL)* (Stout and Windle 1990), which can also be used with adults using cochlear implants. The Cochlear Corporation has prepared *MiniSystem 22 Rehabilitation Manual* (1992), specifically for the Nucleus 22 implant with the MSP speech processor. It provides training materials graded for levels of difficulty ranging from detection to comprehension and can be used with other cochlear implant systems. In addition, many aural rehabilitation curricula developed for hearing aid users can be used for cochlear implant rehabilitation.

Roles of the Audiologist and Speech Language Pathologist

The audiologist on a cochlear implant team is responsible for diagnostic evaluation of the candidate, hearing aid evaluation, selection and fitting, and counseling of the candidate and family. Additional responsibilities may include advising the team regarding the audiological appropriateness of the candidate for implantation. Postoperative responsibilities include initial and subsequent programming of the electrodes, instructing the client in the use and care of the system, regular follow-up testing, and preparing and disseminating appropriate reports. The audiologist is also responsible for care and basic maintenance of the implant equipment.

The aural rehabilitationist, who may be either a speech-language pathologist or audiologist, performs all necessary auditory, auditory-visual, communication strategies, and speech-language training.

Risks

There are potential risks from cochlear implant surgery related to general surgery conducted under anesthesia. These risks are small for persons in good health. In addition, there is potential for infection from insertion of internal components, but the risk is quite small; should infection occur, it can be treated with anti-biotics. A branch of the facial nerve travels across the middle ear. If the nerve swells during surgery there may be temporary weakness of one side of the face. This tends to resolve itself. Temporary postoperative dizziness may occur because of stimulation of the vestibular system, but this also resolves itself. Few reports of infection or damage to the facial nerve or vestibular system have appeared in the literature (Cohen, Hoffman, and Strosthein 1988). Occasional instances of facial discomfort while using cochlear implants have been remedied by deactivating specific electrodes.

Other potential risks of cochlear implantation include tympanic membrane perforation or perilymphatic fistula at time of surgery. As with other potential risks, few reports of these problems appear in the literature, and successful surgical repair is possible for both problems. The implant user may have to avoid MRI, electrocautery, diathermy, and radiation procedures near the site of the implant.

Some critics of cochlear implants have contended that implantation should await more advanced systems. However, implants can be replaced as indicated by several reports of successful explanation and reimplantation of devices. Jackler, Leake, and McKerrow (1989) reported thirty-one cases of successful removal and reimplantation of the Nucleus 22 device. In addition, thirty-five clients are successfully using the Nucleus 22 system that they received as replacement for malfunctioning 3M single channel systems.

Benefits and Limitations

Cochlear implants do not restore normal hearing; however, a substantial number of postlingually deaf adults have achieved some open-set speech recognition on monosyllabic word or sentence tests with a multichannel implant. Despite the fact that open-set word recognition is possible for a large number of clients, the range of scores is considerable: 0–60 percent for monosyllabic words and 0–100 percent for words in sentences (Osberger 1990). According to Cohen, Waltzman, and Shapiro (1989), approximately 25 percent to 50 percent of all multichannel implant users can understand some speech on the telephone, but the degree of speech understanding varies considerably. It is important for clients to understand that not all cochlear implantees achieve high degrees of word recognition through audition alone, and there is no way to predict whether an individual will achieve a high level of auditory-only speech understanding.

Clients will benefit more from cochlear implants if they function in an auditory environment in which people use spoken language consistently and in which they are expected to speak. A client, particularly an adolescent, who is not interested in spoken language is a poor risk for a cochlear implant.

Almost all clients using multichannel implants demonstrate improved awareness and recognition of environmental sounds, enhanced speechreading, and improved voice monitoring, even if they do not achieve open-set word recognition. These are the claims made by manufacturers. The small number of prelingually deaf adults and adolescents who have received cochlear implants typically demonstrate improved sound awareness and speechreading, but generally do not achieve open-set word recognition.

Tactile Aids

A wearable tactile aid looks like a body-worn hearing aid but delivers vibrotactile or electrotactile signals to the user rather than auditory information. The device may be single or multichannel and, if the latter, may use either a wideband or feature-extraction processing strategy. Currently, a tactile aid is used to help an individual lipread or learn to lipread, given sufficient training. Perhaps in the future, more sophisticated design of systems will allow tactile-only speech recognition.

Description of a Tactile Aid

Microphone The microphone may be located within the speech processor or may be connected to it by a cord. Either way, it must be worn outside the clothing. The microphone transduces speech information into electrical signals that are delivered to the speech processor, where they are coded to be maximally useful to the client's tactile receptors.

Speech Processor With a single channel system, such as the Minifonator (Siemens Hearing Instruments), the entire electrical signal may be compressed and/or frequency transposed, then transmitted to one vibrator or electrode. Tactile receptors cannot differentiate between frequencies above 500 Hz; therefore, in order to present high frequency information, high frequencies are sometimes electronically transposed to a lower-frequency range. Although this strategy does permit awareness of high-frequency sounds, it does not provide sufficient frequency analysis for phoneme recognition.

A multichannel system involves several vibrators or electrodes placed on different skin areas, with different frequencies assigned to different locations. Two processing options are analogous to those used with cochlear implants. The wideband or spectral display (vocoder) filters the entire signal into discrete frequency bands sent to different vibrators or electrodes arrayed on the skin. Examples of vocoders are the Tactaid II+ (Franklin 1986), and the Audiotact, developed by Sevrain-Tech in 1989.

The speech-feature processing strategy extracts the fundamental frequency, and frequencies that provide vowel and consonant information. The Tactaid VII (Franklin 1991) provides outputs relating to first and second formant frequencies as well as the fundamental. The Tickle Talker uses a processing strategy similar to the Nucleus 22 cochlear implant; it extracts fundamental frequency, plus first and second formant frequencies (Blamey et al. 1988). Research has not shown superiority of either vocoder or speech-feature extraction processing strategies. Investigators have demonstrated significant improvement with long-term training with both processing systems (Lynch, Oller, and Eilers 1989; Levitt 1988).

Type and Location of Stimulation Tactile systems are available with vibrotactile (Minifonator, Tactaid II+, Tactaid VII) or electrotactile arrays (Audiotact, Tickle Talker). Electrotactile systems require less power than vibrotactile but tend to have smaller dynamic range. In addition, electrotactile stimulators may result in skin irritation because electrodes must make good contact with the skin.

Stimulators need to be placed in areas of maximum tactile receptivity and convenience of access, such as wrist, palm, sternum, fingers, and abdomen. Tactaid stimulators are placed on the wrist or sternum, the Audiotact on the abdomen, and the Tickle Talker on the fingers.

Selection Criteria

The tactile aid candidate is similar in many ways to the cochlear implant candidate. Tactile stimulation is considered when a hearing loss is so profound that a personal hearing aid is unsuccessful. Other reasons for unsuccessful use of hearing aids include auditory fatigue characterized by fading of the auditory signal, or pain, dizziness, or severe tinnitus induced by amplified sound. People experiencing these hearing aid problems may be candidates for tactile stimulation. A tactile aid can also be used with a hearing aid by clients who have some residual hearing but receive minimal benefit from amplification. Still another use for tactile aids is as a transition device for first time hearing aid users whose thresholds are in the profound range.

Tactile aids are also an option for people with profound hearing loss who are not candidates for cochlear implants for one reason or another (e.g., destruction of the eighth nerve). Unlike cochlear implants, tactile aids are not invasive and can be used on a trial basis. They are considerably less expensive than cochlear implants. The ideal tactile aid candidate is motivated to use the system on a daily basis, accepts its appearance, and is willing to master basic operation and maintenance requirements. In addition, he or she is willing to commit to a long-term training program to learn to interpret tactile information. A support network of family and friends is important.

Tactile aids can be incorporated into a cochlear implant program. Cowan et al. (1991) demonstrated that four hearing-impaired adults who did not meet selection criteria for cochlear implantation did show substantial benefit from the Tickle Talker after a period of training. Mean vowel, consonant, open-set word and sentence identification, and connected discourse tracking scores were significantly higher when the Tickle Talker was used with speechreading and/or hearing aids compared to speechreading and hearing aid alone. Sometimes a cochlear implant candidate is given a trial with a tactile aid to determine whether tactile stimulation is a viable alternative. Tactile aids can also be used to teach clients the tasks needed to program the cochlear implant after surgery. See Miyamoto, Myers, and Punch (1987) for further discussion of the tactile aid in a cochlear implant program.

Training and Rehabilitation

All individuals using tactile aids need extensive training with the device to learn to decode the vibratory or electrotactile patterns. The extent of training needed is unclear because subjects in most research studies have not plateaued in their learning curves. We know that long training times are needed and that learning continues beyond the plateaus. Training procedures and materials such as *Commtram* (Plant 1984) and DASL (Stout and Windle 1990) are similar to those used with cochlear implant recipients. The Mailman Center for Child Development at the University of Miami has developed a curriculum composed of seven tactual goal categories ranging from awareness of tactual stimulation to connected discourse tracking and generalization (Vergara et al. 1992). Tactile aid training, perhaps more than cochlear implant training, needs to focus on integration of tactile and visual input. Continuous discourse tracking is a popular procedure to achieve this type of integration (see chapter 7).

Benefits and Limitations

Research has shown that single-channel tactile aids can provide awareness and sometimes identification of environmental sounds and the prosodic features of speech (Weisenberger and Russell 1989; Weisenberger 1989). Multichannel systems can provide some phonemic information, which can result in some open- and closed-set word recognition after long-term training (Blamey et al. 1988; Cowan et al. 1988, 1989). However, the greatest amount of improvement in closed- and open-set word recognition and continuous discourse tracking occurs when tactile and visual cues are used together (Cowan et al. 1988; Blamey et al. 1988). Comparison of multichannel tactile aid and cochlear implant performance has shown little difference in closed-set tasks, but significantly higher open-set word recognition with implants than with tactile aids and speechreading together (Blamey et al. 1988; Osberger 1990). Some cochlear implant users are able to achieve open-set speech recognition through audition only but many function similarly to tactile aid users. Research evidence indicates the need for both cochlear implants and tactile aids in the rehabilitation of profoundly deaf individuals.

Conclusions

The use of technology must be considered a basic part of communication therapy for deaf and hard of hearing adults. Hearing aids are varied and sophisticated enough to benefit to some degree most people with hearing loss. Assistive listening devices can be helpful in interpersonal or group communication situations (e.g., in noise, with reverberation, or in distance listening) where hearing aids are minimally effective. Deaf people who cannot benefit from hearing aids or assistive listening devices can often be helped by cochlear implants. Deaf people who cannot or do not want to use auditory input often benefit from visual or tactile telecommunication and alerting devices or tactile aids used with visual input. Technology may be considered for all deaf and hard of hearing adults.

References

Abbas, P. J., and C. Brown. 1991. *Assessment of the auditory nerve.* In *Cochlear implants: A practical guide,* ed. H. Cooper. San Diego, Calif.: Singular Publishing Group.

Beaulac, D. A., M. S. Pehringer, and L. F. Shough. 1989. Assistive listening devices: Available options. *Assistive Devices: Seminars in Hearing* 10(1):11–30.

Bentler, R. A. 1991. Clinical implications and limitations of current noise reduction circuity. In *The Vanderbilt hearing aid report 11,* ed. G. A. Studebaker et al. Parkton, Md.: York Press.

Berkey, D. A., M. W. Marion, M. E. Robinson, and D. D. Van Vliet. 1992. New technology: Programmable hearing aids. *Seminars in Hearing* 13(2):105–188.

Berliner, K. I., W. M. Luxford, and W. F. House. 1985. Cochlear implants: 1981–1985. *American Journal of Otology* 6:173–186.

Blamey, P. J., R. S. C. Cowan, J. I. Alcantara, and G. M. Clark. 1988. Phonemic information transmitted by a multichannel electrotactile speech processor. *Journal of Speech and Hearing Research* 31:620–629.

Braida, L. D., et al. 1979. Hearing aids: A review of past research on linear amplification, amplitude compression and frequency lowering. *ASHA Monograph,* no. 19.

Brandt, F. D. 1995. Basic configuration of a hearing aid. Washington, D.C.: Gallaudet University, Department of Audiology and Speech-Language Pathology.

Bratt, G. W., and C. A. Sammeth. 1991. Clinical implications of prescriptive formulas for hearing aid selection. In *The Vanderbilt hearing-aid report 11,* ed. G. A. Studebaker et al. Parkton, Md.: York Press.

Byrne, D. 1981. Clinical issues and options in binaural hearing aid fitting. *Ear and Hearing* 2:187–193.

Byrne, D., A. Parkinson, and P. Newall. 1991. Modified hearing aid selection procedures for severe/profound hearing losses. In *Vanderbilt hearing-aid report 11,* ed. G. A. Studebaker et al. Parkton, Md.: York Press.

Causey, D., and D. Bender. 1980. Clinical studies in binaural amplification. In *Binaural Hearing and Amplification,* ed. E. Libby. Chicago: Zenetron, Inc.

Cohen, N. L., R. A. Hoffman, and M. Strosthein. 1988. Medical complications related to the Nucleus multichannel cochlear implant. *Annals of Ontology, Rhinology, and Laryngology* 97 (suppl. 135):8–13.

Cohen, N. L., S. B. Waltzman, and W. Shapiro. 1989. Telephone speech comprehension with use of the Nucleus cochlear implant. *Annals of Otology, Rhinology, and Laryngology* 98:8–11.

Cole, W. 1993. REM: A multipurpose tool for fitting, selling, and ordering. *Hearing Instruments* 44(7):9–11.

Compton, C. L. 1991a. Clinical management of assistive technology users. In *The Vanderbilt Hearing-Aid Report 11,* ed. G. A. Studebaker et al. Parkton, Md.: York Press.

———. 1991b. Use of remote microphone and direct connect hardwire systems with television. In *Assistive devices: Doorways to independence.* Annapolis, Md.: Vancomp Associates.

———. 1992. Assistive listening devices: Videotext displays. *American Journal of Audiology* 1(2):19–20.

Compton, C. L., and F. D. Brandt. 1986a. Advantage of the remote microphone for listening in noise. In *Assistive listening devices: A consumer-oriented summary.* Washington, D.C.: Gallaudet University.

———. 1986b. An induction loop system and how it interfaces with the telecoil of a hearing aid. In *Assistive listening devices: A consumer-oriented summary.* Washington, D.C.: Gallaudet University.

———. 1986c. Infrared system and three ways it can input to a listener's ear. In *Assistive listening devices: A consumer-oriented summary.* Washington, D.C.: Gallaudet University.

Compton, C. L., L. Van Middlesworth, and L. DiPietro. 1992. *All about the new generation of hearing aids.* Washington, D.C.: Gallaudet University, National Information Center on Deafness.

Cooper, H. 1991. Selection of candidates for cochlear implantation: An overview. In *Cochlear implants: A practical guide,* ed. H. Cooper. San Diego, Calif.: Singular Publishing Group.

Cowan, S.C., J. I. Alcantara, P. J. Blamey, and G. M. Clark. 1988. Preliminary evaluation of a multichannel electrotactile speech processor. *Journal of the Acoustical Society of America* 83:2328–2338.

Cowan, S. C., J. I. Alcantara, L. A. Whitford, P. J. Blamey, and G. M. Clark. 1989. Speech perception studies using a multichannel electrotactile speech processor, residual hearing, and lipreading. *Journal of the Acoustical Society of America* 85:2593–2607.

Cowan, S. C., P. J. Blamey, J. Z. Sarant, J. I. Alcantara, L. A. Whitford, and G. M. Clark. 1991. Role of a multichannel electrotactile speech processor in a cochlear implant program for profoundly hearing-impaired adults. *Ear and Hearing* 12(1):39–46.

Dermody, P., and D. Byrne. 1975. Loudness summation with binaural hearing aids. *Scandinavian Audiology* 4:23–28.

Fabry, D. A. 1991. Programmable and automatic noise reduction in existing hearing aids. In *The Vanderbilt hearing aid report 11*, ed. G. A. Studebaker et al. Parkton, Md.: York Press.

———. 1993. A clinical procedure described for evaluating compression hearing aids. *Hearing Journal* 46(11):25–30.

Fabry, D. A., and D. J. Van Tasell. 1990. Evaluation of an articulation-index-based model for predicting the effects of adaptive-frequency response hearing aids. *Journal of Speech and Hearing Research* 33:676–689.

Five types of hearing aids. 1988. In *Hearing aids: What are they?* Washington, D.C.: Gallaudet University, National Information Center on Deafness.

Franklin, D. 1986. *Tactaid II+*. Somerville, Mass.: Audiological Engineering.

———. 1988. Tactile aids: What are they? *Hearing Journal* 41(5):18–22.

———. 1991. *Tactaid VII*. Somerville, Mass.: Audiological Engineering.

Gilmore, R. A. 1991. 3-D vs. conventional induction loop assistive listening systems. Poster session presented at the American Academy of Audiology Convention, Denver, Colorado.

———. 1992. Assistive listening systems: How ASHA members fit in. *ASHA* 34:44–47.

Gray, R. 1991. Cochlear implants: The medical criteria for patient selection. In *Cochlear implants: A practical guide,* ed. H. Cooper. San Diego, Calif.: Singular Publishing Group.

Harkins, J. E. 1991. Visual devices for deaf and hard of hearing people: State of the art. *GRI Monograph Series*, series A, no. 2. Washington, D.C.: Gallaudet Research Institute.

Hawkins, D., and W. Yacullo. 1984. Signal-to-noise ratio advantage of binaural hearing aids and directional microphones under different levels of reverberation. *Journal of Speech and Hearing Disabilities* 49:278–286.

Hawkins, D. B., L. B. Beck, G. W. Bratt, D. A. Fabry, H. G. Mueller, and P. G. Stelmachowicz. 1991. Vanderbilt/VA hearing aid conference 1990 consensus statement. *ASHA* 37–38.

Hearing aid telecoil illustration (EIA 504). 1993. Washington, D.C.: Electronic Industries Association.

Hickson, L. M. H. 1994. Compression amplification in hearing aids. *American Journal of Audiology* 3(3):51–65.

Hochberg, I., A. Boothroyd, M. Weiss, and S. Hellman. 1992. Effects of noise and noise suppression on speech perception by cochlear implant users. *Ear and Hearing* 13: 263–271.

Hochmair, E. S., and I. J. Hochmair-Desoyer. 1985. Aspects of sound processing using the Vienna intra- and extracochlear implants. In *Cochlear implants,* ed. R. A. Schindler and M. M. Merzenich. New York: Raven Press.

House, W. F., and K. L. Berliner. 1991. Cochlear implants: From idea to clinical practice. In *Cochlear implants: A practical guide,* ed. H. Cooper. San Diego, Calif.: Singular Publishing Group.

House, W. F., K. L. Berliner, W. G. Crary, M. L. Graham, R. Luckey, N. Norton, H. Tobin, J. Urban, and M. Wexler. 1976. Cochlear implants. *Otolaryngology Clinicians of North America* 85 (suppl. 27).

Humes, L. E. 1991. Prescribing gain characteristics of linear hearing aids. In *The Vanderbilt hearing-aid report 11,* ed. G. A. Studebaker et al. Parkton, Md.: York Press.

Jackler, R. K., P. A. Leake, and W. S. McKerrow. 1989. Cochlear implant revision: The effects of reimplantation on the cochlea. Proceedings of the American Otological Society Meeting, San Francisco, California.

Johnson, W. A. 1993. Beyond AGC-O and AGC-I: Thoughts on a new default standard amplifier. *Hearing Journal* 46(11):43–47.

Kessler, D. K., and R. A. Schindler. 1993. Progress with a multi-strategy cochlear implant system: The Clarion. Proceedings of the Third International Cochlear Implant Conference, Innsbruck, Austria.

Killingsworth, C. A. 1989. Using assistive devices in the hearing health care practice. *Assistive Devices: Seminars in Hearing* 10(1):90–103.

Killion, M. C. 1990. A high fidelity hearing aid. *Hearing Instruments* 41(8):38–39.

———. 1993a. The K-Amp Hearing Aid: An attempt to present high fidelity for persons with impaired hearing. *American Journal of Audiology* 2(2):52–74.

———. 1993b. Transducers and acoustic couplings. In *Acoustical factors affecting hearing aid performance,* ed. G. A. Studebaker and I. Hochberg. Boston: Allyn and Bacon.

Killion, M. C., and S. Carlson. 1974. A subminiature electret-condenser microphone of new design. *Journal of the Audiological Engineering Society* 22:237–243.

Killion, M. C., and S. Fikret-Pasa. 1993. The three types of sensorineural hearing loss: Loudness and intelligibility considerations. *Hearing Journal* 46(11):31–36.

Killion, M. C., and E. Villchur. 1993. Kessler was right—partly: But SIN Test shows some aids improve hearing in noise. *Hearing Journal* 46(9):31–34.

Letowski, T. R. 1993. Nonlinear signal processing: Classification of amplitude-compression systems. *Hearing Journal* 46(11):13–18.

Levitt, H. 1988. Recurrent issues underlying the development of tactile sensory aids. *Ear and Hearing* 9(6):301–305.

Luxford, W. M. 1994. Who is a good candidate for a cochlear implant? *SHHH Journal* 15(1):12–13.

Lynch, M. P., D. K. Oller, and R. E. Eilers. 1989. Portable tactile aids for speech perception. *Volta Review* 91(5):113–126.

Madison, R., and D. Hawkins. 1983. The signal-to-noise ratio advantage of directional microphones. *Hearing Instruments* 34(2):18.

McKay, C. M., and H. J. McDermott. 1993. Perceptual performance of subjects with cochlear implants using the Spectral Maxima Sound Processor (SMSP) and the Mini Speech Processor (MSP). *Ear and Hearing* 14:350–367.

McKay, C. M., H. J. McDermott, A. E. Vandali, and G. M. Clark. 1992. A comparison of speech perception of cochlear implantees using the Spectral Maxima Sound Processor (SMSP) and the MSP (MULTIPEAK) Processor. *Acta Otolaryngolica* 112:752–61.

Mecklenburg, D., and E. Lehnhardt. 1991. Development of cochlear implants in Europe, Asia, and Australia. In *Cochlear implants: A practical guide,* ed. H. Cooper. San Diego, Calif.: Singular Publishing Group.

Michelson, R. P. 1971. Electrical stimulation of the human cochlea. *Archives of Otolaryngology* 93:317–323.

MiniSystem 22 rehabilitation manual. 1992. Englewood, Colo.: Cochlear Corp.

Miyamoto, R. T., W. A. Myres, and J. L. Punch. 1987. Tactile aids in the evaluation procedure for cochlear implant candidacy. *Hearing Instruments* 38(2):33–37.

Mueller, H. 1981. Directional microphone hearing aids: A ten-year report. *Hearing Instruments* 32(11):18–20, 66.

———. 1994. Update on programmable hearing aids. *Hearing Journal* 47(5):13–20.

Mueller, H., and A. Grimes. 1987. Amplification systems for the hearing impaired. In *Rehabilitative audiology: Children and adults,* ed. J. G. Alpiner and P. McCarthy. Baltimore: Williams & Wilkins.

Mueller, H., A. Grimes, and S. Erdman. 1983. Subjective ratings of directional amplification. *Hearing Instruments* 34(2):14.

Mueller, H., D. Hawkins, and R. Sedge. 1984. Three important options in hearing aid selection. *Hearing Instruments* 35(11):14.

Mueller, H., D. B. Hawkins, and J. L. Northern. 1992. *Probe microphone measurements.* San Diego, Calif.: Singular Publishing Group.

Nabelek, A., and D. Mason. 1981. Effects of noise and reverberation on binaural and monaural word identification by subjects with various audiograms. *Journal of Speech and Hearing Research* 24:375–383.

NIH. 1988. NIH Consensus Development Conference Statement: Cochlear Implants, 2–4 May, NIH Conference, Bethesda, Maryland.

————. 1995. NIH Consensus Development Conference Statement: Cochlear Implants in Adults and Children, 15–17 May, NIH Conference, Bethesda, Maryland.

Olsen, W. O. 1986. Physical characteristics of hearing aids. In *Hearing aid assessment and use in audiologic habilitation*, 3rd ed., ed. W. R. Hodgson. Baltimore: Williams & Wilkins.

Osberger, M. J. 1990. Audiological rehabilitation with cochlear implants and tactile aids. *ASHA* 32(4):38–43.

Patrick, J. F., and G. M. Clark. 1991. The Nucleus 22-Channel Cochlear Implant System. *Ear and Hearing* 12(4) (suppl.): 3S–9S.

Pence, P., D. R. Cunningham, and I. M. Windmill. 1993. Objectivity vs. subjectivity: Does REM improve the fit? *Hearing Instruments* 44(7):16–17.

Plant, G. 1984. *Commtram: A communication training program for profoundly deafened adults*. Sidney, Australia: National Acoustic Laboratories.

Ross, M. 1982. Communication access for the hearing impaired. *Hearing Instruments* 33(1):7–9.

Schindler, R. A., and D. K. Kessler. 1993. Clarion Cochlear Implant: Phase 1 investigational results. *American Journal of Otology* 14(3):263–272.

Simmons, R. B. 1966. Electrical stimulation of the auditory nerve in man. *Archives of Otolaryngology* 84:24–76.

Stout, G. G., and J. Windle. 1990. *The developmental approach to successful listening*. Houston, Tex.: Houston Oral School for the Deaf.

Strauss, K. P. 1992. Nationwide relay services. *ASHA* 34:48–49.

Stuckless, E. R. 1994. Developments in real-time speech-to-text communication for people with impaired hearing. In *Communication access for persons with hearing loss*, ed. M. Ross. Baltimore, Md.: York Press.

Stypulkowski, P. H. 1993. Advances in technology necessitate new terms and specifications. *Hearing Journal* 46(11):19–24.

TDD with telephone receiver in the modem. 1988. Washington, D.C.: Gallaudet University, National Information Center on Deafness.

Tecca, J. E. 1993. Two ways you can use REM to verify hearing aid performance. *Hearing Instruments* 44(7):12–15.

Tyler, R. S., and N. Tye-Murray. 1991. Cochlear implant signal-processing strategies and patient perception of speech and environmental sounds. In *Cochlear implants: A practical guide,* ed. H. Cooper. San Diego, Calif.: Singular Publishing Group.

Vaughn, G. R., and R. K. Lightfoot. 1992. Assistive listening devices and systems for adults with hearing impairments. In *Aural Rehabilitation,* ed. R. Hull. San Diego, Calif.: Singular Publishing Group.

Vergara, K. C., L. W. Miskiel, D. K. Oller, R. Eilers, and T. Balkany. 1992. Hierarchy of goals and objectives for Tactual Vocoder training with hearing-impaired children. Proceedings of the Second International Conference on Tactile Aids, Hearing Aids, and Cochlear Implants, Stockholm, Sweden.

Weisenberger, J. 1989. Tactile aids for speech perception and production by hearing-impaired people. *Volta Review* 91(5):79–100.

Weisenberger, J., and A. F. Russell. 1989. Comparison of two single-channel vibrotactile aids for the hearing-impaired. *Journal of Speech and Hearing Research* 32:83–92.

Wilson, B. S. 1993. Signal processing. In *Cochlear implants: audiological foundations,* ed. R. S. Tyler. San Diego, Calif.: Singular Publishing Group.

PART

3

Communication
Skill Areas

Introduction

Each chapter in this section will discuss a different skill area. Included in each chapter will be a review of formal and informal assessments, followed by a discussion on therapy strategies. Client-centered decision making based on each individual's assets, aspirations, and environment will be discussed in relation to each of the skill areas. Examples of integrating each skill area with others in this section will be prevalent throughout these chapters. Chapters 7 and 8 focus on receptive skills; chapters 9 and 10 emphasize expressive skills; and the chapter on language, chapter 11, discusses both receptive and expressive areas.

Auditory skills are discussed in chapter 7. Redinger proposes a broad focus to training auditory skills and emphasizes the importance of technology in working with culturally Deaf adults and adolescents.

Chapter 8 reviews speechreading, with emphasis on analytic and synthetic methods. Kaplan discusses the application of speechreading skills to other skill areas and to the integrated therapy approach.

Mahshie and Allen, in chapter 9, discuss articulation and voice therapy, with specific emphasis on culturally Deaf individuals. They pro-

vide guidelines and suggestions for evaluation and therapy within the framework of the integrated communication model.

Chapter 10 presents information on pronunciation skills, an area many deaf and hard of hearing individuals choose to work on. Bally presents guidelines for assessing pronunciation and strategies for therapy in an integrated setting.

Chapter 11 presents information on teaching language skills, with specific emphasis on vocabulary, figurative language, written language, and pragmatics. Nichols and Moseley discuss refinement of these skills, with particular emphasis on a classroom setting with Deaf adolescents.

7

Auditory Skills

Bobbi Redinger

■　■　■　■

Starting with Paleolithic man and the initial utterance for the purpose of communication, there has been some form of "auditory training." Auditory training can encompass everything from refinement of vocal patterns early in life to the intense training sometimes needed to benefit from a tactile aid. In 1961, Carhart called auditory training "taking full advantage of sound cues" (Chermak 1981, 146); Durity (1982) defined it as "maximiz[ing] use of residual hearing for greater participation in the auditory environment" (296). As far back as 1894, Mabel Hubbard Bell, wife of Alexander Graham Bell, strongly favored the use of synthetic auditory training over analytic training (Hartbauer 1975). Strong advocates exist today for specific methods of auditory training.

The goal of this chapter is to expand traditional auditory training methods to include therapy options appropriate for culturally Deaf adults as well as deafened and hard of hearing individuals. This chapter starts with a brief historical review of traditional auditory training methods. These methods are familiar and have numerous references; therefore, they will only be summarized here. Next, the evaluation and development of auditory perceptual skills will be explored, followed by a discussion of different types of technology available to enhance auditory signals for communication. Finally, rehabilitation models incorporating hearing aids, assistive devices, cochlear implants, and tactile aids will be presented using the Integrated Therapy Model. The emphasis of this book is to provide another perspective of therapy—therapy that can be used with persons who have all types of hearing loss and who use all modes of communication.

History of Auditory Training

From the time of the pioneers in audiology, there has been an accepted definition of auditory training: to teach the hearing-impaired person the most effective use of their residual hearing (Newby 1964). Carhart (1947) was one of the first in the field of audiology to propose a systematic approach to auditory training in children. His program had four stages: Sound Awareness, Gross Discrimination, Broad Discrimination, and Fine Discrimination. In 1966, Hirsch also identified four stages: (1) Detection, awareness of the presence or absence of sound; (2) Discrimination, determining a same/difference relationship between two sounds; (3) Identification, where sound is labeled; and (4) Comprehension, where sound meaning is derived (Van Tasell 1981). Despite the nearly twenty years difference, the similarities between Hirsch's and Carhart's stages are striking. Both seem to suggest that the purpose of auditory training stages is to break down the listening/communication process for analysis and remediation. Thirty-some years after Carhart's introduction of his auditory training stages, Erber (1982) used these same stages as a basis for his auditory skills training course.

These well-established stages of auditory training programs may, however, exclude some populations of persons with hearing loss. Thus, the advent of new technology now allows these populations, previously not candidates for auditory training, to manipulate sound to their communicative advantage. The traditional definition of auditory training has now become much broader than Durity's definition of "maximizing residual hearing." The goal is to enhance communication, whether through acoustic signals or through technology. Kelly (1973) explains that listening takes place in two stages: the conveyance of an acoustic signal to the receiving station (the ear) and the recognition and interpretation of that signal by the brain. For people who cannot use their auditory systems, the reception of that acoustic signal may be intercepted and transduced for use by the visual or tactile sensory systems. Thus auditory training may maximize residual hearing as well as train individuals to use devices that translate acoustic signals for reception by an alternative sensory system, such as an alerting system for the telephone. Therefore, an inclusive definition of auditory training is proposed:

> Auditory training is the process by which the individual learns to optimize communication by using technology that can (1) receive clues intended for the auditory system and (2) deliver the information in an enhanced way to the auditory system or (3) modify the acoustic signal and deliver the information to an alternative sensory system.

The above definition will be used in this chapter to denote training for both those who use residual hearing for communication and those who use technology in order to be connected to the auditory world. The unique qualities of each client will directly impact the decision about appropriateness of auditory training and integrated therapy. Qualities that will have a direct impact on auditory skill development and use of alternative technologies include the degree, configuration, and etiology of the hearing loss; residual hearing capabilities; age of onset and amplification; preferred mode of communication; and the client's sociocultural environment.

Assessment of Auditory Skills

The basis for any auditory training, be it in the use of hearing aids or an assistive alerting device, is an accurate assessment of the person's auditory skills. It is essential that clinicians continue to expand their pool of test materials to include relevant, accurate assessment tools. As part of the overall evaluation process, the client's self-assessment is important to consider for successful implementation of integrated therapy. Currently, the typical auditory assessment includes pure tone audiometry, immittance, and word recognition tests. For culturally Deaf individuals, some test procedures will need to be adapted or enhanced to assess their auditory skills. Because many references exist on auditory skill assessment (Katz 1994; F. N. Martin 1981; Newby and Popelka 1985; Rintelmann 1991), only brief summaries will appear here along with adaptations for use with culturally Deaf adults.

Pure Tone and Immittance Testing

Measurement of auditory acuity through a pure tone test is valuable information in that it provides threshold values for specific frequencies for each ear. This information is useful for quantifying the degree and configuration of the hearing loss. By the time a person with a congenital hearing loss reaches adulthood, it is likely that he or she has endured numerous hearing tests, possibly hundreds. It is important to engage this adult in the testing process—to explain the purpose of each step and, ultimately, to show why sequential audiograms are useful in documenting and tracking a hearing loss.

Similarly, immittance testing provides objective information about the integrity of the middle ear. This information along with the pure tone threshold results provides etiologic clues toward diagnosis of the hearing loss.

Word Discrimination Testing

Information about the client's understanding of monosyllabic words in quiet and noise is obtained using word discrimination materials. However, the value of percentage correct scores from monosyllabic word lists is limited, and completion of these tests may not be possible for some people with severe or profound hearing losses. Martin and Morris (1989), reporting on current audiological practices in the United States, tallied the responses of 468 certified, practicing audiologists.

They reported that 91 percent of audiologists assess speech discrimination using monosyllabic word lists, presented by monitored live voice. Phonetically balanced word lists, the bases for monosyllabic word lists used in clinical practice, were initially developed for use in communication systems during World War II (American National Standard Institute 1989). Henoch (1991) points out that, although audiologists are not in the business of evaluating radio and telephone communication systems, they *are* in the business of assessing how a person with a hearing loss will perceive speech in a variety of environments given the degree of hearing loss in both ears. These word discrimination tests do not take into account the fact that two individuals with the same audiogram and word recognition scores may function differently and need different rehabilitative services. Yet, McCarthy and Culpepper (1987) note that, regardless of the benefit to the client, rehabilitation determinations are often made on the basis of these percentage scores along with the pure tone audiogram. Assessment of the client's auditory perception skills may be more appropriate in determining the direction of rehabilitation.

Auditory Perceptual Testing

Auditory perceptual skills may include speech discrimination as well as functional listening skills. One of the first batteries that addresses the assessment of functional skills of deaf and hard of hearing individuals is the Minimal Auditory Capabilities (MAC) Battery (Owens et al. 1985). Initially developed for use with postlingually deaf adults, who are candidates for cochlear implants, the MAC Battery has also been used to evaluate the speech perception abilities in prelingually deaf adults. The MAC Battery was originally designed to give a comprehensive picture of the client's speech reception abilities. It consists of fourteen subtests ranging from the discernment of intonation patterns of speech to the recognition of words in sentences. Each subtest is included in the battery because it assesses a different feature or parameter of speech. Fifer, Stach, and Jerger (1984) compared the MAC Battery scores of pre- and postlingually deaf adults and concluded that the degree of hearing loss, not the age of onset, determined scores on the MAC Battery. The authors also state that parts of the MAC Battery can be used in hearing aid selection procedures for persons with severe to profound hearing losses.

Another tool for assessing auditory skills with adults is the Test of Auditory Comprehension (TAC) (Trammell and Owens 1977). The TAC was originally designed to investigate the speech reception skills of young children on a linguistic rather than phonetic level. The TAC provides information about the hierarchical auditory skills such as the ability to discriminate between linguistic and nonlinguistic sound, word identification, comprehension of speech phrases varying in complexity, comprehension of stories in quiet, and comprehension of stories against competition. The TAC provides a scaled profile meant to determine where young children fall on an auditory skill development continuum.

Finally, the Monosyllable, Trochee, Spondee Test (MTS) provides information about the client's ability to identify words in a closed-set format. The MTS scoring scheme evaluates not only identification skills but pattern perception (monosyllable versus multiple syllables) and stress pattern perception (trochees versus spondees) (Erber and Alencewicz 1976).

Considerations for Testing Multicultural Populations

The TAC is a viable alternative to word recognition tests for some adults, especially those with limited previous use of auditory skills, those who may have low English language levels, or those who cannot complete most of the MAC Battery. The first two subtests of the TAC can be completed without use or knowledge of English. These two subtests provide information about discrimination skills of suprasegmentals. This information, although limited, is more helpful to the audiologist in determining functional hearing abilities than any 0 percent score obtained on a speech discrimination test. The information obtained using these first two subtests can be helpful in determining realistic expectations of amplification for the individual and can help establish auditory training goals within integrated therapy. Thus, although not designed or normed for these adult populations, the TAC assists in determining where such adult clients fall on the English auditory skill development continuum.

For those clients who can perform speech discrimination tests, standardized materials for non-English speaking or multicultural deaf adults are not readily available in mainstream audiological settings. McCullough, Wilson, Birck, and Anderson (1994) use new technology to assess the client's functional auditory skills. The Spanish Word Identification Test (McCullough et al. 1994) is a picture-pointing, computer-controlled multimedia test developed from the Picture Identification Task (PIT) (Wilson and Antablin 1980). The audiologist uses an audiometer connected to a computer to present words for identification, and pictures appear on a computer monitor in front of the client as a four-picture selection paradigm. The target word is pictured with three rhyming alternatives. The client simply points to the picture to identify the digitally recorded word presented through the audiometer. Use of picture pointing for identification does not require the audiologist to be fluent in a variety of languages. The audiologist scores the picture-pointing test by knowing the correct response pattern. These tests make the audiologist more effective within an increasingly diverse society by providing tools for use with a wider range of clients. This test format is a prototype for word identification tasks in a variety of languages: currently materials are being developed in Arabic, Russian, Mandarin, Cantonese, and Tagalog. Psychometric functions for the Spanish Word Identification Test are being established (McCullough et al. 1994). These tests provide speech understanding materials in the form of an identification task. The next area of test development is in evaluating the client's discrimination skills in linguistic contexts such as sentences or paragraphs. The presentation of visual cues for the assessment of speechreading skills can also be useful information in determining auditory training skills in integrated therapy.

Less sophisticated adaptations of speech materials may include the use of a modified Ling 5 Sound Test (Ling 1976), repetition of digits, and same/different tasks in the client's native language. Informal assessments using interpreters or family members can help the clinician obtain information about the use of visual cues in speech understanding. Although the information from these adaptations is limited, it can provide preliminary information for the development of therapy goals for some multicultural clients. Knowledge of simple adaptations to speech assessment materials will allow the audiologist to evaluate more effectively the abilities of a particular client and the benefits derived from amplification and auditory training.

It is clear that more research is necessary, and more test materials that are culturally and linguistically appropriate must be made available to the audiologist in order to assess accurately the total auditory capabilities of the client. In light of world mobility, cultures continue to meld, so therapy approaches must change to meet these needs. If the goal of integrated therapy is to benefit the whole person, factors that impact that person must be part of the overall therapy plan.

Summary of Auditory Skill Assessment

A comprehensive assessment protocol that includes pure tone, immittance, and functional auditory testing allows a complete communicative picture of the individual. Results from auditory skill assessments are the basis for selecting an amplification configuration. Auditory perceptual skill results provide information about the functional communication skills of the client. If these tests are conducted in conjunction with visual cues, additional information will be available about the client's speechreading skills and communication strategies, and the results will be used in negotiation process in determining goals for integrated therapy.

Cochlear Implant and Tactile Aid Assessment

In addition to auditory-perceptual skill evaluation, further assessments may be necessary for alternative rehabilitation methods. The assessment protocols for cochlear implants and tactile aids are very similar; however, they result in different rehabilitation paths.

Cochlear Implant Assessment

In 1957, Djourno and Eyries implanted an electrode into a deaf patient's cochlea, thus starting one of the most researched and controversial areas of auditory rehabilitation: cochlear implants (Lancet 1988). This topic has created great differences of opinion, which may not allow an open discussion of the use and benefit of cochlear implants for some people in today's society. Some of the greatest differences in opinion come from within the research and medical communities, and some differences stem from the lack of clear, standardized criteria for cochlear implantation and assessment batteries for determination of cochlear implant candidacy.

A general criterion for many cochlear implant programs is a statement similar to the following: the person must have a profound, bilateral, sensorineural hearing loss and demonstrate no benefit from hearing aids. However, many implant teams do not agree on what "benefit from hearing aids" means. The team may ask questions such as "How is hearing aid benefit determined and measured? Is it aid to speechreading? Or is it awareness of environmental sounds?" Often, cochlear implant teams compare the benefit from a hearing aid with the proposed benefit from a cochlear implant by measuring the aided soundfield results of the two devices. This information may not be enough to make a decision about rehabilitation options. King (1991) states that some assessment protocols for a cochlear implant is a process of "who qualifies" rather than "what treatment do they need." Whatever decision is made, however, if a person is going to enter into evaluation for a cochlear implant, he or she should have tried or have knowledge of standard alternative treatments such as hearing aids, sensory aids (tactile), and/or signal processing hearing aids. Information about technology, such as assistive alerting systems and telecommunication equipment, should be part of any cochlear implant assessment program. A comprehensive assessment process must include not only assessment of auditory skills and hearing aid trials, but also evaluation of the status of the auditory nerve, other medical criteria, and psychological variables.

The critical elements of an accurate, comprehensive, and relatively time efficient test battery includes assessing a range of speech perception skills, including intonation, syllable number, segmental abilities, and open-set recognition. The purpose of each of the tests listed in table 7.1 is to assess these parameters in some way. Kessler (1993) states that most cochlear implant teams use part of the MAC Battery, but few use all of it. King (1991) proposes a hierarchical test protocol ranging from identification of syllable number and stressed syllables in words in a closed-set format to word recognition in sentences and discourse tracking skills. Research continues to develop standardized, taped versions of a comprehensive assessment battery. Auditory skills tests are used in combination with other auditory, medical, psychological, and speech-and-language assessments to determine candidacy for the cochlear implant.

In addition to information derived from appropriate formal assessment tools, decisions about the implanting of pre- and postlingually deaf individuals should be based on thorough information in two other major areas: medical/audiological and social/cultural considerations. Medically and audiologically, there is virtual agreement among related professions regarding the use of cochlear

Table 7.1 Standard Test Batteries to Evaluate Cochlear Implants

Test Name	Authors
Minimal Auditory Capabilities (MAC)	Owens et al. (1981)
Speech Pattern Contrast Test (SPAC)	Boothroyd (1986)
Iowa Test Battery	Tyler, Tye-Murray (1988)
HIPPS Profile	Cooper et al. (1990)
NAL Lipreading Test	Plant and Macrae (1987)
Sound Pattern Test	King (1987)
5 Linguistic Level Profile	Risberg and Agelfors (1986)

Source: Cooper 1991.

implants by postlingually deaf adults and adolescents, assuming that the candidate meets all preimplant criteria (Luxford 1989). However, controversy stems from the implantation of prelingually deaf adults or adolescents. Tyler and Lowden (1992) look at two concerns when considering implant candidates: (1) the individual's previous exposure to speech and language through audition and (2) the individual's benefit from hearing aids. They argue that postlingually deafened adolescents and adults remember speech sounds and are motivated to regain the use of that sense, but that "pre-lingually deafened individuals have no memory for speech" (Tyler and Lowden 1992, 119). For those individuals, the cochlear implant may provide sound awareness and some identification of environmental sounds, but there is a limited potential for word understanding. These authors admit that they rarely implant prelingually deafened individuals for precisely this reason.

Owens, Kessler, Raggio, and Schubert (1985) state that although prelingually deaf adults may not benefit from hearing aids, the cochlear implant may provide them with a choice they never had before. Cooper (1991a) reports that "the provision of a cochlear implant to congenitally deaf older children and teenagers has generally been found to give a very poor outcome and high incidence of non-use" (95). Cooper attributes the outcome to lack of motivation to use sound and to peer pressure. Menapace (1992) reiterates the high non-user rates of prelingually deaf individuals who receive cochlear implants. She reports one case of a highly motivated prelingually deaf adult who went through two years of preimplant therapy. After the implant, the individual was able to achieve limited word recognition in a closed-set format before the speech processor of the implant unit was stolen. The individual decided not to replace the speech processor because, upon reflection, the device did not meet her expectations, and aural rehabilitation for this client took a different course.

Social and cultural perspectives may contribute to the success of cochlear implants in adults. For example, in a study done with six prelingually deaf adults, Clark, Busby, Roberts, Dowell, Blamey, Mecklenberg, Webb, Pyman, and Franz (1987) list educational choice as one indicator of consistent postimplant use. Deaf individuals who were educated using an oral/aural method were more motivated to use the implant and participate in the postimplant rehabilitation training required for benefit from the implant. Clark et al. (1987) report on two clients who used sign language as their primary mode of communication. They recount that these clients were less motivated during auditory training. The authors state that the clients' auditory receptive language was poor, making communication with them difficult. In the Clark study, the implantation and rehabilitation process that followed may have tried to change the clients' method of communication from a manual language to an oral/aural language. Social and cultural pressures may have separated the clients from their friends and families, causing their resistance to continued rehabilitation.

It is evident that the criteria for candidacy for cochlear implants must include not only new, relevant speech-understanding tests, but social and cultural considerations as well. These considerations are especially valuable during the rehabilitation negotiation process. Keeping social, cultural, medical, and audiological factors in mind allows the clinician and client to discuss openly all rehabilitation options. Cochlear implants may continue to be controversial, but with these factors for consideration, more people will benefit from appropriate rehabilitation.

Tactile Aids Assessment

Assessment criteria for tactile aids are very similar to those of cochlear implants. A selection process for tactile aids at National Acoustics Laboratories (NAL) in Australia looks at audiometric thresholds, speech discrimination and lipreading scores, aided versus unaided results, and subjective responses from the adult users and their significant others (Plant 1992). M. C. Martin (1992) states that research into the assessment and use of tactile aids by adults does not have the high profile that cochlear stimulation research has. This low profile may add to the perception that these devices may be less than optimal for adult aural rehabilitation. However, tactile aids may provide considerable benefit to profoundly deaf individuals, many of whom may not have the benefit of the use of cochlear implants or hearing aids.

Comparison of Cochlear Implants and Tactile Aids

The assessment process of cochlear implants and tactile aids must include a discussion or comparison of alternative types of technology. Rihkanen (1990) compared typical audiological test results and questionnaire responses of three groups of postlingually deaf adults who had been using hearing aids, cochlear implants, or vibrotactile aids for a period of two years. Although the audiological test results were similar for all three types of technology, better discourse tracking skills were obtained by hearing aid and cochlear implant users. The subjective responses about their devices were the most positive for the cochlear implant group and their families; this did not, however, correlate to significant improvements in audiological test results when compared to the results based on the use of other types of technology. The author of the study speculates that this positive subjective response result may be due to the dedication of the cochlear implant users to their choice of technology, rather than to measurable auditory benefits. Blamey and Cohen (1992) look at the benefit and cost effectiveness of tactile aids as compared to cochlear implants. Table 7.2 contains a summary of their findings.

Table 7.2 illustrates the positive and negative issues associated with cochlear implants and tactile aids for different groups of adults. The use of cochlear implants with postlingually deaf adults has the advantage of using the adults' well-established knowledge of sound for rehabilitation. Although a cochlear implant may not be appropriate for an adult with severe hearing loss, it would make use of the adult's listening skills. A tactile device may give aid to visual information for this population, but the amount of training is extensive and most probably prohibitive. Lastly, for prelingually deaf adults, the benefit of using a tactile device on an unimpaired tactile system, as opposed to using a cochlear implant used on an auditory system with limited listening skills, makes the tactile device more attractive.

As assessment procedures for cochlear implants and tactile aids continue to develop and be refined, the controversies about these alternative technologies will also continue. Determining the appropriateness of rehabilitation and benefit from a device can be done only when options are available to the client. When the client is engaged in the decision-making process with the clinician, meaningful and relevant therapy will occur.

The need for auditory training becomes clear when the results from the assessment materials indicate potential benefit from the training and when the client is committed to auditory training. The use of cochlear implants and tactile aids may require intensive training to use effectively the information provided by these devices (Gagne et al. 1991).

Rehabilitation

Appropriate rehabilitation depends on a thorough understanding by the client and the clinician of the client's auditory reception abilities. This section will discuss the selection of an appropriate device (hearing aid, cochlear implant, assistive device, or tactile aid), orientation to that device, and counseling about realistic expectations, and the place of an auditory training program in integrated therapy. Information on traditional approaches in each of the following areas is available from several sources to the reader. Specific emphasis will be given to rehabilitation options for culturally Deaf adults.

Hearing Aids and Rehabilitation

Hearing aids are one of the most widely accepted rehabilitation devices in use. However, as discussed in chapter 1, some populations have a predisposition against hearing aid use. Respect, culturally appropriate materials, and frank discussions about what the hearing aids can and cannot do, are essential in working with individuals on integrated therapy goals.

Rapport Building Sanders (1988) outlines a hearing aid orientation program that starts with rapport building. He asserts that the hearing aid orientation goes beyond the technological expertise of the clinician; the clients' emotional needs, not just their audiological needs, must be met during the therapeutic process. Sanders refers to three important axioms of good counseling skills: accurate empathy, unconditional positive regard, and genuineness. Meeting emotional needs means facilitating solutions by working in partnership with the client. The first step in this process, as explained by Sanders, is to build rapport for a trusting relationship by simply explaining the client's audiogram in terms and language that she understands and in light of her cultural perspective. Explanation of the audiogram will help the client understand her hearing loss, how and why a hearing aid is recommended, and how communication is affected. This simple process builds trust because both the client and clinician are defining the problem and looking for solutions. As Sanders states, the goal is to form a team approach to rehabilitation: the clinician does not know everything. Professionals should listen and learn from their clients. For example, a client who has tried hearing aids before should be encouraged to share with the clinician the perceived shortcomings of the hearing aids. Together, the clinician and client can then search for solutions or alternatives.

Some culturally Deaf adults, working in conjunction with an audiologist, may explore the use of hearing aids. Amplification is an option relatively inexpensive to try that can provide valuable information to the client and the clinician. High motivation and realistic expectations are essential going into the trial period. Many Deaf adults may be hesitant to try amplification because of bad experiences in the past with improperly fit hearing aids. With the new hearing aid technology and advances in fitting practices, proper amplification for a person with a severe to profound hearing loss is easier to obtain.

Selection and Fitting The client/clinician partnership allows a new approach to the selection and fitting of hearing aids. This new approach may incorporate Henoch's (1991) three goals for hearing aid fitting: (1) improvement of audibility and intelligibility of speech while preserving acceptable quality; (2) improvement

Table 7.2 Comparisons between Tactile Aids and Cochlear Implants for Different Population Groups

Hearing Acuity	Tactile Aids		Cochlear Implants	
	Positives	Negatives	Positives	Negatives
Postlingually Deaf adults	Type of hearing loss may not qualify for cochlear implant Can achieve open-set recognition with lipreading	Remember "sound"; more rehabilitation is needed to process tactile information and to show benefit	Gives the client "sound," an auditory signal Open-set word and sentence recognition without lipreading	
Adults with severe hearing loss	Can give high frequency information in noise, supplements vision and hearing			Not appropriate, most do not meet candidacy requirements

Does not destroy residual hearing	Requires extensive training for success	Uses the auditory system that may have developed some listening skills	Surgery costs and more rehabilitation needed due to limited auditory skill development
Can use with hearing aids	Fewer research dollars, fewer subjects, only recently available commercially	Commercial benefit, increased sales, sophistication, and increased research dollars	Increased cost of rehabilitation (10 times that of tactile aids)
Prelingually Deaf adults	No medical risk with the same benefit, less expensive with similar benefit		
	Benefit derived through undamaged tactile system, rather than auditory stimulus through damaged or atrophied system		

of audibility and quality of nonspeech stimuli without the degradation of speech perception; and (3) reduction of the self-perceived hearing handicap of the individual. The hearing aid fitting process can consist of formal and informal testing. Informal assessments may be in the form of subjective responses to listening with hearing aids. Formal testing—functional gain, probe tube measurement systems, and electroacoustic analysis—ensures that the hearing aid provides adequate gain relative to the degree of hearing loss. Using these assessment materials, the client and clinician work together to select the appropriate hearing aids and determine goals for hearing aid use.

In addition to the formal hearing aid measures available, information about the client's everyday functioning with the hearing aid in his or her own environment is needed. Self-report, or a hearing aid diary, can be of some assistance to the audiologist and client for solving difficult listening situations. Participation of the client's significant others in the selection, fitting, and orientation of hearing aids provides an opportunity to glean more information about the client's communication style. It can also be a chance to educate involved people about the limitations and realistic expectations of amplification and the need for adjustments by all parties in the communication situation. Providing all of this information in a form and language that the client and family understand is the key to success in hearing aid use.

Orientation The hearing aid orientation is the next step in the integrated therapy process. It continues building a working relationship between the client and clinician and assures that the hearing aid is fit properly and is used to its fullest potential. Lastly, the hearing aid orientation involves the significant others to ensure functional benefit from the rehabilitation process. Sanders (1988) provides a step by step approach to hearing aid orientation.

The auditory training that follows the hearing aid orientation may be analytic or synthetic. Using different environmental situations will help determine the need for analytical training in environmental sounds. Synthetic training may involve the use of the hearing aid with significant others in everyday communication situations. (See the section on auditory training programs in this chapter for a further explanation of synthetic and analytic auditory training.) Additionally, the use of guided listening exercises with the hearing aids may increase in difficulty from one-to-one communication to listening in groups or in noise. Auditory training with hearing aids may include speechreading, communication strategies, and telephone and assistive devices practice in order to integrate therapy and optimize communication.

Assistive Devices and Rehabilitation

Complete aural rehabilitation often includes utilization of assistive devices alone or as part of a total integrated rehabilitation. Implementation of the Americans with Disabilities Act has increased the need for audiologists and consumers to be informed experts in the area of assistive technology. Palmer (1992) explains that most assistive device protocols are not considered until after the discovery that the hearing aid does not work in all communication situations. To integrate assistive devices into the mainstream audiology practice, Palmer suggests a protocol that considers assistive devices at the time of the hearing aid evaluation. In this model, the assistive device is not an afterthought, but an integral part of the rehabilitative plan for the client. From needs assessment to orientation, the aural rehabilitationist works with the client to optimize the communication process through assistive devices use.

Needs Analysis The first step in this rehabilitation plan is to assess the client's needs. Some of this assessment is done during the hearing aid evaluation. A needs assessment allows evaluation of the communication and alerting needs of the individual, provides a guideline for a streamlined demonstration by the audiologist, and establishes an avenue for follow-up. The needs analysis should be complete enough to determine whether simple detection of auditory signals is needed and/ or if more sophisticated assistance in amplifying the signal for communication in different environments is a requirement.

The format for the needs analysis can be a verbal interview, a written questionnaire, or a computer software program. Verbal needs assessments may be an integral part of the hearing aid evaluation process and may provide the audiologist with their own guidelines for demonstration and follow-up. A written questionnaire completed before the devices demonstration may spur the client into self-evaluation of his or her communication needs and provide a tangible reminder for follow-up contact. Vaughn and Lightfoot (1992) and Compton (1989b) give examples of needs analysis forms. These questionnaires have several things in common that should be included in any needs analysis. They determine difficult listening/understanding situations with respect to environment, alerting needs in a variety of environments, the client's use of amplification and sensory devices, community assistive devices and resources, and projected affordability of a device.

Computer software programs have also been developed to aid in the selection of assistive devices. Interactive Product Locator (Palmer, Garstecki, and Rauterkus, 1990) is a computer program that provides a needs analysis, an interactive questionnaire for specific device selection, and complete device, distributor, and patient databases.

Selection and Fitting Following the needs analysis, selection and fitting of the device(s) occur. The first concern in selecting an assistive device is the sensory modality to be used. Assistive devices are designed to provide an increased auditory signal, visual or tactile stimuli and are designated as assistive listening, telecommunication, and alerting devices. For individuals who process language auditorily or with the assistance of hearing aids, an increased auditory signal is sufficient for most situations. However, those same individuals will not be wearing their amplification while sleeping and therefore may need to employ another sensory channel for the awareness of environmental sounds, e.g., the smoke alarm. The person who does not process language auditorily may utilize visual or tactile signals. Persons with both hearing and visual problems may use tactile signals exclusively.

The choice of sensory mode is a matter of personal preference, and the choice will be made easier with a device trial. A well-stocked demonstration room may allow an initial trial period. However, if a small stock of assistive devices prohibits trials, a good relationship with manufacturers or distributors can make trials a reality.

For the computer-generated demonstration, the completion of the needs analysis in the Interactive Product Locator (Palmer 1992) provides a summary of the product database that matches the client's needs. A display of selected devices includes a picture of the device as well as distributor and other pertinent information.

When a device is selected, either through computer software or a trial use, the device is dispensed or ordered. Depending on the distributor and/or manufacturer, there may be a fairly short product return date, usually thirty days. Making certain of the desired device prior to ordering is time and cost effective for both the audiologist and the client. For stock items, the fitting and orientation procedure continues directly from the demonstration.

The evaluation of the assistive device starts when the device arrives in the audiologist's office. As with hearing aids, evaluation of assistive devices consists of informal and formal testing procedures. Informal testing requires initial listening check of an assistive listening device or trial of an alerting device. This ensures that the device is indeed working properly.

Formal assessment of assistive listening devices can be done using one or all of the following test methods: functional gain, probe tube microphone, and 2cc coupler measures. These test formats may provide comparison data such as frequency response, harmonic distortion, and preferred listening level information for personal amplifiers and FM systems. Determining the type of information needed will determine the formal test procedure to employ.

Functional gain is a threshold measure showing the difference between aided and unaided results. The goal of functional gain testing with a personal amplification device may be to match the functional gain of the device to that of an appropriately fit hearing aid. Functional measures do not mean gain measures alone. Sandlin (1990) asserts that soundfield test procedures can provide information such as preferred listening level, uncomfortable listening level, speech discrimination testing, determination of binaurality, and speech understanding in noise. However, Seewald and Moodie (1992) and Lewis, Feigin, Karasek, and Stelmachowicz (1991) list the limitation of soundfield testing for FM systems as being the difference between aided thresholds and realistic input levels found in the environment. Seewald and Moodie state that "for a majority of FM systems, soundfield aided threshold data obtained with an FM system will overestimate the gain that the system will provide under normal operating conditions" (93). Hawkins (1987) agrees, stating that the difference between input levels in the soundfield and realistic input levels at the microphone of the FM system may vary as much as 15 dB SPL. Soundfield testing is also time consuming and requires the participation of the client. Sandlin (1990) finds client participation to be a positive aspect of testing and uses the measurement of preferred listening level at subsequent office visits. However, functional gain measures do not provide information about the output of the assistive devices or the harmonic distortion of the system. Therefore, clinical application of soundfield functional gain testing of personal amplification devices provides limited information about the system and makes alternative testing methods more attractive.

Real ear probe tube measures with assistive listening devices provide objective information that can be readily compared to the same measures done with a hearing aid. Measures of frequency response, output limiting characteristics, insertion gain, and input/output functions can be obtained through probe tube microphone measures (Mueller, Hawkins, and Northern 1992). Problems with input equivalence in functional gain testing can be corrected in probe tube microphone measurements, allowing for the measurement of more realistic system input levels. The set-up procedures for probe tube measurements depends on the real ear system being used. Lewis et al. (1991) describe these differences. Real ear probe tube microphone measurements can be used to validate assistive listening devices fitting and also have been used to evaluate different telecoils, telephones, and telephone amplifier options (Grimes and Mueller 1991a,b). This type of testing is not possible with functional gain or 2cc coupler measures. Probe tube measurements provide useful information, but, like functional gain testing, require client participation.

The use of electroacoustic measurements with assistive listening devices can provide frequency response, SSPL90, and harmonic distortion values, without requiring the client to be present. Although ANSI standards for assistive devices are still in development, many manufacturers do provide some frequency response information for their personal amplification and FM systems. For those devices with no manufacturer specifications, 2cc coupler measures will provide a baseline measurement to be used in subsequent testings during return office visits. Seewald and Moodie (1992) have two assumptions when utilizing 2cc coupler measures with FM systems: that the electroacoustic selection method for hearing aids and FM systems is the same and that differences between hearing aid and FM system performances in the 2cc coupler will hold constant for real ear measurements. To correct for differences between hearing aid and assistive device performance, Lewis et al. (1991) suggest a 75 dB input for FM systems as opposed to the traditional 60 dB input for linear hearing aids. The FM system or personal listening system needs to be evaluated in the 2cc coupler in the manner that it will be used. That is, if the client uses the system with earphones, then the earphones must be used in the 2cc coupler. If the system is to be coupled through the client's hearing aid, then that configuration must be used for the electroacoustic measures. For those devices that will not fit in the 2cc coupler chamber, a quiet testing environment is essential.

Measurement of harmonic distortion is an important feature of electro-acoustic measurements that is not available with all probe tube measurement systems or functional gain measures. For instance, different coupling options for the assistive device, with different hearing aids, can produce different amounts of distortion in the system. Changes in volume control of the assistive device can cause harmonic distortion, and when measured with probe tube measures may reveal only appropriate gain values, not the total distortion present in the system.

Use of these formal testing procedures will depend on the type of instrumentation available, the electroacoustic information desired, and the cooperation of the client in the testing procedures. Just as with hearing aids, testing procedures for assistive devices, be they informal or formal, are essential prior to dispensing of the device. Results from formal testing procedures along with informal procedures will provide fitting and use parameters, such as user volume and acoustic coupling options.

Orientation Orientation to the assistive device presents another rapport-building opportunity. A simple checklist can be helpful. It should include an explanation of proper use, how the device interfaces with hearing aids (if necessary), battery type and size, proper care and maintenance, a purchase receipt, trial period information, warranty information/extended warranties, and a schedule for client follow-up appointments.

Explanation of the functioning of an assistive device can be as simple as how a light flasher works or as complex as how infrared light conducts sound. The explanation should be commensurate with the clients' need level and given in language they can understand. The explanation may be aided by handouts with visual descriptions of devices and their uses. Some manufacturers attempt to provide helpful informational brochures with the equipment. For nonnative English speakers or non-English speakers, easy-to-understand handouts with picture diagrams are recommended. Figure 7.1 is an example of a simplified diagram for Telecaption Decoder hook-up developed at the Hearing Society for the Bay Area, San Francisco.

Explanation of interfacing between the hearing aid and an assistive device should occur during the hearing aid orientation and again during the assistive devices orientation. The range of different coupling options for assistive devices should also be discussed. For instance, a client may purchase an infrared system for the television, coupled to the hearing aid through the telecoil using a neck-loop. An explanation about using the hearing aid's telecoil with a loop system installed at the client's community center encourages that same client to use the hearing aid to its fullest potential in a variety of listening situations.

As with use and care of the hearing aid, a packet of written information about use and care of the assistive device will be a reference for clients once they arrive home. Battery, repair, and warranty information in a concise format will be

Telecaption Decoder Connections

Rule 1: Remember, every television is different. Read these guidelines and adapt the drawings to match your own TV. If you have any difficulties, call the Hearing Society.

Rule 2: The television is always connected to the decoder. All additional components are between the decoder and the outside source (wall connection for cable or antenna).

Rule 3: If you have a separate antenna, it must be connected to the last component in the chain, which is the component that connects to the outside source.

TV without ANTENNA to DECODER

1. The VHF/CABLE IN on the television is connected to the TV OUT on the decoder.

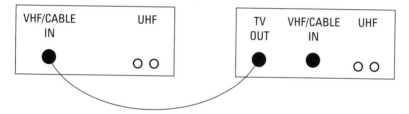

TV with ANTENNA to DECODER

1. The VHF/CABLE IN of the television is connected to the TV OUT on the decoder.
2. The ANTENNA is connected to the UHF plug on the decoder.

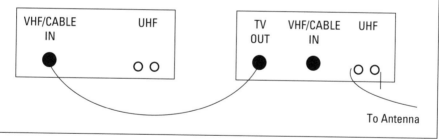

Figure 7.1. Telecaption decoder connections
Source: Hearing Society for the Bay Area 1989.

well utilized by the client. Size, type, and rechargeability information about batteries differ greatly within and between devices; this should be listed in the packet, as well as recharging instructions, if applicable, and where batteries can be purchased. This use-and-care packet should also include proper cleaning instructions for the device. Depending on the device, it may be necessary for the client to return the device to the dispenser for repair or to send the device directly to the company for repair. Warranty policies vary as well; some companies provide repair and extended repair warranties, whereas at some companies all sales are final. The flexibility and availability of a good warranty may be one of the deciding factors in the final selection of an assistive device. The use-and-care packet should make repair and warranty information clear. The option for a trial period with some assistive devices is attractive to the consumer and the dispenser. As stated previously, this trial period may be possible with the use of consignment devices in a well-stocked devices room. However, trial periods may not be available for many devices available through mail-order. Good relationships with manufacturers may make trial periods possible. Proper consideration of options prior to ordering will reduce the number of returned devices. One manufacturer of FM systems keeps a pool of trial systems available for evaluation prior to ordering. This practice has resulted in a return rate of less than 1 percent of FM systems sold by that company (Nelson 1993).

Finally, follow-up appointments can occur within the structure of therapy sessions. These sessions allow for mutual feedback. The clinician can determine if the client is satisfied with the device and if it is meeting his or her needs. The client can clarify any questions he or she may have about warranty responsibilities or additional services for the device. Together, the client and clinician can continue work on therapy goals that involve the use of the assistive device.

The part of integrated therapy most related to assistive devices is not auditory training, but assertiveness training. The client using an assistive-listening system needs to use appropriate communication strategies to employ the cooperation of the speaker or the source of the signal. For example, a client with a personal FM system who needs to hear a lecturer in a small auditorium should educate the speaker about how to use the system and why the system is necessary. This may require helping with microphone placement, reminders not to play with the microphone cord, and the need for the speaker to repeat audience questions through the FM's microphone before answering such questions. Requesting that an appropriate alerting system be installed in an apartment building is another example of learning how to be assertive in the use of assistive devices. By developing and using assistive devices as an integrated service within aural rehabilitation, audiologists and aural rehabilitationists are at the forefront of offering complete rehabilitation services to deaf and hard of hearing individuals.

Cochlear Implants and Rehabilitation

Rehabilitation for clients using cochlear implants starts with preimplant therapy. For adults, these initial sessions may be used to provide informational counseling on realistic expectations for the device. Postimplantation remediation of a cochlear implant begins with fitting the speech processor. As discussed in chapter 6, the initial fitting of the cochlear implant focuses on optimal mapping and informational counseling concerning orientation to as well as use and care of the device.

Proper assessment and results, showing the information available from a cochlear implant, will allow the clinician and client to agree on an appropriate training program. According to Tyler, Tye-Murray, and Lansing (1988), amplification afforded by the cochlear implant is quite different from conventional auditory amplification systems. Although some parameters and acoustical/electrical representations are still not understood, knowledge of how the implant codes information is helpful in determining training materials and appropriate goals. There are two basic distinctions in cochlear implant stimulus processing: wideband or feature extraction. Wideband processing attempts to preserve as much of the original signal or waveform as possible by amplifying, filtering, or compressing the signal. Feature extraction processing changes the original signal considerably by processing only specific speech features. This processing scheme assumes that the designer knows which speech features are the most important. Another distinction between cochlear implants is the number of channels used by the implant. Single-channel units stimulate all neurons in the same way. Multichannel cochlear implants stimulate different parts of the cochlea with different information, much like the ear does.

Single-channel wideband processors supply temporal information, so materials contrasting intonation patterns or length can be part of therapy. Feature extraction by a single-channel device provides information used for the training of voiced/voiceless contrasts or word stress identification. Individual speech sound identification would not be a realistic goal for most clients in auditory training with a single-channel cochlear implant.

Multichannel wideband processors provide a greater range of acoustic information; therefore, therapy materials and goals can include a wider range of speech sound parameters. Multichannel wideband processors may allow the identification of vowels and some consonants. In these wideband processors, environmental stimuli are more appropriate and useable than with feature extraction units. For some multichannel feature extractors programmed to process information unique to human speech, such as the Nucleus unit, training materials using music or environmental sounds would be inappropriate. For all of these processors, the usefulness of the device depends on the client's behavioral responses to the cues provided.

Regardless of the signal processing strategy of the implant, the general goal for the cochlear implant user, in most everyday situations, is the enhancement of visual speech perception (Roberts 1991). The starting point for postimplant rehabilitation therapy is determined by the client's performance during preoperation therapy and by an assessment of the client's needs (see the section on cochlear implant assessment in this chapter). The type of rehabilitation will be different depending on whether the adult's hearing loss occurred before or after language acquisition (Tyler, Tye-Murray, and Lansing 1988). Late-deafened adults and even adolescents will have encoded auditory and visual perceptions into memory. Prelinguistically deaf adults and adolescents do not have that memory, so rehabilitation for this group will include training in auditory and visual perceptions and possibly in word meaning and structure.

Osberger (1990) summarized studies of cochlear implant rehabilitation and determined that half of the postlingually deaf adults with cochlear implants achieved some open-set word recognition, and all but a few of these adults noticed an improvement in environmental sound perception and enhanced lipreading. In addition, the prelingually deaf adults who communicated orally and who were hearing aid users also obtained improved environmental sound perception and increased speechreading skills, although they rarely achieved open-set word recognition. Osberger (1990) reports that greater gains in implant use are achieved when rehabilitation in the form of counseling, sensory training (auditory and/or visual), and communication strategies work starts soon after implantation (within a month). Improvements in environmental sound perception and increased speechreading skills should not be minimized for those clients who might benefit from them.

Some argue that the concentrated rehabilitation associated with cochlear implants contributes to the increase in speech perception abilities. Gagne, Parnes, LaRocque, Hassan, and Vidas (1991) report that postimplant improvements in speech perception are due to increased sensory input and not the intensive rehabilitation program. They note that the greatest benefit from general aural rehabilitation occurred for telephone training and communication strategies use. However, Tyler, Tye-Murray, and Lansing (1988) state that the improvements in the client's communication may be due to specific therapeutic techniques, encouragement from the clinician or significant other, interaction with other cochlear implant recipients, experience with the device, or some combination of the above.

Holden, Binzer, Skinner, and Juelich (1991) report on the benefit provided by a multielectrode cochlear implant to a prelinguistically deaf adult. The adult was highly motivated to use audition for speech reception. He used hearing aids for twelve years before the intense output of the aids caused nystagmus. Educated through high school and three years of college in an aural/oral communication environment, his speech production and speechreading skills were excellent. The client was implanted with a Nucleus 22 Cochlear Implant System, which has a multichannel wideband processor.

Postimplant rehabilitation combined auditory training with the program mapping adjustments of the speech processor. The client demonstrated a normal dynamic range with the cochlear implant, minus the nystagmus. For the first four months, therapy sessions were held twice weekly. Aural rehabilitation consisted of use and care of the device, introduction to music, environmental sound awareness and discrimination, introduction to telephone-coded systems, analytic and synthetic speechreading tasks, and auditory training. The auditory training program was designed to proceed from detection to comprehension. Initial training introduced same/different pairs for discrimination and progressed through identification and recognition skills. At the end of his four-month therapy sessions, he was able to identify closed-set sentences with 85 percent accuracy using the device alone. The combination of his speechreading skills and the auditory signal from the implant allowed the client to achieve 100 percent accuracy on open-set materials. The authors conclude the case presentation by stating that considera-tion of prelinguistically deaf adults for cochlear implants must look at the candi-date's motivation, intelligence, oral skills, support systems, and willingness to be part of the hearing world.

Aural rehabilitation that incorporates cochlear implants concentrates on en-hancing environmental sound perception and increasing speechreading skills; some implant recipients are also able to improve their word recognition skills.

Tactile Aids and Rehabilitation

As with cochlear implants, knowledge of the speech parameters presented by the device will guide the development of therapy goals. Single-channel tactile aids provide prosodic features such as time and intensity variables, as well as aware-ness of environmental signals. Multichannel tactile aids provide some phonemic information. Training for deafened adults with tactile aids focuses on speechread-ing, speech perception skills, and speech production.

Most deafened adults are concerned with both the loss of speech perception and connection to their environment. Analytical training with the tactile aid will isolate those components of training that are to be mastered. Synthetic training reinforces the analytical skill training (see the section on auditory training pro-grams in this chapter for a detailed explanation). Continuous discourse tracking (DeFilippo and Scott 1978) lends itself to tactile and visual training, which in-cludes communication strategy training as well. In the speech tracking proce-dure, the clinician reads to the client from a text. The client then repeats verbatim what was said. Communication strategies such as repetition, rephrasing, or clari-fication may be used to get the client to repeat the segment completely. Auditory connection with the environment is accomplished through environmental sound training. For a deafened adult, the inability to detect events in his or her environ-ment through sound is significant. Training the individual to make use of envi-ronmental sound through technology (assistive devices) is a part of integrated therapy.

As with cochlear implants, an improvement of environmental sound percep-tion and increased speechreading abilities should not be minimized for those cli-ents who benefit from the use of tactile aids, a viable, noninvasive alternative rehabilitation device. For a text dedicated to tactile aids, see *Tactile Aids for the Hearing Impaired* (Summers 1992).

Summary of Cochlear Implant and Tactile Aid Rehabilitation

The Working Group on Communication Aids for the Hearing Impaired (Watson et al. 1991) states that there is a clear distinction between benefit from hearing aids and benefit from cochlear implants. If there is hearing aid benefit (although "hearing aid benefit" is still not defined), a cochlear implant is not recommended. However, there is no distinction between rehabilitation choices concerning coch-lear implant benefit and vibrotactile aid benefit. These decisions depend on the individual—his or her resources and motivation. The Working Group asserts that the largest differences in benefit from these two types of devices is noted in the differing test results of relative "star" cochlear implant users and "star" tactile aids users. The cochlear implant "star" performers are able to outperform tactile aid "stars" on auditory perception tests. The perspective given by mass media stories is that there are many cochlear implant "stars," which contributes to the notion that cochlear implant recipients outshine the best vibrotactile aid users. The reality is that, although 5 to 10 percent of cochlear implant users derive remarkable auditory success, most implant users make more moderate progress, and great variability in auditory skills exists among all cochlear implant users (Watson et al. 1991). The Working Group noted that the small number of tactile aid "stars" is a direct result of the small number of users. They summarize by stating that the way in which some members of the medical community have embraced the cochlear implant supports and encourages increasing numbers of implantations done each year. However, sluggish tactile aid use is attributed to the struggle that research scientists have had in developing a wearable tactile device.

Auditory Training Programs

Traditional auditory training programs and texts usually look at two types of training: analytic and synthetic (Cooper 1991b). (See figure 7.2.) Analytic training is the training of isolated parameters of listening—most typically, individual speech sounds, segments of speech, or words. For example, Ling's phonetic training lessons on the segmentals and suprasegmentals of speech train children to determine the difference between short and long speech signals and between one and two syllables (Ling 1976). Analytic training has also been referred to as a "bottom-up" method, using minimal units to arrive at the intended whole. "Top-down" or synthetic training uses meaningful materials to decipher details for completion of a task. It works to develop conceptual understanding of the speaker's message as opposed to understanding individual words of the message. An example of this type of training would be working on sentence comprehension in a story format. It can simultaneously incorporate language, speechreading, and communication strategy training. For some multicultural clients or culturally Deaf clients, the language training aspect is essential in an integrated therapy model. Tyler, Tye-Murray, and Lansing (1988) state that progress in one area of training may influence performance in another area. For example, work on discourse tracking may improve consonant recognition skills. Often, both analytical and synthetic training is needed as part of an auditory training program.

The development of an auditory training program within an integrated therapy model may look at four areas: therapy components, client characteristics, device parameters, and program evaluation. In an article describing the development of a training program specifically for tactile devices used by children, Gal-

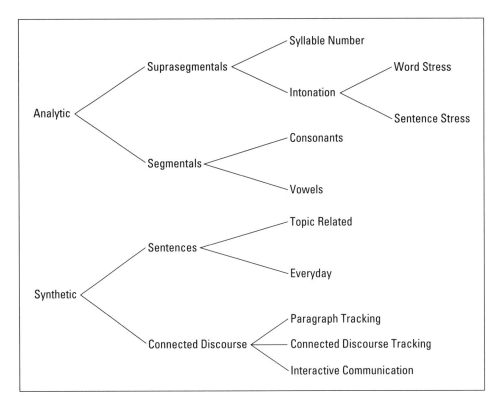

Figure 7.2. Analytic versus synthetic therapy
Source: Cooper 1991.

vin, Cowan, Savant, Blamey, and Clark (1993) describe the seven key components of a training program as follows:

1. Type of training tasks,

2. Amount of training,

3. Motivation and device use,

4. User characteristics,

5. Response formats used in training,

6. Information presented by the device, and

7. Evaluation procedures.

Whether the device used is a cochlear implant, a tactile aid, or any other assistive device, these components can be applied to any adult auditory training program.

The first area of auditory training program development is composed of therapy components, which relate to Galvin's first two factors: the type of training and the amount of training. Therapy materials must also be considered in this area. In auditory training, these materials are analytic and synthetic, including everything from phoneme reception to comprehension of running speech. Erber (1982) specifically emphasizes the use of conversational materials for effective training of adults in most situations. He goes on to state that analytical training is useful for specific tasks, such as telephone training. Relevant, functional therapy materials that motivate adult clients will be the most successful in an auditory training program. Galvin et al. (1993) support the use of close-set and open-set response formats for auditory training because both types of responses are required in everyday communication situations.

The amount of training needed for effective use of a device is the next important component of an auditory training program. The amount of time available for auditory training is different for children and adults. Children often have the opportunity to take advantage of daily auditory training through an educational setting. Adults typically have less time to spare, so a training program may need to be more intensive, concentrating on specific objectives needed for everyday communication. The amount of training time also relates to the adult's motivation. Getting a device that may require long training periods, extensive mapping, and refinement can be a difficult decision for a working-age adult.

The second area of auditory training program development is related to the client traits, which Galvin calls motivation, device use, and user characteristics. The client's motivation and his or her support system (friends and family) will determine the success of any training program. Particularly for adolescents, peer pressure and family support for the amplification choice may be a decisive factor in the ultimate success of the adolescent's use of device. For both adults and adolescents, extensive training programs must be adaptable to simulate everyday listening environments so that the family or support system members can take part in the training process on an informal level. Consistent use will provide experience with the device. This experience is likely to lead to the determination of functional benefit by the client. Other client-related characteristics, such as age, previous knowledge of language, residual hearing, and ability to integrate speech information from more than one modality, will determine the course for the auditory training program.

The third area of consideration in an auditory training program is client knowledge of the parameters of the device. The kind of information available through the amplification device and how it is presented are important in determining training goals and in organizing the order of task presentations. This aspect of the training program is similar to auditory training goal development and the use of cochlear implant speech processor features.

The last component of an auditory training program is evaluation of the client's progress with the device and evaluation of the device itself. Ongoing client evaluation allows analysis of the auditory training program effectiveness, of the client's progress, and of information for use in research. Measurable results are important in any training program. However, for adults who have a choice about therapy options, functional improvement in communication is key for the continuation of therapy. Generally, in the evaluation of the devices in use, if a person consistently uses a device and is dependent on it for communication (i.e., if a hearing aid is used for alerting the user to environmental sounds or a cochlear implant aids in speech understanding), then the device is providing some benefit. Maximizing this benefit is the goal of integrated therapy. Device evaluation can also provide information about the long-term safety of each device.

Examples of Auditory Training Programs for Prelingually Deaf Adults

Auditory training programs for adults may be examined by keeping the above program components in mind. One program for auditory training with adults is used at the House Ear Institute, which implants adults and children. Eisenberg (1985) developed the auditory training program for prelingually deaf adults with cochlear implants. The goal of the program is to introduce sound to the new implant recipient. Although specifically designed to be used with an implant, techniques in this program may be generalized for use in introducing any prelingually deaf adult to sound through a variety of devices. The program consists of two basic parts: the Music Therapy Program and the Environmental Sounds Program. The goal of the Music Therapy Program is to promote an understanding and interest in basic sound parameters. The Environmental Sound Program builds on the Music Therapy Program to incorporate meaning into newly learned sound parameters. Most of the lessons at the Institute use both the Music Therapy Program and the Environmental Sound Program; however, the Environmental Sound Program can be used as an independent auditory training program. Each lesson plan includes concepts, goals, equipment and materials, procedures, and extended lesson ideas. Because each individual demonstrates different strengths and weaknesses throughout the program, each lesson can be condensed or expanded to meet the individual's needs.

The Music Therapy Program uses a "fun" medium to teach different sound parameters, encouraging the use of sound as meaningful and applicable to everyday life. Duration, intensity, and tempo are natural parts of music and useful concepts for introducing sound. The music-based training reinforces the concept that sound is pleasurable. These concepts are used to help the client separate random noise from meaningful sound. The Environmental Sound Program takes the parameters learned in the Music Program and organizes them using specific situations. For example, Music Therapy Lesson Plan 2 introduces the concept of musical beat and varying tempos. The corresponding Environmental Therapy Lesson 2 on timing relates different tempos to varied energy levels. "People-made" sounds may vary depending on the person's energy level. For example, an excited person may speak quickly; thus, his voice may contain a lot of energy and be associated with a quick tempo. In contrast, the voice of someone who is having a relaxed conversation may contain less energy and may be associated with a slower tempo. Finally, Home Assignments are used to reinforce concepts learned in therapy and to encourage implant use outside of the clinical setting. The program flexibility allows client-based progress to drive the program. This combination of analytic and synthetic tasks, music as a motivator, and functional environmental information has the ingredients for a successful adult auditory training program. The overall goal is to foster curiosity and interest in sound, be it for enjoyment or benefit. Success in this program is if the individual uses the device daily, regardless of the reason. As discussed earlier, consistent use of the device suggests benefit.

Example of an Auditory Program for Hard of Hearing Adults

Another auditory training program for adults was designed at the National Technical Institute for the Deaf (NTID). Snell (1992a) outlines the components of a successful auditory training program for adults:

> Several characteristics appear common to the more successful programs in training adult auditory perceptual skills. These include motivated, enthusiastic listeners and teachers, opportunities to listen many, many times to invariant productions of each stimulus, listener controlled pacing of stimuli, repetition rate and presentation level, segmentation of training in appropriately sized chunks, and immediate feedback about correct recognitions and error patterns. (1)

These characteristics are the bases for the auditory training programs for students at NTID. Starting in 1972, students at NTID were offered courses to help maintain or improve the listening skills they developed prior to coming to college. As part of the curriculum, all students at NTID are profiled according to their auditory perceptual skills, and given a profile number from 1 to 5. Profile 1 designates students who do not process auditory signals for communication; Profile 5 students can use audition alone for understanding. Courses are recommended depending on the profile.

These elective courses require the students' active participation through analysis of their own listening skills and exploration of techniques and equipment for independent listening. Profile 1 and 2 students characteristically obtain very limited information through audition alone. The course outline for these students encourages the use of prosodic features as an aid to speechreading. The class for Profile 3 students focuses on obtaining the main idea of the message through listening and structural cues. The course for Profile 4 and 5 students stresses the acquisition of "listening fluency," the ability to fully use the auditory message in combination with communication strategies for understanding. In the Profile 4 and 5 course, listening situations encountered outside of the classroom and homework assignments are noted and shared with the instructor through a notebook system. The notebook is used to help the students analyze their listening skills and evaluate their communication behavior in different situations. A music lab is also part of the curriculum, employing popular songs and famous speeches, not only for motivational reasons, but as a clever way to introduce tracking skills. Using the lyrics printed on record jackets or from music stores, lab sessions require students to track songs for understanding. This very energetic program motivates both the students and the teachers (Snell 1992b).

Case Study: Integrated Therapy Plan
for a Multicultural Deaf Adult

Using the components outlined by Galvin et al. (1993), an adult auditory training program can be developed for any client. These components and a broad definition of "auditory training" can be used to integrate auditory training into any therapy situation. For example, an immigrant from Nicaragua, Ed is an adult client with a profound congenital hearing loss. With limited educational opportunities in his native country, he relied on his family for basic necessities and communicated with "home signs." Upon arrival in the United States, his cousin taught him how to paint houses and brought him to a clinic for "help." The first considerations for integrated therapy were the type and amount of training and the training materials. Ed was scheduled for therapy sessions twice weekly, one hour in a group setting, another hour with one-on-one instruction. The therapy materials needed to be functional, motivating topics.

Ed's auditory training goals included environmental sound training. The first objective toward this goal was use of an alarm clock, which would ensure he got to work on time. We include this as auditory training in that Ed had to use technology in order to be connected to important auditory information—his alarm clock. The motivation for this type of auditory training was economically based: if Ed did not get up on time, he would not be paid for the whole day. The second objective in this area was the use of the client's residual hearing for safety on the job. Economics dictated the selection and fitting of a power hearing aid. Ed was oriented to his auditory environment through a trial period in varying situations. Auditory training consisted of experience with the hearing aid. From daily use, Ed became aware that noises can be directly related to events that he sees and actions that he takes. For example, the discovery that closing a door creates sound was a surprise to Ed. However, Ed was able to detect environmental sounds with only limited discrimination abilities. Therefore, optimizing Ed's use of his residual hearing meant further exploration of environment sound rather than discrimination of those sounds.

Although sign language was used as the communication mode for therapy, Ed required further sign instruction to integrate home signs into a structured sign system. This instruction was provided by a skilled signer. Along with sign language instruction, other language skills such as reading were included in therapy. Identification of color names in printed English and sign language, plus the concept of addresses and city locations, were included in therapy and were very important concepts for a house painter. Ed understood neither spoken nor written Spanish. Therefore, Spanish language work was not included in the goals with this client. His main goal was integration into American society, so American Sign Language (ASL) and basic English were the languages chosen for therapy.

Analysis of the components of this training program reveals: (1) the materials selected for therapy were functional, motivating topics for Ed; (2) the materials were presented in a mode of communication that he understood (gestures, basic ASL, basic English); (3) the use of the realistic information from the device (hearing aid) was developed and improved; and (4) evaluation of therapy materials and of Ed's success was ongoing. Eventually, Ed's house painting work increased to the point that he had little time for therapy. For Ed and the clinician, this was considered therapeutic success.

Summary

Optimizing communication is the goal of an integrated model of therapy and of auditory training. The integrated approach to communication therapy, as discussed in this book, has the whole person and his or her needs as the focus of any intervention process. Van Tasell (1981) specifically states that auditory training should be an integral part of a total communication skills program. This statement is based on the premise that auditory management is the development of the use of residual hearing. As evident in this chapter, auditory training can now be defined in broader terms to incorporate not only auditory events (sound) for use in communication but also the use of technology for the manipulation of sound for communication.

Paramount in this new perception of rehabilitation is an accurate assessment of the communication skills of the client coupled with a partnership in rehabilitation between the client and clinician. This partnership will lead to the development of therapy goals relevant to the life of our most important colleague, our client. The low number of auditory training programs for adults and adolescents attests to the need for research into the development of successful training programs. Whether the auditory training is for use of a tactile aid or an alerting device, when it is meaningful, it will be appropriate rehabilitation.

References

Alpiner, J., ed. 1982. *Handbook of adult rehabilitative audiology*, 2d ed. Baltimore: Williams & Wilkins.

American National Standards Institute. 1989. Method for measuring the intelligibility of speech over communication systems (S3.2). New York: American National Standards Institute.

Blamey, P., and R. Cowan. 1992. The potential benefit and cost-effectiveness of tactile devices in comparison with cochlear implants. In *Tactile aids for the hearing impaired,* ed. I. Summers. London: Whurr Publishers.

Carhart, R. 1947. Auditory training. In *Hearing and deafness;* a guide for laymen, ed. H. Davis. New York: Murray Hill Books.

Chermak, G. D. 1981. *Handbook of audiological rehabilitation.* Springfield, Ill.: Charles C. Thomas.

Clark, G., P. Busby, S. Roberts, R. Dowell, P. Blamey, D. Mecklenburg, R. Webb, B. Pyman, and B. Franz. 1987. Preliminary results for the Cochlear Corporation Multielectrode Intracochlear Implant in six pre-linguistically deaf patients. *American Journal of Otology* 8(3):234–239.

Cochlear implantation for the profoundly deaf. *Lancet,* 26 March (1):686–687.

Compton, C., ed. 1989a. Assistive listening devices. *Seminars in Hearing* 10(1).

———. 1989b. *Assistive devices: Doorways to independence.* Columbia, S.C.: The Academy of Dispensing Audiology.

Cooper, H. 1991a. Selection of candidates for cochlear implantation: An overview. In *Cochlear implants: A practical guide,* ed. H. Cooper. San Diego, Calif.: Singular Publishing Group.

———. 1991b. Training and rehabilitation for cochlear implant users. In *Cochlear implants: A practical guide,* ed. H. Cooper. San Diego, Calif.: Singular Publishing Group.

DeFilippo, C., and B. Scott. 1978. A method for training and evaluating the reception of ongoing speech. *Journal of the Acoustical Society of America* 63:1186-1192.

Durity, R. 1982. Auditory training for severely hearing impaired adults. *Deafness and communication: Assessment and training,* ed. D. Sims, G. Walter, and R. Whitehead. Baltimore: Williams & Wilkins.

Eisenberg, L. 1985. *Introduction to sound for pre-lingually deaf adults,* 2d ed. Los Angeles: House Ear Institute.

Erber, N. P. 1982. *Auditory training.* Washington, D.C.: Alexander Graham Bell Association for the Deaf.

———. 1988. *Communication therapy for hearing-impaired adults.* Abbotsford, Australia: Clavis Publishing.

Erber, N. P., and C. M. Alencewicz. 1976. Audiological evaluation of deaf children. *Journal of Speech and Hearing Disorders* 41:256–267.

Fifer, R., B. Stach, and J. Jerger. 1984. Evaluation of the Minimal Auditory Capabilities (MAC) Test in prelingual and postlingual hearing-impaired adults. *Ear and Hearing* 5(2):87-90.

Gagne, J., L. Parnes, M. LaRocque, Rassan, and S. Vidas. 1991. Effectiveness of an intensive speech perception training program for adult cochlear implant recipients. *Annals of Otology, Rhinology and Laryngology* 100:700–707.

Galvin, K., R. Cowan, J. Savant, P. Blamey, and G. Clark. 1993. Factors in the development of a training program for use with tactile devices. *Ear and Hearing* 14(2):118-127.

Grimes, A. M., and H. G. Mueller. 1991a. Using probe-microphone measures to assess telecoils and ALDs, part 1: Assessment of telecoil performance. *The Hearing Journal* 44(6):16–21.

———. 1991b. Using probe-microphone measures to assess telecoils and ALDs, part 2: Assessment of ALDs, telephones, and telephone amplifiers. *The Hearing Journal* 44(7):21–29.

Hartbauer, R. E. 1975. *Aural habilitation: A total approach.* Springfield, Ill.: Charles C. Thomas.

Hawkins, D. 1987. Assessment of FM systems with an Ear Canal Probe Tube Microphone System. *Ear and Hearing* 8(5):301-303.

Hearing Society. 1989. Telecaption decoder connections. San Francisco: Hearing Society.

Henoch, M. 1991. Speech perception, hearing aid technology, and aural rehabilitation: A future perspective. *Ear and Hearing* 12(6):S187-S191.

Hodgson, W. R., ed. 1986. *Hearing aid assessment and use in audiologic habilitation,* 3rd ed. Baltimore: Williams & Wilkins.

Holden, L., S. Binzer, M. Skinner, and M. Juelich. 1991. Benefit provided by a multi-electrode intracochlear implant to a prelingually deaf adult. *Missouri Medicine* 88(3):143–148.

Katz, J., ed. 1994. *Handbook of clinical audiology,* 4th ed. Baltimore: Williams & Wilkins.

Kelly, J. C. 1973. *Clinician's handbook of auditory training.* Washington, D.C.: Alexander Graham Bell Association for the Deaf.

Kessler, D. 1993. Personal communication. University of California, San Francisco.

King, A. 1991. Audiological assessment and hearing aid trials. In *Cochlear implants: A practical guide,* ed. H. Cooper. San Diego, Calif.: Singular Publishing Group.

Knutson, J., H. Schartz, B. Gantz, R. Tyler, J. Hinricks, and G. Woodworth. 1991. Psychological change following eighteen months of cochlear implant use. *Annals of Otology, Rhinology, and Laryngology* 100:877–882.

Lewis, D., J. Feigin, A. Karasek, and P. Stelmachowicz. 1991. Evaluation and assessment of FM systems. *Ear and Hearing* 12(4):268–280.

Ling, D. 1976. *Speech and the hearing impaired child: Theory and practice.* Washington, D.C.: Alexander Graham Bell Association for the Deaf.

Luxford, W. 1989. Cochlear implant indications. *American Journal of Otology* 10(2):95.

Martin, F. N. 1981. *Introduction to audiology,* 2d ed. Englewood Cliffs, N.J.: Prentice Hall.

Martin, F. N., and L. Morris. 1989. Current audiologic practices in the United States. *The Hearing Journal* 42(4):25–44.

McCarthy, P., and N. B. Culpepper. 1987. The adult remediation process. In *Rehabilitative audiology: Children and adults,* ed. J. Alpiner and P. McCarthy. Baltimore: Williams & Wilkins.

McCullough, J., R. Wilson, J. Birck, and L. Anderson. 1994. A multimedia approach for estimating speech recognition of multilingual clients. *American Journal of Audiology* 3(1):19–22.

Menapace, C. 1992. Personal communication. Englewood, Colo.: Cochlear Corporation.

Mueller, H. G., D. Hawkins, and J. Northern. 1992. *Probe microphone measurements: Hearing aid selection and assessment.* San Diego, Calif.: Singular Publishing Group.

Nelson, K. 1993. Personal communication. Minneapolis, Minn.: Telex Communications, Inc.

Newby, H. 1964. *Audiology,* 2d ed. New York: Appleton-Century-Crofts.

Newby, H. A., and G. R. Popelka. 1985. *Audiology,* 5th ed. Englewood Cliffs, N.J.: Prentice-Hall.

Osberger, M. J. 1990. Audiological rehabilitation with cochlear implants and tactile aids. *ASHA* 32 (April): 38–43.

Owens, E., D. Kessler, M. W. Raggio, and E. Schubert. 1985. Analysis and revision of the Minimal Auditory Capabilities (MAC) Battery. *Ear and Hearing* 6(6):280–290.

Palmer, C. 1992. Assistive devices in the audiology practice. *American Journal of Audiology* 1(2):37–57.

Palmer, C., D. Garstecki, and M. Rauterkus. 1990. An interactive product locator for the selection of assistive devices. Paper presented at the American Speech-Language-Hearing Association Convention, Seattle, Washington.

Plant, G. 1992. Selection and training of tactile aid users. In *Tactile aids for the hearing impaired,* ed. I. Summers. London: Whurr Publishers.

Redinger, B., and Friedman, J. 1990. Communication therapy for foreign-born deaf adults: Issues for consideration. Paper presented at the Academy of Rehabilitative Audiology 1990 Summer Institute, Orlando, Florida.

———. 1992. Complete assistive devices management. Paper presented at the California Speech-Language-Hearing Association Convention, San Francisco.

Rihkanen, H. 1990. Subjective benefit of communication aids evaluated by postlingually deaf adults. *British Journal of Audiology* 24:161–166.

Rintelmann, W. F. 1991. *Hearing assessment,* 2d ed. Austin, Tex.: Pro-Ed.

Roberts, S. 1991. Speech-processor fitting for cochlear implants. *Cochlear implants: A practical guide,* ed. H. Cooper. San Diego, Calif.: Singular Publishing Group.

Sanders, D. 1988. Hearing aid orientation and counseling. In *Amplification for the hearing impaired,* 3rd ed. ed. M. Pollack. New York: Grune & Stratton, Inc.

Sandlin, R. 1990. Clinical application of sound field audiometry. *Handbook of hearing aid amplification, vol. 2: Clinical considerations and fitting practices.* Boston: College-Hill Press.

Seewald, R. C., and K. S. Moodie. 1992. Electroacoustic considerations. In *FM auditory training systems: Characteristics, selection and use,* ed. M. Ross. Timonium, Md.: York Press.

Snell, K. 1992a. Efficacy of training in auditory vowel recognition. Paper presented at Academy of Rehabilitative Audiology Summer Institute, Rochester, New York.

————. 1992b. The sounds of English: The acquisition of aural language. Auditory Training Curriculum, Rochester, New York.

Summers, I., ed. 1992. *Tactile aids for the hearing impaired.* London: Whurr Publishers.

Trammell, J. L., and S. L. Owens. 1977. The Test of Auditory Comprehension. Paper presented at the Annual Convention of the American Speech-Language-Hearing Association, Chicago, Illinois.

Tyler, R., and M. W. Lowden. 1992. Audiological management and performances of adult cochlear implant patients. *Ear, Nose and Throat Journal* 71(3):117–122.

Tyler, R., N. Tye-Murray, and C. Lansing. 1988. Electrical stimulation as an aid to speechreading. *Volta Review* 90(5):119–148.

Van Tasell, D. J. 1981. Auditory perception of speech. In *Rehabilitative audiology for children and adults,* ed. J. Davis and E. Hardick. New York: Wiley & Sons.

Vaughn, G., and R. Lightfoot. 1992. Assistive listening devices and systems for adults with hearing impairment. In *Aural rehabilitation,* ed. R. Hull. San Diego, Calif.: Singular Publishing Group.

Watson, C. S., R. A. Dobie, N. Durlack, L. E. Humes, H. Levitt, J. D. Miller, C. E. Sherrick, F. B. Simmons, G. A. Studebaker, R. S. Tyler, and G. P. Widin. 1991. Speech perception aids for hearing impaired people: Current status and needed research. *Journal of the Auditory Society of America* 90(2):637–685.

Wilson, R. H., and J. K. Antablin. 1980. Picture identification task as an estimate of word-recognition performance of nonverbal adults. *Journal of Speech and Hearing Disorders* 45:223–228.

8

Speechreading

Harriet Kaplan

■ ■ ■ ■

The purpose of this chapter is to provide information about the nature and process of speechreading, its benefits and limitations to communication, as well as evaluation and methods of training as they apply to adults and adolescents. Although goals may be different in some cases, speechreading issues and methodologies tend to be similar with culturally Deaf adults and those who became deaf or hard of hearing later in life. Therefore, the two populations will not be discussed separately, but differences will be noted where appropriate.

Speechreading is a useful supplement to aided residual hearing for most hard of hearing adults and a primary mode of communication for some deaf adults. For some adults, the objective may be to understand basic English vocabulary better and to use communication strategies effectively; for others, the goals involve better understanding of connected speech in a variety of situations. In either case, speechreading training is worth pursuing, given client motivation. Culturally Deaf adults usually prefer to communicate with American Sign Language, which is not compatible with speechreading, rather than English. However, many culturally Deaf individuals are interested in developing their English skills for use in situations where they must communicate with nonsigning individuals. These culturally Deaf people can benefit from speechreading training if they are aware of its benefits to their specific communication needs and are motivated to develop their speechreading skills.

Most hard of hearing clients are interested in improving their audiovisual understanding of spoken language in a variety of situations, whereas culturally

Deaf clients who use sign language as their primary mode of communication might be interested in better understanding of vocabulary important for specific situations. For example, a Deaf client might wish to focus speechreading therapy on spoken language specific to vocational needs. It is especially important with this clientele to use materials relevant to their communication situations and to integrate speechreading with other aspects of communication training, such as the use of English idioms, pragmatic and linguistic structures, and communication strategies. As with other aspects of aural rehabilitation, speechreading is part of the integrated therapy model. It is rarely taught alone, but is usually combined with training of auditory skills, communication strategies, and English language.

What Is Speechreading?

The terms "speechreading" and "lipreading" are frequently used interchangeably. To most people, these terms mean the ability to understand speech by observing movements of the lips, tongue, and jaw. Nitchie has defined the process as "the art of understanding a speaker's thought by watching the movements of his mouth" (Jeffers and Barley 1971, 4). This definition implies that a skilled speechreader can receive a complete message from speech movements and thereby substitute vision for hearing. There are oral deaf people who are able to communicate well using speechreading or lipreading as a primary modality with or without audition as a support sense. However, other deaf or hard of hearing individuals rely on audiovisual input. Audiovisual input is more the norm than the exception, even for many profoundly deaf people. Most speechreaders integrate visual information with whatever auditory cues they are able to receive.

The basis of speechreading is correct interpretation of the movements of the lips, tongue, and jaw. Skilled speechreaders, however, depend on much more than articulatory movements. In addition to these movements, they rely on facial expressions, gestures, body language, linguistic redundancy, and clues available from the communication situation. A better definition of speechreading might be "the ability to understand a speaker's thoughts by watching the movements of the face and body and by using information provided by the situation and the language" (Kaplan, Bally, and Garretson 1987, 1). In accordance with the integrated therapy model, visual perception of the spoken word and meaningful body movements are developed in conjunction with auditory skills, communication strategies, and use of situational and linguistic clues.

Components of Speechreading

Jeffers speaks of a speechreading process that involves (a) sensory reception of speech movement patterns, (b) association of the patterns with meaningful concepts, and (c) mental "filling in" of information not received by the eyes (Jeffers and Barley 1971).

The Analytic Component

The first part of the process, sensory reception or visual proficiency, constitutes the analytic component. It involves reception and correct interpretation of all speech sounds that are at least partially visible. Although there are limitations to the visibility of the sounds of spoken English, speechreading instruction must address this component of the process to ensure that the individual is using all possible information present on the lips, tongue, and jaw.

The Synthetic Component

The association and "filling in" parts of the process constitute the synthetic component. Synthetic ability is an important part of speechreading because so many of the speech movements are not visible on the face. The ability to "guess correctly" often differentiates the poor from the skilled speechreader. The synthetic component involves the interpretation of gestures and body language as well as linguistic and situational redundancy.

Gestures and Body Language Gestures and body language are used in all cultures and may substitute for speech or supplement what the speaker says. Berger, Martin, and Sataloff (1970) and Popelka and Berger (1971) demonstrated that understanding of speech improves significantly when appropriate gestures are used and deteriorates when gestures are inappropriate (e.g., distracting movements).

Body movements and facial expressions convey mood as well as linguistic information. Raised eyebrows indicate questioning; a puzzled look suggests lack of understanding. The more expressive a speaker and the better the speechreader can interpret the nonverbal cues, the better the understanding of the message.

Linguistic and Situational Redundancy Speechreading is strongly associated with ability to use the redundancy of the language provided by the rules of the language learned as children. These rules determine which sounds are present in the spoken message, how the sounds are combined into words, and how words are combined into sentences. For example, sentences beginning with words such as *what, where, who* are often questions. Because nouns and pronouns must agree, the presence of the pronoun *she* in an utterance indicates that a subsequent word is *mother* rather than its homophene (visually similar word) *brother*. The importance of linguistic information in a communication situation increases as the amount of sensory information decreases, as in the case of the speaker who articulates poorly. The individual who knows the language does not have to receive visually all components of the spoken message in most situations to be able to understand. The mind fills in the information and does so rapidly and at an unconscious level.

Language comprehension is strongly related to speechreading ability, especially in children (Jeffers and Barley 1971; Boothroyd 1988). The relationship between language comprehension and speechreading ability does not usually hold in hard of hearing adults because a high level of language comprehension is not required to speechread average conversation (Jeffers and Barley 1971, 128). However, adults may not always use the clues provided by linguistic redundancy in communication situations.

Situational factors also provide communication redundancy. Language can be predicted to some degree based on the situation and the roles of the communicators. In a restaurant, for example, the waiter can be expected to use different language than a dinner companion. Pragmatic constraints influence what is likely to be said, thereby limiting the possibilities in a visually ambiguous situation. Specific language forms for starting and ending conversations and for turn taking are customarily used and are predictable. Some deaf individuals are not familiar with English pragmatic constraints and appropriate language forms and are limited in their ability to use these forms of communication redundancy. With such individuals, speechreading goals may include improvement in the use of English pragmatics.

Speechreading is a combination of what the eye can see (analytic skills) and what the mind can correctly fill in, based on use of linguistic and situational cues (synthetic skills). It is necessary to develop both components. A skilled speechreader is able to use whatever speech information is visible on the face (analytic) and combine it with facial expression, body language, linguistic and situational redundancy, communication strategies, and whatever auditory information is available to understand a message.

Relationship to Audition

The ability to hear some sound helps most people speechread. With properly fitted hearing aids, many deaf and hard of hearing people are made aware of the presence of sound, pauses in the flow of speech, differences in duration and stress of utterances, intonation differences that signal a question or statement, and some vowel sounds. All of these auditory features are important to meaning and produce no visible markers. When the visual and audible aspects of language are combined, there is significant increase in information. There has been a fair amount of research on the effects of hearing on speechreading by adults and older children. The research strongly supports the use of audition and speechreading together (Berger 1978; O'Neill and Oyer 1981; Sanders 1982; Garstecki 1988).

Phoneme Visibility

The sounds or phonemes of speech vary in their visibility. Some can be clearly identified by the eye (e.g., b, p, m), whereas others are not visible at all (e.g., k, g). The following discussion addresses this issue.

The Sounds of Speech: Vowels and Consonants

Vowels are stronger, longer in duration, and generally have more energy in the low frequencies than some consonants, particularly unvoiced consonants. Although vowels are easier to hear, they are more difficult to differentiate from each other on the lips. Three major lip and two major tongue positions are involved in producing the vowel sounds of English. The lip opening may be narrow as in the word *feet,* wide as in the word *far,* or puckered as in the word *too.* Lip opening may be vertical as in the word *law* or horizontal as in the word *sat.* The tongue may be raised in the front of the mouth as in the word *sit* or in the back of the mouth as in the word *suit.* Although the lip movements are visible, the tongue movements are not.

Differences between the lip and tongue movements of specific vowels of English are minimal and not dependable, particularly during rapid speech. In addition, the exact way vowels are made varies from person to person, depending on personal habits and the individual's home region or country. For all these reasons, most speechreaders use audition, if possible, or context to identify vowels.

Consonants are more difficult to hear than vowels because they are shorter in duration and weaker in sound, but as a group tend to be more visible on the face. Some consonants, however, are not visible or only partially visible because tongue movements are often not clearly visible. Consonants are particularly important for understanding of speech.

For the following discussion, sounds are written orthographically. Some consonants are made in the front of the mouth, others in the middle, and some in the back of the mouth. Some involve only the lips (e.g., p, m, w), others involve lips and teeth (e.g., f, v), and a large group involves the tongue (e.g., d, t, s, l, k). The sounds made in the front of the mouth are quite visible. Those made in the middle of the mouth may be partially visible depending on the speaker, rate of speech, lighting and distance conditions, and the specific word in which the sound occurs. For example, the l in the word *like* is more visible than the l in the word *tall* because the open mouth position allows a view of the tongue. The consonants made in the back of the mouth (k, g, h, y, ng) are not visible at all and must be inferred from context.

Some consonant movements are stable across speakers whereas others vary; for example, some speakers place the tongue between the teeth for the *th* sound, whereas others keep the tongue behind the teeth. Visibility of consonants varies with the rapidity of the speech, the precision of the speaker's articulation, and viewing conditions (lighting and distance). Sounds that are visible under ideal conditions may not be visible under more typical communication conditions in which the talker speaks at a fairly rapid rate and does not attempt to articulate precisely.

The following consonant movements tend to be more visible and more stable under typical viewing conditions:

1. *f,v*
2. *p,b,m*
3. *w,r* at the beginning and middle of words
4. the voiced and voiceless *th* sounds (e.g., *think* and *this*)
5. *sh,ch,j* as in *joke, zh* as in *measure*

The other consonants (t,d,s,z,l,r,n,k,g,h,y) and consonant blends are far more difficult to see on the lips; the speechreader must rely on context.

Homophenes and Visemes

Homophenes are sounds that look alike (e.g., p, b, m). Homopheneity further complicates visibility of spoken English. Because many sounds look alike, it is not always easy to identify the specific word a speaker is saying. For example, without context or audibility, it is impossible to distinguish between the words *pay, bay, may.* The only way to distinguish between homophenous sounds or words is by using context, either the specific sentence or the larger conversation. Consonant sounds tend to cluster into groups of homophenes. Each of these groups is called a viseme, a term coined by Fisher (1968). It is possible for a viseme to contain only one speech sound, but that is unusual. Although the members of a viseme are not visually distinctive, visemes tend to be visually distinctive from each other.

Researchers have sought to define viseme groups for years, but there is no one universal descriptive system that includes all phonemes in all contexts and visual communication settings. Factors that influence the way speechreaders assign phonemes to visemes include talker differences (Kricos and Lesner 1982; Lesner and Kricos 1981), viewing conditions (Jeffers and Barley 1971), and effects of different phonemic environments, such as consonant in word-initial position (CV), consonant in word-final position (VC), or consonant between two vowels (VCV) (Binnie, Montgomery, and Jackson 1974; Binnie, Jackson, and Montgomery 1976; Owens and Blazek 1985). For example, different phonemes look similar on the lips when comparing syllables such as *la* and *da* than when comparing syllables such as *al* and *ad.* Although studies show varying numbers of visemes and differences in the composition of specific visemes, several visemes appear to be common to all studies. Labial visemes *(b,p,m/; /f,v)*, the voiced and voiceless *th,* and *sh,ch,j,zh* seem to be relatively stable. Other viseme groupings vary widely from study to study (Jackson, 1988). Training seems to affect viseme composition. Walden, Erdman, Montgomery, Schwartz, and Prosek (1981) found significant differences between pre- and post-therapy viseme groupings, including clustering of unassigned phonemes into visemes as a function of training.

Obviously there is no one viseme grouping constant for all talkers and communication environments. Therefore, it is well to perform analytic training using a variety of talkers having different visual characteristics in a variety of communication situations. It might be well, at least early in therapy, to select a descriptive system that represents typical viewing conditions. Jeffers and Barley (1971) present a system consisting of the following six clusters:

1. p,b,m
2. f,v
3. w,r

4. voiced and voiceless *th*

5. sh,ch,j,zh

6. s,z,t,d,n,l,y,k,g,h,ng

When a speechreader becomes proficient in differentiating between these visemes, differences between *k,g,h,ng* and the remainder of viseme number six can be trained.

Although the viseme concept can be extended to vowels, Jeffers and Barley (1971) point out that most vowels look similar enough to be practically homophenous. There are only two or possibly three speech movements sufficiently stable to be of value in identifying vowels and diphthongs. These are movements that identify high front (e.g., *e* as in *feet*), high back (e.g., *u* as in *shoe*), and low back (e.g., *a* as in *far*) vowels. For the most part, vowel perception needs to depend on context.

Information Available through Speechreading

It is not possible, even for the best speechreader, to see every word on the face. There are problems related to the nature of speech, the speech habits of the talker, the speechreading environment, and the characteristics of the speechreader. Despite the fact that articulatory movements are limited by these factors, many speechreaders communicate quite well by using linguistic and situational information.

The Speech Signal

At best, articulatory movements are only partially visible. Woodward and Barber (1960) found that under typical viewing conditions approximately 60 percent of all speech sounds are either invisible or difficult to see because many speech movements occur inside the mouth. Other research has shown that under usual viewing conditions vision provides approximately one-fifth of the information available through hearing (Jeffers and Barley 1971).

In addition, homophenous words are frequently responsible for breakdowns in understanding. Berger (1972) looked at a sample of 25,000 words used in conversation and found that 33 percent had one or more homophenes. Another source of difficulty is the rapidity of normal speech. Ordinary speech averages about thirteen speech sounds per second while the eye is capable of seeing only eight to ten movements per second. When a talker speaks faster than normal, even more of the message is missed. Nevertheless, it is important to train clients to identify those components of speech that are visible and to make them aware of which sounds are homophenous so that they may better use contextual clues.

The Talker

Lip movement and the amount of mouth opening are very important factors in ease of speechreading. Some people barely move their lips, and sometimes produce careless, indistinct speech that is difficult to hear as well as to speechread. People with thin lips are generally harder to understand than those with fuller lips because speech movements are less distinctive. It is possible for a talker to barely move the lips and still produce speech that can be understood auditorily. It is also possible to produce intelligible speech using nonstandard lip movements. Irrelevant head and body movements, anything in the mouth of a person who is talking, and facial hair that covers the articulators interfere with speechreading. The talker who is easiest to speechread talks a little more loudly and little more slowly than usual without exaggerating, has clear speech movements, and uses much expression and appropriate gestures. Regardless of the difficulty a client may have speechreading a specific talker, the process becomes easier as the talker becomes more familiar. Therefore, it is advantageous to train clients to speechread a variety of talkers, including, if possible, people with whom they frequently interact.

The Environment

Environmental conditions can create problems. The farther away the talker is from the speechreader the more difficult the understanding of speech. Although distance is generally not a problem in one-to-one conversation, it can be a problem in the classroom, at a meeting, in church, or in the theater. Poor lighting impedes speechreading. The light source should be in front of the speaker but not in the eyes of the speechreader. Visual distractions such as activity occurring behind or to the side of the talker can interfere with visual concentration needed for speechreading.

Following a conversation visually as it moves from talker to talker in a group presents special difficulties because by the time the deaf person identifies the new speaker some of the information may be lost. The speechreader may not be aware of sudden change of topic. Furthermore, not all speakers in a group may be visible. Group conversation often challenges the hearing person; it is one of the most difficult situations for a person with hearing loss unless all participants are using sign language.

It is important for the speechreader to be aware of communication problems created by environmental conditions because communication strategies can be planned to overcome some of the problems. For example, distance problems can sometimes be overcome by the use of assistive listening devices (chapter 6) or by such strategies as positioning oneself close to the talker to facilitate speechreading. Other communication strategies discussed in chapter 3 can address the problems of group conversation.

The Speechreader

Visual attention is very important for speechreading; a momentary shift of attention may result in loss of important information. People vary in their ability to concentrate on the speaker's face for long periods of time. Familiarity with the language of the speaker and the topic of conversation are also important. Speechreading becomes more difficult if, for example, the speechreader's English vocabulary and grammar are limited or if the subject of conversation is unfamiliar.

Many of these limitations can be overcome by the use of the anticipatory and repair strategies discussed in chapter 3. It is wise for speechreading and communication strategies to be taught together. Use of context clues and residual hearing can compensate for visual limitations to some degree. Hearing and speechreading can be considered valuable supplements to each other.

Evaluation of Speechreading

Speechreading assessment is performed for a variety of reasons. First, it is important to determine the client's general level of functioning—e.g., whether he or she is a good, fair, or poor speechreader. A second purpose is to monitor change as a function of training; typically, tests are given at the beginning and the end of therapy. A third purpose of assessment is to provide information about proper subgrouping of individuals when speechreading training is performed with a group. A fourth assessment function is to determine which teaching methods might be most useful for a student. For example, not all students need viseme training; some students require audiovisual training using full voice, whereas others do better with minimal amounts of voice, perhaps against a background of noise. The factors to consider in speechreading assessment are discussed below.

Validity

Test validity may be defined as whether that test actually measures what it is designed to measure. A good speechreading test should evaluate how well a person speechreads in real-life situations; however, we do not know the most appropriate type of material or test format to achieve this goal. In actual conversation, one sentence logically follows another, providing contextual clues. Yet, most speechreading tests do not provide contextual cues because they consist of lists of unrelated sentences. It is possible that a person may score poorly on such a speechreading test, but use context cues and communication strategies well enough to function well during actual conversation.

Sentence speechreading tests are usually scored by giving credit for every word or every key word identified correctly. Neither word order nor understanding of sentence meaning are considered. In real life, however, it is unnecessary for a speechreader to understand every word, only enough of the material to grasp the meaning. A test that requires literal repetition may be evaluating memory rather than speechreading skill.

It is possible to construct tests that require the speechreader to view a story and then answer questions about it. This procedure is more representative of actual communication. However, examiners must agree on what makes an answer correct or whether to give partial credit.

Other issues involved in developing connected speech tests for speechreading evaluation include choosing topics and vocabulary that are universally acceptable, materials that best evaluate what a speechreader must do every day, and the appropriate language to teach. The language of most of the sentence tests is appropriate for most adults; the vocabulary is colloquial and is comparable to a third-grade reading level. However, these tests may not be suitable for adults who are unfamiliar with English idioms or English sentence structure.

Assessment of Skill Level

One purpose of speechreading assessment is to determine whether a person is a poor or a skilled speechreader. In order to do so, it is necessary to use a tool that is normed on a representative population so that it is clear what the scores demarcating the categories of poor, fair, good, and excellent mean. None of the commonly used speechreading tests are normed on hearing or hard of hearing populations, although local norms for deaf adults have been developed for the CID Everyday Sentences Test at the National Technical Institute for the Deaf (NTID) (Johnson 1976; Jeffers and Barley 1971, 115, 116, 337). Therefore, defining an individual's level of skill based on the test is questionable. When administering a test to a group, however, individuals may be rank ordered for purposes of grouping, provided the test is considered reliable.

Talker Differences

Some people are easier to speechread than others. These differences have been documented by research (Kricos and Lesner 1982; Montgomery, Walden, and Prosek 1987). There are many questions, however, concerning the proper use of speaker differences. In a testing situation, is it more appropriate to use a talker who is easy to speechread or one who is more difficult to understand? Is it better to use a male speaker, a female, an elderly person, or a child? Which type of speaker best represents the speechreading requirements of daily conversation? Perhaps a speechreading test should incorporate several different talkers.

Environmental Conditions

As with talker differences, it is unclear which environmental conditions provide the best approximation of everyday speechreading requirements. Is it best to use full-face presentation, profile or both? Should lighting and distance factors be optimal when real life situations may be less than optimal? Should live or taped testing be performed? Although live testing is more similar to real life communication, it is very difficult to maintain the consistency of presentation needed for repeated evaluations.

Measurement of Change

An important use of speechreading tests is to measure improvement as a function of therapy. Typically, comparable sentence tests are given at the beginning of therapy and at the end of the training program. The amount of improvement is defined by the change in score. Reliability issues must be considered when tests are used in this way. Test-retest reliability must be statistically established and the critical difference score (the minimal difference score that can be considered a real, rather than a chance, difference) must be known. All the other validity issues previously discussed must also be considered. When a test reveals improvement as a function of therapy, that improvement should be reflected as real life communication. Only if a test samples actual speechreading tasks that occur in real life can we feel confident about results of therapy. Following is a discussion of commonly used speechreading tests.

Sentence Tests

The most commonly used speechreading tests for adults consist of lists of unrelated sentences containing vocabulary comparable to a third-grade reading level. The sentences that vary in length from two to ten words use colloquial, everyday language. Each test has at least two highly correlated forms that allow comparison of performance under different conditions. Research has shown, however, that the various sentence tests correlate highly with each other only when they are presented by the same talker under the same conditions (Jeffers and Barley 1971). Therefore, test lists may be used interchangeably.

The oldest of the sentence tests is the Utley, consisting of two comparable forms (Utley 1946). The Utley was developed as a film test, but is commonly presented live-voice. Other comparable sentence tests are the Barley, based on CID Everyday Sentences (Barley 1964) and the John Tracy Film Test of Lipreading (Taaffe 1957). A more complete description of these tests can be found in chapter 7 of *Speechreading* (Jeffers and Barley 1971).

Another sentence speechreading test is the CID Everyday Sentences Test, which consists of comparable forms, each consisting of ten sentences scored on a keyword basis. The CID Everyday Sentences Test was originally developed as a test of auditory skills and was later adapted for visual use. Dancer et al. (1994) have been using Harris's Revised Central Institute for the Deaf (CID) Everyday Sentence Lists A and B (Harris, Haynes, Kelsey, and Clack 1961). Wilson, Dancer, and Stamper (1984) found the lists to be statistically equivalent with high inter-correlation coefficients. The CID Everyday Sentence Test correlates well with the other speechreading sentence tests (Davis and Silverman 1970; Johnson 1976). Test norms have been developed for a prelingually deaf adult and adolescent population at the National Technical Institute for the Deaf (Johnson 1976). The following functional descriptors have been given to each score range:

100–75 percent—student understands the complete message

74–54 percent—student understands most of the content of the message

53–33 percent—student understands, with difficulty, about half of the message

32–11 percent—student understands little of the content of the message, but does understand a few isolated words or phrases

10–0 percent—student cannot understand the message

The Jacobs Test (Sims and Jacobs 1976) was developed at NTID for assessment of the results of training because it was less difficult than the CID Everyday Sentences Test and seemed to be more sensitive to change. It consists of four forms of twenty sentences each that correlate well with each other.

Viseme Tests

The Binnie Test (Binnie, Jackson, and Montgomery 1976) is a consonant identification task using CV syllables (the vowel is always *a* as in *far*). The client is given an answer sheet with twenty nonsense syllable response choices; each nonsense syllable represents one of the twenty consonant stimuli used in the test. Each of the consonant stimuli is presented five times in random order, and the client must place a mark under the response option considered correct.

An item is considered correct if the response falls into the proper viseme. For example, correct responses for the stimulus *ba* would be *ba, pa,* or *ma.* The purpose of this test is to determine whether the student can differentiate between and identify visemes correctly. If a student scores highly, viseme training is probably not necessary. The Binnie Test can also identify the specific visemes in which the student needs training.

There are several problems with this procedure. First, only CV stimuli are used; performance cannot be assumed to be the same in other contexts (e.g., VC, CVC, VCV). Second, the test is generally presented under ideal viewing conditions and cannot be assumed to generalize to less ideal conditions. Third, the procedure is lengthy.

Erber (1988) developed an abbreviated form of the Binnie that he calls the Modified Binnie. Its purpose is to identify unusual lipreading errors because most people can differentiate between visemes. The Modified Binnie consists of eight consonant stimuli (j,w,b,v,voiced th,l,d,g) in a VCV context using the vowel *a* (e.g., aba). Each consonant, representing a different viseme, is presented five times in random order for a total of forty stimuli. Responses are recorded on an eight-by-eight matrix and interpreted in a manner similar to the original Binnie Test.

Continuous Discourse Tracking

An evaluation procedure called continuous discourse tracking was developed by DeFilippo and Scott to evaluate speechreading with and without a tactile aid (DeFilippo and Scott 1978; DeFilippo 1988). It is being used for receptive and expressive evaluation and therapy. Following is a description of the process used for evaluation of speechreading. The talker says part of a sentence, which the client is required to repeat verbatim. If the client makes a mistake, the talker uses a hierarchy of communication strategies until the communication breakdown is resolved. The process is timed, usually for five or ten minutes. A word-per-minute score is computed by dividing the total number of words repeated correctly by the number of minutes. The higher the score, the better the client understands.

A major advantage of the tracking procedure is that it uses connected material that provides language content. In addition to evaluation, it can be used for training of speechreading, auditory skills, audiovisual communication, and communication strategies. It can be used for pre- and post-therapy evaluation provided that similar materials and the same talkers are used. It is important that materials be motivating and within the language capability of the client.

Continuous discourse tracking has limitations, however. Scoring reflects not only the client's skill, but also the speechreadability of the talker and the difficulty of the material. The tracking procedure requires a verbatim response, which is not a natural way of communicating. Verbatim response not only presents validity issues, but also tends to reinforce analytic behavior that may be detrimental to good speechreading. Owens and Raggio (1987) developed a modified tracking procedure that accepts nonverbatim or "gist" responses. This is desirable for training purposes, but is questionable for evaluation purposes because of the difficulty maintaining consistent scoring criteria.

Other issues concerning continuous discourse tracking are: (1) written, rather than spoken language is evaluated; (2) comprehension of the message is not generally evaluated, although the tracking procedure can be modified to probe comprehension when it is used for training; (3) use of commercial material is questionable for some prelingually deaf clients because of their lack of familiarity with the English language; however, it is possible for the clinician to write material at an appropriate language and interest level, which has been done at Gallaudet University for specific clients; and (4) tracking rate may be affected if the client has poor speech because the talker may not be able to determine response accuracy. However, an alternate response system such as typing or signing can be substituted for speech.

Speechreading Training

There are three approaches to speechreading training: analytic, synthetic, or a combination of the two. Analytic training focuses on recognition of the visible movements of speech phonemes. Synthetic training emphasizes the prediction of meaning by using linguistic and situational constraints present in the communication situation.

Early speechreading methods developed in Europe and the United States in the latter half of the nineteenth and early part of the twentieth centuries were primarily analytic in nature, although all contained some synthetic components (Bunger 1952; Bruhn 1949; Nitchie 1950; Kinzie and Kinzie 1931, 1936). Many, if not most, of the speechreading training procedures have their roots in these early systems. Discussions of the history of speechreading training can be found in Jeffers and Barley (1971), French–St. George and Stoker (1988), and Kaplan, Bally, and Garretson (1987).

Analytic Methods

Most analytic activities focus on differentiation between and identification of visemes. The goal is to recognize visible movements quickly and accurately. A typical analytic exercise might start with a description of the movements for a viseme (e.g., for *ba, pa, ma* the lips come together and part quickly), follow with practice words containing the viseme, and end with a contrast between those practice words and other words containing previously taught visemes. The practice words can then be used in sentences.

Jeffers and Barley (1971) developed an exercise called "Quick Recognition Exercise" for consonant viseme discrimination, based on six consonant visemes in the initial position of words and five in the final position. Minimally paired words representing each viseme are written on the board. The teacher speaks the words in varying order. In order for the client to repeat the words in correct order, the consonants must be correctly identified.

Some speechreading teachers and clinicians feel that analytic training should be de-emphasized in favor of synthetic, language based activities. Some clinicians choose to eliminate all analytic training, whereas others include but spend relatively little time teaching visemes.

Other analytic activities involve drill, frequently in the form of games or competition, of frequently used words or phrases such as numbers, days of the week, or question words. Crossword puzzles provide a popular activity for this purpose. Such activities can be used within the same therapy program for auditory training if the client has sufficient residual hearing or for training in the linguistic use of question words. Some prelingually deaf clients can benefit from the latter type of therapy. Combining these therapy goals with speechreading is one example of integrated therapy.

Synthetic Methods

Synthetic training includes all activities involving connected speech, such as conversations, stories, or skits. The goal is to train the client to use linguistic and situational clues. Typically, proper nouns and other key words are taught in advance and the theme of the story might be discussed. After the presentation of the language material, the student responds with nonliteral or "gist" repetition, answers to questions, or the performance of some appropriate action. Literal repetition should be discouraged.

Ability to recognize and understand idioms is frequently included in speechreading training. Such activities are usually integrated with language training according to the integrated therapy model. For example, the client identifies idioms encountered during everyday experiences. The meaning of these idioms is taught, after which practice in visual and/or audiovisual recognition occurs. The client and clinician can then role play situations in which these idioms are used.

Homophene identification is part of synthetic training. Because homophenous words look identical on the face (e.g., *bay, pay, may*), students are taught to use context in selecting the correct homophene. Jeffers and Barley (1971) developed an activity called "Quick Identification Exercise" for this purpose. First, the students identify a small group of homeophenous words while observing the teacher's utterance. They must then select the word spoken by the teacher from this group by using information presented in sentences spoken by the teacher.

The constellation concept, designed as an anticipatory strategy, is an excellent approach to speechreading training (Kaplan, Bally, and Garretson 1987). A situation, either one which creates communication difficulty or one which is of interest to the client, is selected. Spoken words and phrases expected to be encountered in that situation are identified. This spoken material is used for speechreading practice. The language is then sequenced logically and presented in a dialogue by the teacher or with students participating in role plays. Speechreading training may be integrated with work on communication strategies by incorporating discussion of the dynamics of the situation (e.g., roles of the communicators, expected sequence of language, expected problems and ways of dealing with these problems). Training may take place primarily visually using minimal voice, audiovisually in quiet, or audiovisually in noise.

At the National Technical Institute for the Deaf (NTID), connected discourse exercises focus on vocabulary, sentences, and short paragraphs related to a student's academic curriculum. Materials relevant to on-the-job situations such as interviews or staff meetings are also included. Face-to-face therapy is supplemented with self instructional videotaped exercises (Jacobs 1982; Johnson and Crandall 1982)

Continuous discourse tracking, discussed earlier in this chapter as an evaluation procedure, can also be used for speechreading and communication strategies training. Relevant, appropriate materials are presented during each session and also used for homework. The tracking rate measure serves as a way of monitoring improvement. When used for training purposes, the Owens and Raggio modification (1987) requiring "gist" rather than verbatim repetition is preferable because it is a more motivating, less frustrating procedure and is more similar to typical conversation. However, a tracking rate should not be established when nonverbatim response is accepted.

Several other modifications to the traditional tracking procedure are possible. First, the student can be required to ask for strategies rather than receive them from the teacher. This procedure facilitates the teaching of communication strategies by forcing the student to use strategies as he or she would use them in actual conversation. Second, the teacher may perform a variety of pretracking activities such as:

1. Teaching all proper nouns, key words, and new vocabulary

2. Teaching the mechanics of using the various strategies

3. Having the client generate the material by using a constellation or some other procedure

4. Giving the student the topic, title, first line, or theme of the material before the tracking activity

5. Allowing the client to read through the material before initiation of tracking

Speechreading Materials

Whatever the objective of an activity, materials should be appropriate to the client's needs and interests. Language should be within the client's linguistic capability, should be related to work, academic curricula, hobbies, and current events, and should deal with difficult communication situations. The most relevant materials are written by the teacher or generated by the client. With prelingually deaf adults, it is especially important to pay attention to the appropriateness of the materials. Because their English language skills are sometimes limited, materials must be written at the proper level. In addition, they should reflect the client's experiences.

Technology Interactive video, whether in the form of videotape or videodisc, is inherently motivating. It is usually used to supplement classroom instruction or individual therapy, but can also be used by clients for home study. A clinician need not be present, and training can be scheduled at times convenient to students. Although many programs tend to be analytic in nature, there have been attempts to develop real-life simulation activities (Tye-Murray, Tyler, Bong, and Nares 1988).

Computer technology provides the versatility to control complex protocols tailored to individual needs. It makes possible an interactive learning situation in which successive stimuli are determined by previous responses. A range of stimuli (e.g., simple, overlearned utterances to more complex sentences and stories) and a variety of response formats (e.g., multiple-choice closed-set tasks and open-set identification) can be made available.

Currently, videotape instructional programs are more available than videodisc materials, probably because of the high cost of videodisc equipment and development of videodisc masters. Videodisc programs will probably become more available, however, because the type of interactive programming needed for effective training in speechreading, auditory skills, and communication strategies requires videodisc technology.

Videodiscs Tye-Murray, Tyler, Bong, and Nares (1988) developed three programs to train speechreading and assertive communication.

The goal of Program l is audiovisual consonant speechreading training using consonant vowel syllables, single syllable words, and words embedded in carrier phrases. Male and female talkers present the stimuli. An incorrect response results in repetition of the stimulus, whereas a correct response produces a visual reinforcer.

Program 2 provides synthetic audiovisual speechreading training and development of communication strategies. One of ten talkers presents a sentence. The student responds by touching one of four picture response options presented on a touchscreen. If the response is not correct, the student may select one of five repair strategies. The procedure continues until the sentence has been identified correctly.

Program 3 provides situation-specific speechreading training, using eleven exercises based on real-life situations. First, the student views a film clip establishing the setting. Then, a talker presents sentences audiovisually in closed-set format similar to that used in Program 2. If the student responds incorrectly, she selects repair strategies until she correctly identifies the sentence. Some of the talkers deliberately create difficult communication situations (e.g., chew gum, make noise).

The concepts used in Program 3 are similar to the Morkovin-Moore Training Films (Morkovin and Moore 1948). These films present conversations that might occur in daily life (e.g., the family dinner, at the bank). The films have not been widely used because they are technically poor, the talkers are not easy to speechread, and some of the scenes do not seem natural. Nevertheless, these films introduced the concept of using technology for role-playing life situations to teach speechreading.

The Dynamic Audio Video Interactive Device (DAVID) program (Sims 1988) provides speechreading drill materials dealing with familiar expressions and job-related sentences. Depending on level of performance, a student uses a multiple-choice, fill-in-the-blanks, or open-set format. Materials can be presented with or without sound. The student can request repetition or clues about sentence content.

The Auditory-Visual Laser Videodisc Interactive System (ALVIS) (Kopra et al. 1985) was developed for postlingually deaf adults. It consists of five- to eight-word sentences presented in order of speechreading difficulty. Each sentence is presented a maximum of five times, with each presentation accompanied by different auditory or visual clues.

Computer-Assisted Tracking (CAST) (Pichora-Fuller and Cicchelli 1986) is a tracking program developed for adventitiously deaf adults. It consists of paragraphs, each loaded with a particular viseme. The speechreader views the paragraph in its entirety, then types each phrase as it is viewed. The computer provides feedback, displaying the correct portion of the response and leaving blanks for misidentified words. The student has the option of asking for a replay of the phrase or going on to the next phrase in hopes of using context clues to identify the initial one. The program allows for the inclusion of other communication strategies. After a maximum of ten trials on a phrase, the missing words are filled in. The program provides positive reinforcement for a good guess based on identification of a homeophenous sound, even if the sound is not the correct phoneme.

Videotapes *Lipreading Made Easy* (Greenwald 1984) is a two-hour tape providing analytic training. It shows a speaker pronouncing words full face and profile view. It consists of eighteen lessons that may be used with a textbook of the same title.

Read My Lips (1987) is a six-tape series consisting of words, phrases, and everyday sentences. A pencil-and-paper response format is suggested. Responses in the form of open captions appear shortly after the stimuli are presented.

I See What You're Saying (1990) consists of two tapes containing words, sentences, and connected speech presented by a variety of talkers. Lessons proceed from easy to difficult, and clues are presented as needed. The tapes focus on identification of basic visible speech movements and also present strategies for understanding speech in difficult communication situations.

Speechreading Series (1990) is a series of self-instructional videotapes providing connected speech materials for speechreading practice. Materials relevant to a variety of everyday and on-the-job situations are included. Each videotape includes worksheets, scoring directions, and suggestions for individualizing instruction.

Speechreading Strategies (Palmer and Scott 1988) teaches speechreading strategies in three real-life situations: (1) checking out books in the library, (2) meeting someone for the first time, and (3) purchasing an airline ticket. Each segment is captioned and dramatized to show the consequences of not using strategies in these situations. This is followed by repetition of the same situations using appropriate communication strategies. A Teacher's Guide is included.

Speechreading videodiscs and videotapes can easily be used for integrated therapy. For example, the Tye-Murray et al. videodiscs or the Palmer and Scott videotapes use the language of real-life situations and are programmed to teach not only synthetic visual and audiovisual perception, but also communication strategies appropriate to these situations.

Summary

Speechreading is a complex skill involving more than visual perception of sound movements. It is related to knowledge and use of language redundancies, to ability to use situational clues, and to familiarity with communication strategies. Therefore, although not neglecting the analytic component, speechreading training should be primarily synthetic in nature and should be integrated with training of communication of strategies, language, and residual hearing.

References

Barley, M. 1964. CID Everyday Sentences Test of Speechreading Ability. In *Speechreading* (1971), ed. J. Jeffers and M.Barley. Springfield, Ill.: Charles C. Thomas.

Berger, K. W. 1972. Visemes and homophenous words. *Teacher of the Deaf* 70:369–399.

———. 1978. *Speechreading: Principles and methods,* 2d ed. Kent, Ohio: National Educational Press, Inc.

Berger. K. W., J. Martin, and R. Sataloff. 1970. The effects of visual distractions on speechreading performance. *Teacher of the Deaf* 68:384–387.

Binnie, C. A., P. L. Jackson, and A. A. Montgomery. 1976. Visual intelligibility of consonants: A lipreading screening test with implications for aural rehabilitation. *Journal of Speech and Hearing Disorders* 41: 530–39.

Binnie, C. A., A. A. Montgomery, and P. L. Jackson. 1974. Auditory and visual contributions to the perception of consonants. *Journal of Speech and Hearing Research* 17: 619–630.

Boothroyd, A. 1988. Linguistic factors in speechreading. *Volta Review* 90(5):77–87.

Bruhn, M. E. 1949. *Mueller-Walle method of lipreading,* 7th ed. Washington, D.C.: Volta Bureau.

Bunger, A. M. 1952. *Speech reading: Jena method,* 2d rev. Danville, Ill.: Interstate Co.

Dancer, J., M. Krain, C. Thompson, P. Davis, and J. Glenn. 1994. A cross-sectional investigation of speechreading in adults: Effects of age, gender, practice, and education. *Volta Review* 96:1, 31–40.

Davis, H., and S. R. Silverman 1970. Central Institute for the Deaf Everyday Sentences. In *Hearing and Deafness*, appendix. New York: Holt, Rinehart, and Winston.

DeFilippo, C. 1988. Tracking for speechreading training. *Volta Review* 90(5):215–239.

DeFilippo, C., and B. Scott. 1978. A method for training and evaluating the reception of ongoing speech. *Journal of the Acoustical Society of America* 63:1186–1192.

Erber, N. P. 1988. *Communication therapy for hearing-impaired adults.* Abbotsford, Victoria, Australia: Clavis Publishing.

Fisher, C. 1968. Confusions among visually perceived consonants. *Journal of Speech and Hearing Research* 11:796–804.

French-St. George, M., and R. Stoker. 1988. Speechreading: An historical perspective. *Volta Review* 90(5):17–32.

Garstecki, D. 1988. Speechreading with auditory cues. *Volta Review* 90(5):161–178.

Greenwald, A. B. 1984. *Lipreading made easy.* Washington, D.C.: Alexander Graham Bell Association for the Deaf.

Harris, J., H. Haines, P. Kelsey, and T. Clack. 1961. The relation between speech intelligibility and electroacoustic characteristics of low-fidelity circuitry. *Journal of Auditory Research* 1:357–381.

I see what you're saying. 1990. New York: New York League for the Hard of Hearing.

Jackson, P. L. 1988. The theoretical minimal unit for visual speech perception: Visemes and coarticulation. *Volta Review* 90(5):99–115.

Jacobs, M. A. 1982. Visual communication (speechreading) for the severely and profoundly hearing-impaired young adult. In *Deafness and communication,* ed. D. G. Sims, G. G. Walter, and R. L. Whitehead. Baltimore: Williams & Wilkins.

Jeffers, J., and M. Barley. 1971. *Speechreading (lipreading).* Springfield, Ill.: Charles C. Thomas.

Johnson, D. D. 1976. Communication characteristics of a young deaf adult population: Techniques for evaluating their communication skills. *American Annals of the Deaf* 121: 409–424.

Johnson, D. D., and K. E. Crandall. 1982. The adult deaf client and rehabilitation. In *Handbook of adult rehabilitative audiology,* 2d ed., ed. J. G. Alpiner. Baltimore: Williams & Wilkins.

Kaplan, H., S. J. Bally, and C. Garretson. 1987. *Speechreading: A way to improve understanding.* 2d ed. Washington, D.C.: Gallaudet University Press.

Kinzie, C. E., and R. Kinzie. 1931. *Lip-reading for the deafened adult.* Philadelphia: John C. Winston Co.

———. 1936. *Lip-reading for children.* Washington, D.C.: Volta Bureau.

Kopra, L. L., R. J. Dunlop, M. A. Kopra, and J. E. Abrahamson. 1985. Computer-assisted instruction in lipreading with a laser videodisc interactive system. Paper presented at the Computer Conference of the American Speech-Language-Hearing Foundation, New Orleans, Louisiana.

Kricos, P. B., and S. A. Lesner. 1982. Differences in visual intelligibility across talkers. *Volta Review* 86:219–225.

Lesner, S. A., and P. B. Kricos. 1981. Visual vowel and diphthong perception across speakers. *Journal of the Academy of Rehabilitative Audiology* 14:252–258.

Montgomery, A. A., B. E. Walden, and R. A. Prosek. 1987. Effects of consonantal context on vowel lipreading. *Journal of Speech and Hearing Research* 30:50–59.

Morkovin, B. V., and L. M. Moore. 1948. *Life-situations speechreading through the cooperation of senses,* 2d ed. Los Angeles: University of Southern California Press.

Nitchie, E. H. 1950. *New lessons in lipreading.* Philadelphia: J. B. Lippincott Co.

O'Neill, J. J., and H. Oyer. 1981. *Visual communication for the hard of hearing,* 2d ed. Englewood Cliffs, N.J.: Prentice Hall.

Owens, E., and B. Blazek. 1985. Visemes observed by hearing-impaired and normal-hearing adult viewers. *Journal of Speech and Hearing Research* 28:381–393.

Owens, E., and M. Raggio. 1987. The UCSF tracking procedure for evaluation and training of speech reception by hearing-impaired adults. *Journal of Speech and Hearing Disorders* 52:120–128.

Palmer, L., and L. Scott. 1987. *Speechreading strategies.* Portland, Ore.: Educational Productions.

Pichora-Fuller, M. K., and M. Cicchelli. 1986. *Computer-Aided Speechreading Training (CAST): Owner's manual.* Toronto: University of Toronto Department of Otolaryngology, Mount Sinai Hospital.

Popelka, G. R., and K. W. Berger. 1971. Gestures and speech reception. *American Annals of the Deaf* 116:434–436.

Read my lips. 1987. Mustang, Okla.: Speechreading Laboratories.

Sanders, D. A. 1982. *Aural rehabilitation,* 2d ed. Englewood Cliffs, N. J.: Prentice Hall.

Sims, D. G. 1988. Video methods for speechreading instruction. *Volta Review* 90(5):273–288.

Sims, D. G., and M. A. Jacobs. 1976. Speechreading evaluation and the National Technical Institute for the Deaf. Paper presented at the convention of the Alexander Graham Bell Association, Boston.

Speechreading series. 1990. Portland, Ore.: Educational Productions.

Taaffe, G. 1957. A film test of lip reading. *John Tracy Clinic research papers,* no. 11. Los Angeles: John Tracy Clinic.

Tye-Murray, N., R. S. Tyler, B. Bong, and T. Nares. 1988. Computerized laser videodisc programs for training speechreading and assertive communication behaviors. *Journal of the Academy of Rehabilitative Audiology* 21:143–152.

Utley, J. 1946. A test of lip reading ability. *Journal of Speech Disorders* 11:109–116.

Walden, B. E., S. A. Erdman, A. A. Montgomery, D. M. Schwartz, and R. A. Prosek. 1981. Some effects of training on speech recognition by hearing-impaired adults. *Journal of Speech and Hearing Research* 24:207–216.

Wilson, S., J. Dancer, and J. Stamper. 1984. Visual equivalency of Harris's revised CID everyday sentence lists. *Volta Review* 86:267–273.

Woodward, M. F., and C. G. Barber. 1960. Phoneme perception in lipreading. *Journal of Speech and Hearing Research* 3:212–222.

9

Speech and Voice Skills

James J. Mahshie and Antoinette S. Allen

■   ■   ■   ■

A main focus of this book is culturally Deaf individuals whose hearing loss occurred early in life (prior to significant language development) and whose primary contact with the hearing world is through vision rather than hearing. Although those people who lose their hearing later in life also experience significant speech and voice difficulties, these result from a gradual loss of voice and speech skills, rather than from a failure to develop them. Accordingly, the aims of intervention will often be quite different for these two groups of individuals. This chapter will focus primarily on those whose hearing loss occurred early in life. The reader working with clients having a late onset hearing loss is referred to a number of excellent resources, such as Alpiner and McCarthy (1987) and Hull (1982).

Aims and Orientation in Speech Mastery

The level of speech mastery attained by a deaf or hard of hearing person depends on a number of factors, including hearing status, quality of speech instruction, attributes of the language environment, degree of parental support, and cogni-

We are grateful to Lynn Rowland for her assistance in typing the tables and Melanie Glass for proofreading drafts of the manuscript.

tive/motor skills. It is not surprising, therefore, that the extent of spoken language mastery achieved by Deaf adolescents/young adults varies.

The varied skill levels of Deaf adolescents and adults is but one of a series of client attributes that clinicians must consider when developing a speech communication intervention plan. For example, when developing a therapy plan, the clinician typically considers the learner's motivation and attitude, particular speech goals, and existing skill level. Unfortunately, many of the speech-teaching strategies currently available are designed for young children. Although such instruction may be useful for the younger Deaf child, these procedures often fail to be adequate (or appropriate) for the older student or young adult.

This chapter describes a number of variables to be considered when providing useful and relevant speech instruction to Deaf adolescents and adults. In addition to providing an overview of principal factors involved in establishing the speech and voice skill goals for particular adolescents or young adults, the chapter examines the important elements of spoken language acquisition and describes a number of strategies for both evaluating proficiency and facilitating improvement.

Most current clinical models for facilitating the spoken language of Deaf individuals were developed for children. The sequence of tasks with which the child is presented is based more or less on normal development (for example, Ling 1976; Calvert and Silverman 1975). The assumption is generally made that these children will be working simultaneously on speech skills (voice, articulation, respiration, etc.) and on language skills (syntax, semantics, phonology, morphology, and pragmatics) that will ultimately be expressed through speech.

The situation is typically quite different for a deaf adolescent or adult. The intelligibility of Deaf adults' speech will range broadly, from very understandable to extremely unintelligible. Moreover, the individual's skills may not reflect the orderly acquisition suggested in the literature on teaching speech to Deaf children (for example, Ling 1976; Calvert and Silverman 1975; McGinnes 1963). The Deaf adolescent/adult may have some later-occurring skills, but not earlier ones. The individual may have fairly sophisticated understanding of certain grammatical rules (such as for plural production), but not the articulatory skills needed to express such knowledge.

In addition, many Deaf adolescents or adults have received prior aural rehabilitative services, perhaps for a significant part of their lives. In most cases, the student is approaching the later stages of therapy, with services most likely ending (or being much less accessible) in the foreseeable future. This results in a certain immediacy concerning outcomes. Whatever is taught needs to be of use in the near rather than distant future.

Because the skills and abilities of Deaf adults and children differ significantly, it is understandable that clinicians working with adult clients find approaches developed for children to be less than adequate. The adult has knowledge of and abilities in spoken communication, plus the need for more immediate use of what is taught. Thus, the approach used to teach speech skills to adult clients typically employs top-down strategies in which meaningful words and phrases are used to teach both production level skills (such as the motor patterns for articulation of /s/) as well as phonological usage skills (such as the pronunciation of various plural forms). Furthermore, the focus of intervention with adults is typically toward teaching skills and information that will facilitate more immediate, functional spoken communication. For example, a client may be travelling by plane during an upcoming holiday and may wish to improve her ability to ask a few questions concerning the flight, seating arrangements, etc. A clinician can choose vocabulary appropriate to air travel and incorporate work on production of specific speech features determined to be difficult for the client. In addition to working on the specific speech production tasks targeted for improvement, the client can also work on increasing vocabulary and the use of communication strategies. This approach thus enables work on a number of integrated therapy goals that have direct relevance to the client's life experiences.

There are circumstances, however, in which focusing on speech teaching may not be appropriate or advisable. Perhaps the most common reason for de-emphasizing speech teaching with a Deaf adolescent or adult is that the student has a low likelihood of using oral/aural communication. Should the client have minimal need for or interest in aural/oral communication in her daily life, there appears to be no professional or ethical need to provide such service. The Deaf client who reports using sign language as a primary means of communication at work, home, or during recreation, or whose speech intelligibility is low, may not be a candidate for services focusing on speech and/or voice. In instances where the prognosis for significant improvements in speech is poor, focusing on speech development activities may not be warranted. As suggested throughout this book, other skill areas can be addressed in working with the minimally or nonspeaking Deaf adult that can benefit her communication with hearing people. In working with individuals for whom the prognosis or motivation for speech development is poor, the communication professional will best serve the client by being aware not only of the individual's communication need, but also of the person's values, attitude, and motivation regarding the use of speech for communication.

An additional factor contraindicating speech intervention is lack of interest. Just as many adult Deaf individuals are interested in seeking assessment and services in the area of speech and voice, many also have no interest in such services. It is our responsibility as communication professionals, both ethically and professionally, to respect those decisions and work with each client on her own terms. This perspective suggests that, regardless of the professional's opinion concerning how a particular client may benefit from service, consideration should be given not only to the client's communication needs and assets, but also to her values, attitudes, and motivation regarding using speech and voice as a means of communication. The culturally Deaf client will often make a communication decision, as well as other life decisions, from a different cultural viewpoint than other deaf or hard of hearing clients. The individual may or may not have a desire to use spoken communication with the hearing world regardless of the oral/aural skills possessed. These individuals may feel that their communication base, rooted in a visually oriented sign/gesture language, is adequate for their anticipated life needs. Providing speech services to a client with this perspective is destined to be nonproductive and will likely alienate the adolescent so that services will less likely be sought in the future when the client's communicative needs might change or motivation to work on speech skills might be greater.

A dilemma can sometimes result for the adolescent if her stated need and motivation are at odds with school system requirements or parental wishes. More and more academic programs are beginning to recognize that speech therapy may not be for everyone and that it is of little value to force such activities on the individual. Alternatively, it may be desirable to meet with the student to discuss the motivation level for continued speech activity. Often, such activity can result in demonstrating instances in which elements of what the student can currently do (such as produce certain words important for emergencies) can be further developed. If the client is presented with a broader range of activities than may have been typical of earlier speech therapy, she may be more inclined to continue receiving services, especially with a focus more appropriate to her needs. If the adolescent is attending speech classes primarily because others (such as parents or employers) have pressured her, it may be necessary to talk with the parent or employer about his or her expectations. It may also be desirable to discuss the issues involved among the speech-language pathologist, the student, and the third party in order to establish reasonable expectations and acceptable goals for intervention. Before therapy directed at speech skill development can be expected to progress, the student or adult must be adequately motivated and must see the potential benefit. Without adequate student motivation to work on the skill areas involved in therapy, the prognosis for improvement is poor.

Assessment in Speech Mastery

As previously suggested, speech mastery by Deaf adolescents and adults can range broadly. Accordingly, the goals for speech improvement for an individual with minimal speech intelligibility will differ significantly from the goals established for an individual with highly intelligible speech. Furthermore, individuals with different degrees of speech intelligibility may find themselves in vastly different communication circumstances, resulting in quite different goals for speech. To determine an appropriate set of speech-related goals for the client, it is necessary to consider the Deaf person's present speech skill level as well as her communication contexts and needs. Assessment of skills and abilities as well as examination of the client's attitudes and motivation for speech and voice work are thus essential.

Evaluating Skills and Abilities

The aim of speech assessment is to establish: (1) the client's communication strengths and weaknesses; (2) whether attitudes and motivation are consistent with the aims of speech improvement; and (3) a set of reasonable and realistic speech teaching goals. Among the specific questions that direct an evaluation are:

1. To what degree does the speech or voice pattern demonstrated by the Deaf adult impact on the naturalness or intelligibility of her speech? (Sims, Walter, and Whitehead 1982)

2. Does the client's speech or voice pattern have a significant effect on communication?

3. What is the client's perception of the voice or speech pattern (i.e., does the client see it as a problem)?

4. Is the client truly interested in therapy or is he seeking assessment and/ or service because of parental pressure or because he has "always had speech therapy"?

5. What are the attributes of the client's residual hearing? Is the client's residual hearing adequate for development of targeted speech skills through audition? Will alternate sensory modalities need to be explored?

6. Is the client using amplification? If so, is it adequate?

7. What is the relationship between the clients' perception of speech and voice, and their production of speech and voice? (Sims, Walter, and Whitehead 1982.)

8. Which sounds/features can the client produce consistently? Inconsistently? Not at all? (Sims, Walter, and Whitehead 1982.)

9. Does the client know and use English pronunciation rules?

10. Does the client have realistic goals and expectations for speech improvement given her current skill level, motivation, time commitments, etc.?

A variety of formal and informal procedures can be used to address these questions. The following sections describe standardized and nonstandardized instruments for evaluating speech and voice skills, along with a set of informal procedures useful for evaluating the attitudes and motivation of the client as well as the client's speech and voice skills in less-structured settings.

Oral Mechanism Exam It is apparent that many of the speech and voice difficulties experienced by deaf or hard of hearing individuals are the result of their hearing loss. It's also possible, however, that other problems involving the structure and function of the speech production mechanism may contribute to and be a causative factor in the presenting speech and voice patterns of the deaf client.

The accurate differential diagnosis of speech and voice difficulties thus requires an oral mechanism examination (Creaghead, Newman, and Secord 1989). Careful examination of the oral mechanism enables the clinician to establish whether the client's speech and voice characteristics are the result of hearing loss, organic/functional deviations, or both.

Common among various published approaches to conducting an oral mechanism examination (for example, St. Louis and Ruscello 1981) is the systematic inspection of the oral structures during both speech and nonspeech activities. Examined are the structural and postural attributes of facial characteristics, the lips, teeth, tongue, and the palatal, velar, and pharyngeal regions during rest, nonspeech, and speech activities. In the event that abnormalities are observed, a medical, dental, or neurological referral is indicated.

The client's ability to produce various diadochokinetic tasks should also be assessed. Interpretation of Deaf speaker diadochokinetic rates, however, can sometimes be problematic because deaf and hard of hearing speakers often exhibit speaking rate and articulatory difficulties that prohibit production of "normal" diadochokinetic rates. That is, hearing loss often results in diadochokinetic speech patterns similar to those resulting from motor deficits. One study by Robb, Hughes, and Frese (1985) examined diadochokinetic rates of thirty adolescents ranging in age from 15;1 to 18;9 years of age with moderately severe to profound hearing loss. The subjects performed significantly slower than normal on all speech-timing tasks. In addition, the subjects showed within-group differences that appeared related to speech intelligibility and degree of hearing loss. Although Robb, Hughes, and Frese's data can be used to compare obtained diadochokinetic rates (see table 9.1), it is generally necessary to interpret diadochokinetic findings carefully and to judge deviations in these rates as significant only in cases where there are observed structural or postural difficulties that would further indicate concerns about motor intactness.

Standardized Tests Although clearly limited in number, several standardized tests have been developed to evaluate the speech skills of Deaf individuals. Other tests, though not specifically intended for use with deaf clients, can be adapted for use with this population. Table 9.2 lists a representative group of standardized tests that can be used with Deaf adolescents/adults, along with a brief indication of the information that can be obtained from each test.

Articulation. Few standardized articulation tests exist that provide adequate information about the speech production skills of deaf and hard of hearing adult clients. Many tests are designed for younger children (Goldman and Fristoe 1972), and none have been normed on Deaf students. Moreover, many "traditional" articulation tests fail to evaluate suprasegmentals, evaluate only a limited subset of vowels, and evaluate consonants in only limited contexts.

The most commonly used speech (articulation and voice) evaluative tools for the Deaf population are Ling's Phonetic and Phonologic Assessments (Ling 1976). These instruments are primarily used with children and purport to ad-

Table 9.1 Syllable String Production Time (in Seconds) and Mean Syllable Duration Values (in Milliseconds) for Thirty Hearing-Impaired Adolescents

Syllable	Total Time (sec) (SD)	Syllable Duration (msec) (SD)
pʌ	5.2 (1.7)	25.8 (10.2)
tʌ	5.7 (1.9)	28.1 (9.8)
kʌ	6.2 (1.3)	30.9 (11.2)
pʌtʌ	9.7 (2.8)	64.6 (18.9)
pʌtʌkʌ	10.8 (3.7)	107.9 (37.6)

Note: Scores represent time required for twenty repetitions of monosyllables (pʌ, tʌ, kʌ), fifteen repetitions of a bisyllable (pʌtʌ), and ten repetitions of a trisyllable (pʌtʌkʌ).
Source: Robb, Hughes, and Frese 1985.

dress sounds segment acquisition from a developmental perspective. The goal for a Deaf adult, however, may be production of a restricted vocabulary or speech that can serve functional needs for the individual. Focusing solely on developmental sequences of sounds without reference to the segment's impact on speech intelligibility may not be most appropriate for adult clients. It is possible, however, to use already established tools (not necessarily normed on the Deaf population) to assess the articulation and voice skills of the adolescent and adult Deaf population. Although norms from these tests obviously cannot be used, the instruments do provide an organized and systematic way of sampling and analyzing speech.

The Fisher-Logemann Test of Articulation Competence (FLTAC) (1971) provides an easy-to-use format for evaluating articulation, and permits analyses of speech errors in several different ways. The test permits assessment of consonants and vowels, at both the word and sentence level, and allows the clinician to delineate error patterns by manner, place, and/or voicing at both the word and sentence levels. This provides useful information about error patterns and possible sources of articulation difficulties (at the word or sentence level) that might need attention during therapy. The test further enables examination of errors by

Table 9.2 Formal Speech Measures That Can Be Used with Deaf Adolescents and Adults

Test	Information
Andrew's Voice Evaluation (1988)	Parameters of voice including intensity, pitch, quality, environmental factors
Fisher-Logemann Test of Articulation Competence (1971)	Production of consonants and vowels at the word and sentence level
Fundamental Speech Skills Test (1990)	Breath control, voice quality, pitch control, suprasegmental production, and overall intelligibility Developed specifically for deaf and hard of hearing populations
Goldman-Fristoe Test of Articulation (1972)	Production of consonants in words and short passages; for use with the KLPA to determine phonological patterns
Khan-Lewis Phonological Analysis (1986)	For use with the GFTA to determine phonological patterns and their degree of severity
Ling Phonetic Level Speech Evaluation (1976)	Production of suprasegmentals and segmentals of speech Developed specifically for deaf and hard of hearing populations
Ling Phonologic Level Speech Evaluation (1976)	Use of suprasegmentals and segmentals at the phonological level Developed specifically for deaf and hard of hearing populations
National Technical Institute for the Deaf Voice and Speech Examination (1975)	Parameters of voice including intensity, pitch, quality, prosody, rate, breath support, and overall intelligibility Developed specifically for deaf and hard of hearing populations

production features (manner, place, and voicing) that can be of value in identifying patterns of misarticulations across different phoneme segments or contexts (for example, deletion of final plosives or overocclusion of fricative consonants). Knowledge of such patterns can subsequently be used to develop efficient intervention strategies.

The Goldman-Fristoe Test of Articulation (GFTA) (1972), although not normed on an adult or Deaf population, provides information on errors during production of isolated words and a means of evaluating those same segments at the conversational level (during a story-telling activity). This again enables the clinician to compare production patterns in both isolated words and in sentences. Furthermore, when the GFTA is used in conjunction with the Khan-Lewis Phonological Analysis (KLPA) (1986), the clinician can determine what phonological processes are present, to what degree (limited, within normal limits, excessive) they are used in the oral language production, and what effect use of that process has on overall intelligibility.

Voice. Voice and prosodic speech skills can be evaluated using measures that have been standardized on this population. The National Technical Institute for the Deaf (NTID) Voice and Speech Examination (Subtelney, Orlando, and Whitehead 1981) permits evaluation of a number of different speech attributes by a trained listener. Based on a reading of the Rainbow Passage (Fairbanks 1960), the listener assigns a 1 (severe problem) to 5 (no problem) rating to describe the client's ability to control pitch, loudness, breath stream, prosody, rhythm, nasal resonance, and overall intelligibility. Although norms for deaf speakers are not provided, results from the NTID Voice and Speech Examination can be used to establish goals for nonsegmental aspects of speech, as well as other fundamental aspects of speech production, such as breath stream support and control.

More recently, the Fundamental Speech Skills Test (FSST) (Levitt, Youdelman, and Head 1990) has been developed to permit standardized sampling and evaluation of deaf individuals' "fundamental" speech skills. The test is divided into four sections designed to assess general production skills (such as breath control, voice quality, etc.), pitch control (variability and overall pitch level), suprasegmental production (stress, intonation patterns, etc.), and spontaneous speech (evaluation of all skills during less-structured activities). Although norms are provided for children and adolescents to age twenty, the test can also be used as a criterion referenced test. (See table 9.2.)

Nonstandardized Assessment Instruments *Articulation.* Although certain formal tests are structured to obtain articulatory information during more- and less-structured speaking tasks, it is often the case that formal testing offers a somewhat different picture of speech production ability than is observed during conversational speech. For this reason, it is necessary to examine speech patterns during less-structured, more spontaneous speech activities. These can involve reading of standard or phonetically balanced passages such as the "Grandfather" (VanRiper

Table 9.3 Sample Scoring Worksheet for Speech Stimulus Material

Name:
Date:

Bob goes to the same vacation place every summer. He sleeps in a tent in his sleeping bag. He gets up at five-thirty in the morning to see the sunrise and go fishing at the trout pond. If the fish are biting well, he catches about ten fish in one day. After lunch he rides his bicycle to the top of Fossil Mountain. He believes he can see for more than fifty miles. After Bob gets back to camp he takes a nap under the tall oak tree. When he wakes up he cleans his fish and cooks them over the fire. After dinner he drinks his coffee with sugar and thinks about his good day.

√	Bob	√	about
√	goes	d/n	ten
mb/m	same	√	fish
√	vacation	√	day
√	place	ʃ/tʃ	lunch
√	every	√	top
d/s; mb/m	summer	√	Fossil
√	sleeping	√	believes
√	bag	√	camp
√	at	dn/n	nap
√	five	√	under
√	morning	√	tall
√	sunrise	√	oak
√	fishing	θ/ð	them
√	pond	√	dinner
v/f	if	v/f	coffee
√	biting	√	sugar
t/tʃ	catches	√	thinks
		√	good

Note: Client's errors include those involving difficulty with velopharyngeal control, manner of production, and voicing.

1954), "Rainbow" (Fairbanks 1960), or "Bob Goes on Vacation" (see table 9.3 appendix 9A) passages; describing a picture sequence, or producing spontaneous speech.

The clinician can examine samples of less-structured speech and can note patterns of articulation that might be consistent or inconsistent with more formalized assessment instruments. For example, the client might produce final /s/ patterns appropriately in isolation or on a formal articulation test, but omit final /s/ segments in less-structured speech. For this client, the focus of intervention might be on phonological usage of the articulatory patterns. Articulatory errors that are consistent between the two tasks, however, would suggest working on basic motor production skills as a precursor to activities aimed at teaching appropriate linguistic use of that pattern.

Pronunciation. One of the difficulties in evaluating the articulation abilities of Deaf clients is the confounding of assessment of articulation skills and the individual's knowledge of English pronunciation rules. For example, a Deaf client may experience difficulty producing /ʒ/ in the utterance "measuring cup" when the target is presented as a written word. The difficulty may be due to the individual's limited ability to articulate that segment or to a limited understanding of the rules for pronouncing the "s" in this word. It is thus extremely important to evaluate the client's skills and, if needed, establish appropriate goals for improving pronunciation skills (see chapter 10 for a detailed description of the evaluation and teaching of pronunciation skills).

Voice. It is important to evaluate voice and suprasegmental speech skills both during structured or rehearsed speaking activities and during spontaneous speech. (More will be said later about procedures that can be used to elicit spontaneous speech.) Such speech samples can be informally evaluated for various voice qualities using the NTID Speech and Voice Evaluation (Subtelney, Orlando, and Whitehead 1981) or other more ad hoc inventories of voice and suprasegmental speech attributes. An excellent framework for evaluating voice and suprasegmental parameters obtained in less-structured settings is the Andrews Voice Evaluation (AVE) (Andrews and Summers 1988). The AVE evaluates respiration, phonation, resonance, rate, high risk factors, and interpersonal factors, including motivational, environmental, and social-emotional factors that may have an effect on voice.

The AVE is particularly useful for evaluating speaking rate. Often, decreased ability to monitor one's own speaking rate through audition will result in a client speaking at an excessively fast rate. It should also be noted that continuous monitoring of rate or focus on "speech skills" over the years can also cause a client to produce spontaneous speech in a very slow and laborious manner, which can have a negative impact on overall intelligibility.

Intelligibility In addition to information about specific articulatory patterns used by a Deaf or hard of hearing adult, measures of overall speech intelligibility are extremely important. Intelligibility ratings provide a barometer of overall speech usefulness and are important in establishing realistic therapy goals for the client. Reading passages or spontaneous speech can be useful for obtaining a crude measure of speech intelligibility (for example, the NTID Speech Intelligibility Scale [Subtelney, Orlando, and Whitehead 1981]). Although ordinal-interval rating scales applied to reading passages or spontaneous speech can be used to obtain a general picture of speech intelligibility, some concern has been expressed about the appropriateness of such scales for rating intelligibility (Schiavetti, Metz, and Sitler 1981). Alternative procedures, involving use of more sophisticated scaling methods, can provide more valid information, but there are currently no formal instruments that incorporate such scaling of intelligibility. It may be necessary to use less than optimal procedures until better instruments are available.

Receptive Skills and Their Role in Speech and Voice Teaching To achieve changes in speech production that are communicatively useful, Deaf or hard of hearing clients must develop both a means of understanding the correct production targets and a means of monitoring her own productions (i.e., feedback). If the client has adequate auditory capabilities, these can be used for speech monitoring. If the client has reduced auditory capabilities, then alternative approaches, such as the use of the sensory aids described below, may be needed. It is thus important to have a fairly comprehensive picture of the client's receptive skills (hearing acuity, ability to perceive speech, speechreading ability, etc.). Of course, a clear understanding of the client's auditory or speechreading abilities will also be useful in developing goals for auditory training or speechreading intervention.

Audiometric evaluation. Developing speech and voice skills will require some means of monitoring production attempts and of developing models of what is to be produced. Although there is no simple or direct relation between the ability to perceive and produce a speech feature, understanding the client's audiogram, and having information about the client's ability to discriminate speech features are important for effective and efficient speech teaching. For example, a client presenting substantial low-frequency hearing but limited high-frequency hearing might be expected to have difficulty hearing and monitoring many consonant segments. Further assessment of speech discrimination ability may reveal significant ability to discriminate certain high-frequency consonants and difficulty discriminating others. The audiometric information can collectively provide the clinician with some insight into the best modality for introducing and facilitating improved production of a particular segment.

It is also important to have a clear idea of the client's potential for use of amplification and to ensure that the adult client is properly fitted with amplification. It is therefore necessary to evaluate the client's perceptual skills and examine how those abilities affect the production of oral language. A recent and complete audiometric evaluation is an essential first step. It should provide information on both hearing acuity and on the client's ability to discriminate and identify speech. If this information is not available, it should be obtained because it will be necessary to establish the extent that audition can be relied on for speech monitoring (see chapter 7).

Many times, the routine audiometric examination does not provide sufficient information for establishing speech-teaching strategies. It may be necessary to obtain additional information about receptive abilities, particularly those skills related to perception of speech stimuli. The Test of Auditory Comprehension (TAC) (1979), though normed on populations age four to seventeen, provides valuable information about auditory-functioning level. The test assesses a range of auditory skills from awareness of sound to comprehension of auditorily presented information in background noise. Earlier subtests assess suprasegmental discrimination, proceeding from gross differentiation between speech and nonspeech stimuli to discrimination among various speech phrases differing in rhythm, stress, and intonation patterns. Subsequent subtests assess discrimination and memory-sequencing abilities for messages containing one, two, and four linguistic elements. Later subtests measure comprehension of simple stories through event sequencing and comprehension of complex stories through detail recall. The final subtests assess auditory figure-ground abilities by presenting simple and complex stories in a background of competing speech noise.

Speechreading. The client's speechreading skills also need to be assessed. This will provide information regarding how much speech information the client can receive via the visual mode. This assessment is also relevant to development of speech and voice production skills because it provides insights about the client's awareness of the visible aspect of how sounds are formed. Standardized measures can be obtained from synthetic tools such as the CHABA Sentences for Speechreading and Auditory Discrimination Evaluation (Alpiner and McCarthy 1987), which assesses comprehension of a series of unrelated sentences. The sentences are typically presented in three ways: visually only, auditorily only, and visually-plus-auditorily. Alternative speechreading tests include the Craig Speechreading Test (1971), which evaluates word and sentence recognition in a format specifically developed for children, and the Binnie Lipreading Test (Binnie, Jackson, and Montgomery 1976), an analytical tool that assesses the client's ability to distinguish differences in basic lip movement patterns. Additional information about the adult client's speech reading abilities can be obtained through nonstandardized techniques such as tracking (DeFilippo 1988), use of constellations (Kaplan, Bally, and Garretson 1987), and informal speechreading assessment involving situation-specific vocabulary, sentences, etc. Additional discussion of speechreading evaluation can be found in chapter 8.

Evaluating Attitude and Motivation through Informal Evaluation

Clients who have indicated that they want their speech and voice skills assessed generally have a reason for seeking services. It is thus important to address the question of what communication needs brought the Deaf client to seek services at this time (see chapter 4 for additional details). Reasons may vary and can have an impact on the overall prospect of speech improvement. Possibly, the client may want to improve communication with hearing family or friends, or she may want a better understanding of her current speech skills.

It is also important that the client receive a clear picture of her current speech intelligibility and a realistic prognosis for the future. It is interesting that many Deaf adolescents and adults have a somewhat distorted view of their speech intelligibility. In some cases, the Deaf adult may view her speech as more intelligible than it really is, whereas in other cases the client may actually view her speech as less intelligible than does the clinician. Overestimating one's own speech intelligibility may be the result of prior therapy experiences in which feedback about improved ability for a specific speech task (such as producing a particular segment or a suprasegmental pattern) was interpreted by the learner as meaning that her speech was intelligible. Clients have often not been given information regarding what their previous speech-language clinician used as the basis for the "good speech" evaluation reported to the client. Alternatively, the client's life experiences may have led her to feel her speech is less intelligible than the clinician suggests.

The above assessment procedures can provide a reasonable picture of the Deaf adult's speech production skills in fairly constrained settings. There may be differences, however, between speech behaviors exhibited during fairly restricted recitation or picture-naming tasks and those observed in speech produced more spontaneously. For this reason, it is extremely important to evaluate speech under conditions in which the student is required to speak with decreasing amounts of structure in the communication interaction. It is also extremely important to obtain information about the client's attitudes, motivation, and expectations about speech therapy. Therapy goals must be reasonable and consistent with the client's availability and motivation.

Given below is a series of approaches that can be used to gain information about the client's skills in less formal settings and to obtain information concerning the client's attitudes about and motivation for speech improvement.

Gathering Information through the Interview Most clinicians rely on an interview to obtain information directly from the client about her motivation and attitudes toward speech that might have an impact on therapy. Questions are directed toward certain background factors such as educational history, therapy history, age at onset, etc. An additional goal of the interview is to establish the client's goals and assessment of her own skills. Equally important during the interview is to establish the client's motivation to focus on spoken English. Finally, the interview provides an opportunity to examine the client's spoken language capabilities in a setting other than the highly structured therapy situation.

Success in developing speech skills requires a positive view toward speech and spoken communication. It is thus important to assess the student's motivation for being in therapy and her perceptions about her own communication strengths.

Clearly, the reason for being in communication therapy varies from person to person. Among the questions that are important for evaluating the student's motivation are:

Why is the student attending therapy?

What are the student's vocational plans?

What does the student see as primary reasons for improving spoken language skills?

How does the student perceive her spoken language skills?

How would the student characterize the reactions of hearing people to her attempts at communicating through spoken language?

In some cases the student may be involved in spoken language classes or therapy because it is required either by the school or because the parent has requested such services. In the event that this is the only reason for enrolling in therapy, it may be necessary to counsel the student and to establish what aspects of spoken language communication might be important to her and what aspects would be consistent with her existing skills, vocational goals, etc. Additional information about informational counseling is offered in chapter 4.

It is also important to establish the student's own perception of her communication via speech. This may involve establishing the degree of success she has experienced in her communication exchanges and her perception of how others react to her attempts to communicate through spoken language. Do others appear impatient, frustrated, or angry when the student attempts to communicate through speaking? Such negative reactions will impact on the student's willingness to use her skills.

Gathering Information through Role Playing Although the information obtained thus far certainly provides a picture of the individual's spoken language, it is an incomplete one, lacking information about how well the individual uses these skills for actual communication in face-to-face interactions. In addition to evaluating skills in isolation, it is necessary to examine speech skills in the context of other skills and in more- or less-structured settings. The discussion below will focus on assessment strategies that examine speech in the context of other communication skills.

Role playing is a useful tool for examining spoken communication skills in a more realistic setting. Through role playing, it's possible to simulate different communication interactions and to structure the interactions so that one is assured that various attributes of the individual's spoken language have been sampled. Thus, role playing permits evaluation of skills and abilities in different settings as well as the use of strategies and discourse rules described elsewhere. The degree of passive or aggressive behavior, the client's perception of his degree of success and comfort with spoken language interactions, and the accuracy and appropriateness of the spoken language produced by the individual during actual interactions can all be evaluated through well-structured role playing.

Several guidelines should be observed in role playing:

1. *The key to successful role playing is selection of realistic situations.* It is important to select situations for role playing that the student is likely to experience. Going to a favorite restaurant, a job interview, or a visit to a doctor are among the kinds of situations that are useful, real-world situations that can be simulated through role playing. Often, the most productive situations can be established by asking the student for situations in which they feel more or less comfortable communicating.

2. *Be clear about the parameters or dimensions to be evaluated during role playing.* Based on the specific aim of the assessment, the clinician should structure the role-playing situation to ensure that an opportunity to use particular skill areas will be provided. For example, if the goal is to establish the extent of assertiveness or for the student to use appropriate repair strategies, then the clinician can set up a situation that will require use of these skills. If the clinician wishes to see how articulation and voice production are affected by communication pressures (an impatient listener, for example), then she can include such elements in the exercise.

3. *Switching roles can help evaluate the client's motivation and attitude.* It's possible to gain insight into the client's feelings by asking her to assume the role of the impatient listener, for example. Through role switching, the clinician gains insight into the client's perception about her own speech and can reflect attitudes that might not be evident through questions or other more direct assessment strategies.

4. *The use of video taping can also be of value.* There is often considerably more diagnostic information available in a role-playing situation than can be evaluated during the actual activity. Video recordings can be examined "off-line" and can serve as a useful self-evaluation tool during subsequent therapy designed to improve communication in these situations.

Summary: Informal Evaluation and Intervention

Informal assessment procedures can provide a picture of speech skills during less-structured speech tasks and also offer a glimpse of the student's attitude and motivation about speech communication and her speech communication skills. The interview and role playing can provide the clinician with an opportunity to evaluate the client's spoken language in a setting less structured than that associated with formalized testing. By recording these interactions it is possible to use the various tools mentioned earlier to assess the voice and articulation patterns evidenced in these less formal settings.

The above section has provided an overview of assessment tools and procedures that can be used to evaluate the articulation and voice characteristics of Deaf adolescents/adults. Particular emphasis has been given to nonstandardized and informal procedures that can provide useful diagnostic information about both the client's attitudes about spoken communication and about her specific skills and abilities in various speech areas across a variety of settings.

Goals and Intervention Strategies

Once the diagnostic information has been obtained, the clinical findings must be translated into reasonable and appropriate clinical goals for the client. The following section examines basic tenets and strategies for developing clinical goals for Deaf adults.

Clinician Considerations in Establishing Goals for Therapy

Following assessment, effective intervention requires establishing goals that are consistent with both the client's reasons for seeking therapy and with her current skills and abilities. Because of the special considerations that exist in working with adolescents and adults, certain basic tenets should be considered in establishing goals for therapy: (1) intervention should be directed toward development of functional speech—language based and directed toward more immediate communication; (2) therapy also should be directed toward refinement of skills for which the student has some demonstrated capability; (3) the student should be aware of how best to use the skills currently acquired; (4) specific skills (speechreading, articulation, voice, etc.) are addressed to the extent that each area impacts on the student's overall communication; and (5) therapy should be ultimately directed toward integrated actual communication. (See figure 9.1.)

These tenets translate into establishing a teaching sequence that focuses not only on which skills are to be taught (and which prerequisite skills the individual already has), but also on the context in which the skills will be used. Thus, therapy directed toward a particular skill area will initially be dealt with in a very structured and predictable context. Drills will be used, but as quickly as possible the student will begin working on that skill at the word or phrase level. The ultimate end-point for therapy, however, is spoken communication in unstructured settings so that the skill will be useful in conjunction with other specific speech and language skills needed for spoken communication (such as speechreading, use of appropriate vocabulary, accurate pronunciation, etc.). Efforts will initially involve individual skills, with skills being integrated and intervention contexts less structured as the student progresses. This intervention framework approaches intervention in an integrated way, yet maintains an understanding of the specific skills ultimately required for communicating.

For example, teaching the client to produce utterances for conveying plurals and possessives would first require establishing the existence of prerequisite skills (such as adequate breath stream support, awareness of articulatory placement for the apical fricatives /s/ and /z/, awareness of continuant versus noncontinuant segments, etc.). Once prerequisite skills are established, the client will work toward production of the segments in isolation, then in VC combinations. Very quickly, the client will be directed toward production of real words in meaningful contexts to express plurality and possession. Once adequate and stable production of the intended articulatory patterns is achieved, the client will be given an

SKILL HIERARCHY AND INTEGRATION

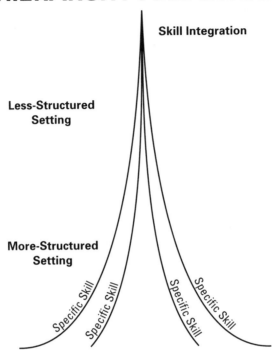

Figure 9.1. Hierarchical relationship between specific and integrated skills
Note: As specific skills are developed, they should then be integrated with other skills and their use in real communication situations facilitated.

opportunity to produce the patterns in settings with decreasing structure, such as those created in script reading, role playing, and assignments outside of the therapy session. This will facilitate self-monitoring and accurate production of the target patterns as the structure of the communication setting decreases. Finally, therapy might also be directed toward teaching the client about the English rules for forming plurals and possessives, as well as the pronunciation rules involved in correctly producing these structures when encountered in a written form.

Client Considerations in Establishing Goals for Therapy

Working with a Deaf adult also provides the opportunity to examine the client's own impressions of her production strengths and weaknesses. The client brings perceptions based both on feedback from previous therapy (such as "good speech") and on her experiences in using speech to communicate. Understanding the client's perception of her speech communication strengths and difficulties and understanding her personal goals for speech improvement can play an extremely important role in motivating the client. For example, findings from voice and speech assessment may reveal difficulties in reception and production of consonant voicing during conversation. These findings can be related to the client's perception that people very often misunderstand certain words that she produces. As the client provides examples of instances in which she experiences difficulty communicating, these should be related to clinical findings, and these "connections" should then be discussed with the client. The clinical evaluation thus has a direct relationship to the client's evaluation of what she is experiencing. It is important to make these connections because the assessment process then becomes a joint venture as opposed to something "being done to/for" the client.

Establishing Congruence of Self-Evaluation and Clinical Evaluation

In establishing realistic goals, it is imperative that the adult client be an active participant in setting the ultimate goals for intervention. It is often a useful activity to have clients describe both their perception of their communication strengths and weaknesses, and their "list" of goals for therapy. The clinician and client can then discuss and compare client aims with the outcome of that assessment. It is the responsibility of the clinician to discuss with clients what they can realistically expect to achieve based on those findings, particularly in the available time frame during which the client will be receiving services. Mutually acceptable goals for therapy that will likely lead to progress can thus be generated.

Individualizing Intervention Strategies

As mentioned earlier, there is much greater variability among Deaf adults' speech skills than one is likely to encounter in younger children. Such variability is due to differences in auditory experiences, English language acquisition, hearing capacity, and the instructional goals that each individual experiences throughout her earlier education. Accordingly, the goals established for a particular client are very much dependent upon her current status.

In addition to considering the adult's current speech production abilities, it is important to examine the likely therapy endpoint for the client before establishing speech goals. If the student is a senior in high school, with marginal speech skills, it's not likely that she will establish fluent, intelligible speech prior to the termination of school-based therapy. Although automaticity may not be the goal for this individual, it is possible that more functional goals aimed at use of limited and practiced vocabulary for specific communication circumstances (emergency situations, going to the doctor's office, etc.) can be achieved in the available time. The goal of intervention for functional speech is thus producing specific utterances rather than being able to accurately produce all sounds in all contexts.

General Approach to Voice and Articulation Therapy

Following establishment of appropriate objectives for speech production, the clinician and client begin to address these objectives through therapy. Although basic skill areas need to be addressed before being applied to more advanced areas, efforts will likely be most productive if they are primarily directed toward functional speech. A "functional" focus does not mean that "prerequisite" skills, knowledge, and ability are not needed before tackling certain aspects of spoken language. For many adult clients, however, drills aimed at establishing automatic speech patterns—those that "take[] conscious attention to produce . . . inaccurately" (Ling 1976, 89)—may have to be abandoned if it appears the Deaf client will not be able to achieve this level of mastery. In such clients, the goal will not be to establish speech skills that can be used for spontaneous conversation, but rather speech skills that will be effective for specific circumstances or situations. For example, if the client expresses interest in using expressive speech to enable use of spoken communication on the job, then efforts will be directed toward vocabulary and speechreading sentences likely to be encountered in this context. Such goals are directed at "functional speech," and will be the focus of much of the discussion that follows.

Articulation

Teaching articulatory skills generally follows three steps: (1) developing cognitive and sensory awareness of the pattern to be produced; (2) eliciting the correct segment in limited contexts; and (3) facilitating more automated and linguistically appropriate use of the articulatory pattern during speech.

Although it is clearly beyond the scope of this chapter to describe in detail the teaching strategies for eliciting production of individual segments, a number of excellent references can be used: Ling (1976) and Edwards (1992). The following provides a general description of activities that can be employed along with a brief description of the rationale for these activities.

Developing Sensory Awareness It is almost always the case that the adult learner must be adequately prepared for the task to be taught. This involves some degree of cognitive preparation, such as description of the articulators involved, the appropriate pattern of breath stream support, explanation of the anatomical bases for production of the target sequence, etc. Consonant sounds can be described in terms of their articulatory features, voicing, manner, and placement (see table 9.4). Such instruction can be extremely valuable because it prepares the

Table 9.4 Voicing - Manner - Placement Worksheet

NAME: AB Client   DATE: _____

	Voicing			Manner			Placement					
	Voice	No Voice	Nasality	Stops	Continues	Glides	Teeth	Lips	Tongue	Hard Palate	Soft Palate	Nose
b	✓			✓				✓				
d	✓			✓					✓	✓		
f		✓			✓		✓	✓				
g	✓			✓							✓	
h		✓			✓				✓	✓		
j	✓				✓				✓	✓		
k		✓		✓					✓	✓		
l	✓				✓				✓	✓		
m	✓		✓			✓		✓				✓
n	✓		✓			✓			✓	✓		✓
p		✓		✓				✓				
r	✓				✓				✓	✓		
s		✓			✓		✓		✓	✓		
t		✓		✓					✓	✓		
v	✓				✓		✓	✓				
w	✓					✓		✓			✓	
y	✓					✓			✓	✓		
z	✓				✓		✓		✓	✓		
ch		✓		✓					✓	✓		
ng	✓		✓						✓		✓	✓
sh		✓			✓				✓	✓		
th		✓			✓		✓		✓	✓		
TH	✓				✓		✓		✓	✓		

Note: Checked areas are used by this client to produce each sound.

Source: Therapy material developed by Scott Bally and Paula Bohn, Gallaudet University.

client (at least in a cognitive sense) to produce the needed attributes for the targeted segment.

In addition, the client should be adequately prepared to perceive in any way possible the target patterns to be achieved. This requires some consideration of the client's auditory capabilities. In the event that auditory perception is unlikely, then alternative sensory modalities (tactile devices or visual displays) should be considered.

Three advantages to the client in beginning work on articulation skill development in this way include:

1. The client develops an appreciation for similarities and differences among different phoneme categories and learns that commonalities can be used as "cues" when trying to produce certain phonemes.

2. The learner is provided a reference point for the future concerning how specific phonemes should or should not be produced.

3. The client is presented a bridge to English pronunciation, which will likely be addressed in the course of improving the client's articulation skills in communicative speech.

Following adequate preparation, activities can be directed at production of the pattern in limited phonetic contexts. For more functionally oriented therapy, the use of real words (that contain the targeted context) is appropriate. Once the pattern is mastered in a limited context, then therapy can be aimed at both expanding the contexts in which that pattern can be produced acceptably and using the segment in less-restricted communication contexts.

Pronunciation and Phonology The ability to produce a correct articulatory pattern is of limited value if the speaker is not aware of the use of that pattern in communicative speech; however, words that will be the target of therapy may have little correspondence between their written and articulated forms. Thus, the word "shoe" is articulated as /ʃʊ/, with four letters corresponding to two sound segments. Pronunciation of vowels can also be confusing when based on the written form (for example, the "a" vowel in "Kate," "cat," and "far" is articulated differently). Very often, differences among the letters "b" or "f" or "g" and the phonemes /b/ or /f/ or /g/ can cause problems for an individual attempting to work on production of these phonemes. It will thus often be necessary to explore the sometimes confusing relationship between graphemes (the written form) and phonemes (the spoken form). Work on pronunciation skills with Deaf adolescent/adult clients will sometimes parallel functional work on articulation; at other times, however, pronunciation should be addressed within its own domain. Although chapter 10 addresses the specifics of pronunciation work with this population, it is important to recognize that articulation improvement and pronunciation activities are inextricably related to each other.

Suprasegmentals and Voice

Suprasegmental or prosodic features can play an important role in producing intelligible speech. In addition to conveying differences among different types of sentences (questions versus statements) and altering meaning through linguistic stress, suprasegmentals also play an important role in the listener's ability to extract meaning from the acoustic stream.

Common suprasegmental and voice-related speech production difficulties experienced by Deaf individuals include production of speech at inappropriate rates, prosodic errors, and abnormal voice quality (Osberger and McGarr 1982). Although rate of speech and prosodic features can be addressed through production of single or multisyllabic words, improvement in production of these suprasegmental features is most effective when it is directed toward actual speaking tasks in real communication situations. As soon as possible, the adult client should be given an opportunity to appropriately utilize rhythm and rate during conversational activities.

Voice Quality Successful remediation of voice difficulties also requires work on both sensory and production learning. Initial sensory learning activities focus on the client identifying what aspects of her voice feel like (using tactile sensations), sound like (using residual hearing), and/or look like (using visual aids).

As was suggested for development of articulation skills, suprasegmental production activities should initially focus on establishing the client's cognitive awareness of production goals. Review of the anatomy and physiology of respiration can provide a useful starting point for improving production. Although this strategy may not be the most appropriate for younger children, it is extremely important that the adult client be provided information about the underpinnings of the patterns to be produced. Clinical experience suggests that breathy or tense voice patterns, or other more postural voice abnormalities, should be addressed first (Stevens, Nickerson, and Rollins 1983). For improvement of breath control and controlled respiration, techniques such as working on diaphragmatic breathing and establishing a supportive posture can be used.

Loudness Production of speech with appropriate loudness is also a common speech production goal for this population. It is important to describe the ways that loudness can be controlled and offer concrete strategies for increasing loudness, such as initiating speech at slightly higher lung volumes than would be used for normal conversational speech. In conjunction with such production skills, work will also involve learning to monitor loudness using combinations of tactile and auditory feedback. Finally, the client can be given information about appropriate loudness levels for various situations and an opportunity to practice speaking using appropriate loudness levels through role playing.

Pitch and Intonation Another common difficulty among Deaf adolescents and adults is appropriate pitch control. This can be manifest as speech that is too high or too low in pitch (Nickerson 1975), that has inappropriate breaks or fluctuations (Martony 1968), or that does not reflect the prosodic use of intonation to signal questions and statements (Phillips et al. 1968).

The average fundamental frequency (f0) of adolescents and adults with hearing loss should be checked periodically. Meckfessel (1965) found that a group of deaf males had a mean f0 of 184 Hz whereas the hearing group had a mean f0 of 130Hz—a significant difference of one-half octave. The hearing group was within what would be expected for that age group (Wilson 1979), but the mean of the deaf group was significantly higher than the norms. Although there was no statistically significant difference between mean f0 of deaf and hearing adolescent girls—256 Hz for deaf girls and 230 Hz for hearing girls (Ermovick 1965), both groups had mean f0s within normal limits (Wilson 1979). There was, however, wide variation among the adolescent deaf girls' productions, with some of them having very high-pitched voices.

An additional common f0 problem among deaf speakers involves the failure to produce intonation patterns that signal questions or statements. In the extreme, this can lead to speech that is perceived as having a monotone quality. As with other areas of intervention, perception should precede production as much as possible. Work may initially focus on the client's ability to listen to or perceive a variety of vocalizations differing in pitch. This activity will lead to perception of pitch differences for vocalizations by others and by the client.

After demonstrating adequate ability to perceive these differences, work can then proceed toward production of intonation patterns. Initial production tasks for improved control of intonation might involve production of discrete vowel vocalizations at different f0 levels (high, mid, low frequency) followed by production of smooth transition between these levels (for example, high-to-mid or low-to-high f0 levels). Once adequate control is achieved for nonmeaningful vocalizations, then work may be directed toward production of these intonation patterns using increasingly meaningful speech material (single syllable words, short phrases, sentences, etc.) in less-structured settings (see Mahshie et al. 1983).

When working on producing an appropriate pitch level and the ability to use appropriate intonation patterns, the use of visual aids, such as the Visi-pitch® or the IBM SpeechViewer®, can be helpful for modeling and providing a visual representation of the client's production pattern. Beginning work should focus on production of vowels (particularly vowels that have already been targeted as part of the articulation program for the client) at a low pitch. Upon success at this task, work can then be directed toward producing a contrast between production of the same vowels at a high and low pitch (given auditory, visual, and kinesthetic feedback). The client may then be asked to produce the vowels with a consonant that can be produced successfully. Segments such as /b/ or /m/ are good candidates because auditory and visual cues can often be attained by even profoundly deaf clients. The choice of consonants, however, should be based on the individual client's repertoire. Following reasonable mastery of these nonmeaningful tasks, the client can then be directed toward production of appropriate pitch levels and patterns in meaningful words, phrases, and sentences.

Resonance   Among common resonance difficulties exhibited by Deaf individuals are hypernasality, hyponasality, and/or, cul-de-sac resonance—a muffled, hollow type of vocal quality (Wilson 1979). Although hypernasality is usually high on the list of voice parameters to be addressed (Wilson 1979), the client will often observe a "switching back and forth" between hypo- and hypernasality, with cul-de-sac resonance consistently present. These resonance patterns are very often quite difficult to remediate because they are well habituated. Intervention focusing on oral-nasal resonance balance should emphasize use of residual hearing along with visual and kinesthetic feedback. Resonance difficulties can also be addressed using a variety of techniques, including visual aids such as the Nasometer® (Kay Elemetrics) or the See-Scape® (CC Publications).

   Ling (1976) suggests that Deaf individuals often produce syllables containing /m/, /n/, and /ŋ/ with excessive nasality throughout the syllable's duration, thus negatively affecting the vowels and consonants. In beginning intervention toward reducing nasality, it is often helpful to use pictures or drawings to demonstrate to the client how the nasal consonants /m/, /n/, and /ŋ/ are produced and how production of these segments differs from oral segments. Within this discussion information can be provided about changes in the velopharyngeal opening when the client is producing speech with inaccurate resonance. Quickest improvements most often occur when perception activities precede work on production. Thus, using auditory, visual, or kinesthetic cues, the client is first made aware of resonance differences in both the clinician and herself. Vowels, syllables, words, phrases, and sentences are produced by the clinician with appropriate oral-nasal coupling and then with excessive or diminished nasal coupling. As the client's skills improve, she may be able to discriminate between adequate and inadequate resonance on specific productions.

   The client may also need to be made aware of the difference between oral and nasal productions. A useful approach to achieve this aim is negative practice involving the conscious use of an incorrect pattern in order to increase the client's awareness of his own incorrect production patterns (Wilson 1979).

   Cul-de-sac resonance quality is believed to result from resonance in the pharyngeal area, possibly related to the retraction of the tongue toward the pharyngeal wall (Subtelny, Whitehead, and Subtelny 1989). Producing consonants and vowels that keep the tongue low and forward (as much as possible) in the mouth, then moving the consonants and vowels higher and back in the oral cavity as the appropriate resonance level is achieved, may thus be useful in reducing this resonance pattern.

Intervention Tools

Cued Speech/Visual Phonics   Methods such as Visual Phonics and/or Cued Speech (Kipila and Williams-Scott 1988) and speech training devices such as the

IBM SpeechViewer© are often useful and appropriate aids to teaching speech skills (Mahshie 1995). Visual Phonics provides a useful connection between the written form and the articulation of a word. Cued Speech is designed to aid speechreading by reducing the ambiguity (through associated hand shapes) of homophonous segments or of segments that have similar lip movements (such as /p/ /b/ and /m/). The IBM SpeechViewer© is one of a small number of computer-based devices that provide the Deaf individual with visual feedback of certain speech patterns.

Such adjuncts to therapy can be most useful for clients as they begin to produce sounds, particularly at the word and phrase level. As the client expands production patterns to more connected speech in less-structured settings, there is usually less reliance on such visual feedback or cues and greater reliance on written words (for signalling a production target) and internal feedback (for monitoring production accuracy).

Amplification and Visual Aids for Speech Teaching Learning to produce speech requires both a model of what is to be achieved and a means of comparing what is produced to what is intended. Both require sensory input. For some, audition may provide a reasonable basis both for developing articulatory modes and for offering feedback for error detection. Use of residual hearing, however, may not be the most viable sensory modality for facilitating skills not yet acquired. This is understandable because most of the skills that could be developed based on auditory (or speechreading) input alone would likely already be acquired.

A number of sensory aids are available that can assist the clinician teaching production of segments or other speech units not readily accessible through residual hearing. Visual displays are useful for demonstrating the intended articulatory patterns and for comparing intended and produced utterances.

Every effort should be made to pair visual sensory feedback with auditory feedback. This permits gradual reduction of visual feedback, with other sensory systems taking greater responsibility for ongoing feedback.

Even when residual hearing is not useful, computer-based visual displays can be of value because they can provide useful information about productions that would otherwise be inaccessible to the speech learner. However, the transfer of learning from the therapy room to actual usage will likely progress much less quickly when alternate sensory modalities (such as residual hearing) are unavailable to the learner.

An additional benefit of computer-based devices, particularly those devices designed to evaluate whole word utterances and to provide an evaluative metric of production accuracy (for example, Kewley-Port et al. 1990), is that they can be useful for drill and practice. These devices provide the learner with opportunities for monitored practice without requiring the clinician's constant attention. This feature is particularly beneficial for the adolescent or adult because it can permit more private practice and can promote more independent work than is possible in clinician-mediated therapy. The benefit of such work is dependent on the ability of the computer to accurately evaluate productions with reference to some target. Recent research (Kewley-Port et al. 1990) has suggested that at least some devices perform nearly as consistently as clinicians in assessing the accuracy of speech productions by Deaf individuals.

Summary

In this chapter we have addressed the primary attributes of Deaf adolescent and adult clients and the special needs that these clients have regarding speech and voice improvement. Because of the high incidence of "fragmented" skills, assessment is shown to be a crucial step in developing appropriate intervention programs and procedures for Deaf adults. A number of formal and informal strategies for assessing the speech and voice characteristics are given, together with a framework for developing appropriate therapy goals and strategies for intervention.

References

Alpiner, J. G., and P. A. McCarthy. 1987. *Rehabilitative audiology: Children and adults.* Baltimore: Williams & Wilkins.

Andrews, M., and A. Summers. 1988. *Voice therapy for adolescents.* Boston, Mass.: Little, Brown.

Binnie, C. A., P. L. Jackson, and A. A. Montgomery. 1976. Visual intelligibility of consonants: A lipreading screening test with implications for aural rehabilitation. *Journal of Hearing and Speech Disorders* 41(4):530–539.

Calvert, D. R., and S. R. Silverman. 1975. *Speech and deafness.* Washington, D.C.: Alexander Graham Bell Association for the Deaf.

Craig Speechreading Test. 1971. In *Speechreading (lipreading),* J. Jeffers and M. Barley. Springfield, Ill.: Charles C. Thomas.

Creaghead, N., P. Newman, and W. Secord. 1989. *Assessment and remediation of articulatory and phonological disorders,* 2d ed. Columbus, Ohio: Merrill Publishing Co.

Davis, H., and S. R. Silverman. 1970. *Hearing and deafness.* New York: Holt, Rineholt and Winston.

DeFilippo, C. 1988. Tracking for speechreading training. *Volta Review* 90(5):215–237.

Edwards, H. 1992. *Applied phonetics: The sounds of American English.* San Diego, Calif.: Singular Press.

Ermovick, D. A. 1965. A spectrographic analysis comparing connected speech of deaf subjects and hearing subjects. Master'sThesis, University of Kansas.

Fairbanks, G. 1960. *Voice and articulation drillbook,* 2d ed. New York: Harper and Row.

Fisher, H., and J. Logemann. 1971. *The Fisher-Logemann Test of Articulation Competence.* New York: Houghton, Mifflin.

Goldman, R., and M. Fristoe. 1972. *The Goldman-Fristoe Test of Articulation.* Circle Pines, Minn.: American Guidance Service.

Hull, R. 1982. *Rehabilitative audiology.* New York: Grune and Stratton.

Jeffers, J., and M. Barley. 1971. *Speechreading (lipreading).* Springfield, Ill.: Charles C. Thomas.

Kaplan, H., S. Bally, and C. Garretson. 1987. *Speechreading: A way to improve understanding,* 2d ed. Washington, D.C.: Gallaudet University Press.

Kewley-Port, D., C. Watson, M. Elbert, D. Maki, and D. Reed. 1990. The Indiana Speech Training Aid (ISTRA) II: Training curriculum and selected cases. *Clinical Linguistics and Phonetics* 5(1):13–38.

Khan, L., and N. Lewis. 1986. *Khan-Lewis Phonological Analysis.* Circle Pines, Minn.: American Guidance Service.

Kipila, E., and B. Williams-Scott. 1988. Cued speech and speechreading. *Volta Review* 90(5):179–189.

Levitt, H., K. Youdelman, and J. Head. 1990. *Fundamental Speech Skills Test.* Englewood, Colo.: Resource Point, Inc.

Ling, D. 1976. *Speech and the hearing impaired child: Theory and practice.* Washington, D.C.: Alexander Graham Bell Association for the Deaf.

McGinnes, M. A. 1963. *Aphasic children: Identification and education by the association method.* Washington, D.C.: Alexander Graham Bell Association for the Deaf.

Mahshie, J. 1995. The use of sensory aids for teaching speech to children who are deaf. In *Speech communication and profound deafness,* ed. K.-E. Spens and G. Plant. London: Whurr Publishers.

Mahshie, J., A. Hasegawa, M. Mars, E. Herbert, and F. Brandt. 1983. Voice fundamental frequency training of hearing impaired speakers. *Journal of the Acoustical Society of America* (suppl. 1) 73:S14.

Martony, J. 1968. On the correction of the voice pitch level for severely hard of hearing subjects. *American Annals of the Deaf* 113:195–202.

Meckfessel, A. L. 1965. A comparison between vocal characteristics of deaf and normal hearing individuals. Master's Thesis, University of Kansas.

Nickerson, R. S. 1975. Characteristics of the speech of deaf persons. *Volta Review* 77:342–362.

Osberger, M. J., and N. McGarr. 1982. Speech production characteristics of the hearing-impaired. In *Speech and language: Advances in basic research and practice,* vol. 8, ed. N. Lass. New York: Academic Press.

Phillips, N., W. Remillard, S. Bass, and W. Pronovost. 1968. Teaching of intonation to the deaf by visual pattern matching. *American Annals of the Deaf* 113:239–246.

Robb, M., M. Hughes, and D. Frese. 1985. Oral diadochokinesis in hearing-impaired adolescents. *Journal of Communication Disorders* 18:79–89.

St. Louis, K., and D. Ruscello. 1981. *Oral Speech Mechanism Examination (OSMSE)*. Baltimore: University Park Press.

Schiavetti, N., D. Metz, and R. Sitler. 1981. Construct validity of direct magnitude estimation and interval scaling of speech intelligibility: Evidence from a study of the hearing impaired. *Journal of Speech and Hearing Research* 24:441–445.

Silverman, S. R., and I. J. Hirsh. 1955. Problems related to the use of speech in clinical audiometry. *Annals of Otology, Rhinology, and Laryngology* 64:1234–1244.

Sims, D., G. Walter, and R. Whitehead. 1982. *Deafness and communication: Assessment and training.* Baltimore, Md.: Williams & Wilkins.

Smith, C. 1975. Residual hearing and speech production in deaf children. *Journal of Speech and Hearing Research* 18:795–811.

Smith, J. D. 1975. Speech and voice therapy at NTID. *Journal of the Academy of Rehabilitative Audiology* 8:117–121.

Stevens, K., R. Nickerson, and A. Rollins. 1983. Suprasegmental and postural aspects of speech production and their effect on articulatory skills and abilities. In *Speech and the hearing impaired: Research, training, and personnel preparation*, ed. I. Hochberg, J. Levitt, and M. J. Osberger. Baltimore: University Park Press.

Subtelney, J. D. 1975a. An overview of the communication skills of NTID students with implications for planning of rehabilitation. *Journal of the Academy of Rehabilitative Audiology* 8:33–50.

———. 1975b. Speech assessment of the deaf adult. *Journal of the Academy of Rehabilitative Audiology* 8:110–116.

Subtelney, J., N. Orlando, and R. Whitehead. 1981. *Speech and voice characteristics of the deaf.* Washington, D.C.: Alexander Graham Bell Association for the Deaf.

Subtelney, J., R. Whitehead, and J. Subtelney. 1989. Cephalometric and cineradiographic study of deviant resonance in hearing-impaired speakers. *Journal of Speech and Hearing Disorders* 54:249–263.

Test of Auditory Comprehension (TAC). 1979. North Hollywood, Calif.: Foreworks Publishers.

VanRiper, C. 1954. *Speech correction: Principles and methods*, rev. ed. Englewood Cliffs, N.J.: Prentice Hall.

Wilson, D. K. 1979. *Voice problems of children*, 2d ed. Baltimore: Williams & Wilkins.

10

Pronunciation Skills

Scott J. Bally

■ ■ ■ ■

Intelligibility of deaf and hard of hearing individuals may be affected by inaccurate articulation as well as voice problems. Research by Bally and Marasco (1991) has noted that significant chronic errors of pronunciation also affect the speech intelligibility of hard of hearing and deaf children or adults. Intervention may be indicated. This chapter will focus on pronunciation skills training. It will describe the reasons that these skills may not always be used or used effectively by deaf and hard of hearing individuals and will discuss relevant assessment and intervention materials—why they may or may not be appropriate to use with this population and how they may be adapted for use by clinicians. Finally, it will include an assessment tool currently being evaluated and utilized with this population.

Professionals in the speech and hearing field may relate training in pronunciation skills to articulation therapy. Articulation focuses on the correct production of speech sounds, whereas pronunciation skills training helps an individual know which sounds should be made and the sequences in which they should be produced based on the written word orthography. Pronunciation skills training also uses an orthographic base to teach rules and contexts that help individuals use appropriate stress and syllabification. Such training includes a working knowledge of the rules of English that use the constructs of the written word (a graphemic system) as a basis for producing the spoken word (a phonemic system).

The study of phonics, extensively researched and discussed in the literature, is another area of training closely related to pronunciation skills. It differs in that it is "concerned with teaching letter-sound relationships only as they relate to learning to read" (Heilman 1993, 1–2). A definition by Scott (1982, 2) provides a more extended definition of phonics as "the application of speech sounds to reading, writing and spelling." Hall (1981, 114) also describes phonics instruction relative to the development of reading skills as "being concerned with the teaching of the association of phonemes (units of sound) with graphemes (units of written language)." Such definitions provide the basis for approaches and programs used primarily to teach reading as an oral skill. The phonic principles and structures of such programs may be readily adapted to pronunciation skills training and will be described later in this chapter.

Challenges for the Professional

A survey of the literature in the area of aural rehabilitation shows that assessment and training for pronunciation skills is one of the least discussed and researched areas of communication relative to deaf and hard of hearing populations. Most related information may be found in programs related to phonics. These teaching approaches focus on learning to read aloud because they presuppose that there is sufficient hearing ability and oral communication skills to effect success. As a result, such phonics programs may have many components that may be useful in teaching pronunciation but are structured in ways that may not be accessible or relevant to deaf and hard of hearing persons.

Other training programs are designed for international populations in English-as-a-Second-Language classes. They use imitation of oral communication rather than an orthographic base for teaching English pronunciation or reducing accents, thereby limiting their use with deaf and hard of hearing clients.

In addition there is a lack of assessment tools for evaluating the pronunciation skills of populations with hearing loss. Oral production of words and sounds is most commonly measured with an articulation test or an analysis of running speech in phonetically balanced passages. Standardized articulation tests currently available were designed for normal hearing populations and do not differentiate articulation errors from pronunciation errors (Bally and Allen 1991). Neither the scoring systems nor the guides for interpretation that accompany such tests recognize the possibility of pronunciation errors. As a result, professionals may overlook the relationship of pronunciation skills to articulation test results or may not think to evaluate pronunciation as an entity separate from articulation.

The Challenges of the English Language

An understanding of the phonetic system of a language is essential for oral production based on orthographic representations (Singh and Singh 1976). Some languages, such as Spanish, French, and German, are "phonetically sound in their orthography—that is, their written system directly represents the spoken system" (Singh and Singh 1976, 215). In contrast, English may be challenging because of the inconsistency of its phoneme-grapheme relationships (Singh and Singh 1976). For example, the grapheme "o" represents a long /ō/ in words such as "go, so, no" but can also be interpreted as /ü/ as in "do" or "to." The reason for this inconsistency is that the English language is composed of words that are from or have evolved from words of other languages. Each written word adopted from another language carries the rules for pronunciation of its parent language and is subject to further modifying influences of the culture into which it comes.

In addition, words that have evolved through scientific origins as well as pop culture may defy logic and/or rules (e.g., the orthographic representations of "sputnik," which might more logically be "sputnick"; "lite" (beverages), evolving from the word "light"; "byte," having no relative precedents in English spelling; or "quiche"). However, when groups of words with similar spellings are adopted from a language, the spelling may become generalized. Subsequently, similar sounding words may be anglicized with parallel spellings and pronunciations (e.g., the "u" in "computer" is pronounced /yü/ as in its Latin predecessors).

Hearing children start to learn to read in the first grade or so, by which time they have already established a functional oral vocabulary. They must then use certain cognitive skills to build associations between the written word and the spoken word. For some children, this may be a challenging task. Words such as "who, ski, and of" or "put" versus "but" may seem to defy reason when their orthographic counterparts are encountered. This may lead to confusion, lack of confidence, and negative attitudes toward the oral reading process. Children must begin to understand the separate but interrelated nature of the graphemic and phonemic systems before they can master oral reading skills. A variety of phonics programs and materials, identified later in this chapter, are available to the educator to assist in training in this area.

Additional Challenges for Deaf and Hard of Hearing Populations

Several additional reasons specific to deaf and hard of hearing populations may explain why they may not have good pronunciation skills. The first is the lack of auditory input needed to imitate speech and subsequently to generalize pronunciation rules. The second is the absence of pronunciation or phonics training in the curricula of many institutions for the deaf where ASL is the preferred language and oral communication skills may not be emphasized. Finally, because there are no assessment tools in published phonics training programs designed or appropriate for these populations, neither assessment to determine a need for such skills may be undertaken nor are programs provided.

Clinicians working with deaf and hard of hearing adolescents and adults should not assume that their clients have a knowledge of the graphemic or phonemic systems. Research by Bally and Marasco (1991) revealed that a small percentage of university students in deaf institutions were unable to recite, write, or fingerspell the English alphabet. A small percent were unable to produce all twenty-six letter components or were unable to generate them in the correct order. In the same study, over 90 percent were unable to identify letters (graphemes) or sounds (phonemes) when modeled by the clinician or explain the difference between the two. As concepts and skills relative to pronunciation became more sophisticated, fewer students in the study demonstrated competency. (See appendix B.)

This study also showed that approximately 85 percent of the deaf university student population had some difficulties producing the English phonemic system, the graphemic system, or both. Many used the systems interchangeably ("a", /b/, "c", etc.) and reported that no one had explained that these were two separate but interrelated systems with separate functions or that they did not always use the same symbols for grapheme and phoneme counterparts ("t" could be /t/ or /th/). Many had had extensive speech therapy throughout their education, but they frequently reported that no one had explained that a "b" could represent the sound /b/ or the alphabet letter /bē/ depending on the context in which it was used. Even at the university level, students had some difficulty understanding that the graphemic system (the alphabet) is designed for writing, that the phonemic system is the basis for speaking, and that the two systems are not always parallel or equivalent. In addition, the study revealed that poor articulation may make it difficult for the clinician to assess the client's ability to distinguish between systems and, therefore, to give accurate feedback to the client.

An additional problem related to the learning of pronunciation skills is that objectives related to oral communication may not be integrated into the curricula of many manually based deaf institutions. A survey of speech-language pathologists in state schools for the deaf (Bally 1991) showed that these institutions adopt nationally available or state mandated programs as components of their curricula in such subjects as math, English, and science. However, reading programs that emphasize reading as an oral skill and relay on auditory input may not be considered for use. When they *are* employed, the oral/auditory components, including pronunciation training, may be eliminated. Therefore, students in these programs may have little or no exposure to pronunciation skill training.

When phonics programs have been part of a student's learning experience, professionals may still note difficulties with pronunciation. Most public schools integrate phonics programs into their reading curricula to help students master the intricacies related to reconciling the dichotomies of the phonemic and graphemic systems (Hall 1981). The systems used are often contrived systems, sometimes merely simplified versions of the International Phonetic Alphabet (IPA) that have no carryover to systems encountered in adulthood (dictionary systems). Even when standardized dictionary systems such as Webster or Thorndike are utilized, they may change from grade to grade or school to school. This inconsistency may confuse students and may result in inaccurate or inconsistent pronunciation skills.

Even when available, phonics programs may still not be appropriate for deaf and hard of hearing populations. Some phonics programs available to parents, educators, and/or the general public today are designed to help children learn to read. Some are marketed as remedial programs for children with delayed or weak reading abilities. *Hooked on Phonics* (1993) has emerged as the best marketed and most widely used of these systems both in home and in remedial school programs. Some additional programs designed to foster reading skills include *Focus on Phonics* (Rice 1980a,b; 1982a,b,c,d; 1983a,b; 1985a,b); *Context Phonetic Clues* (1984); *Word Analysis Cards* (Levels I, II, and III) (1984); *Phonics in Context* (1993); *Picture Cards* (1986), *Pickafit* (1967), *Listen and Do: Consonants* (1963), and *Emphasizing Phonics in Context (EPIC)* (1978). These programs and materials were not designed specifically for deaf and hearing populations. Most use imitation of auditory stimuli as a basis for learning. However, they may easily be adapted for use with this population. In addition, some of these programs are designed for children, so they may not be appropriate for adults and adolescents.

Several programs have been designed for international clients wishing to learn to speak English as a second language or to reduce accents that may impede their intelligibility. These include such programs as Compton's *P-ESL (Pronouncing English as a Second Language) Program* (1987), Catran's *How to Speak English without a Foreign Accent* (1986), and Stern's *The Sound and Style of American English* (1992). All use imitation of spoken models as a basis for mastery of skills. Some use audio tapes, whereas others require modeling by the clinician. Some, such as the P-ESL, do not teach rules that facilitate using a graphemic base for pronunciation. Because these programs are all *based on auditory input,* they may have limited access for deaf and hard of hearing clients. Therefore, none of the available programs is completely appropriate for deaf or hard of hearing people who may not accurately receive auditory input of phonemic information.

Assessment of Pronunciation Skills

The assessment of pronunciation skills for deaf and hard of hearing clients may include, but may not be limited to, the ability to use orthographic information as a basis for the correct production (articulation notwithstanding) of consonant and vowel phonemes and the appropriate use of stress and syllabification. Many of the phonics programs mentioned previously include assessment procedures based on an informal clinical identification and analysis of errors (error count) made in recitations imitated from tapes or generated by test sentences (e.g., Stern 1992; Compton, 1983). This auditory/imitative approach to rehabilitation suggests that a greater number of errors simply calls for more practice to master pronunciation ability. These test procedures do not differentiate between pronunciation and articulation ability, nor do they assess an understanding of the orthographic base for pronunciation.

Similarly, tests designed to measure articulation may not differentiate between articulation and pronunciation errors. A study by Bally and Allen (1991) noted that the results of standard articulation tests often reflect a client's inability to change the graphemic base to a phonemic base when responding to stimulus items. For example, when the stimulus picture of "toes" was presented on the Fisher-Logemann Test of Articulation Competence (1971), many students pronounced the final "s" as /s/ rather than as the appropriately voiced /z/. It would appear that the clients were making a direct transfer from the graphemic to the phonemic base. When the subjects were given other stimulus words such as "jazz" or "buzz" where the final grapheme is a "z," they often produced the equivalent /z/ sound. This suggests that the test response does not result from an articulatory deficit, but rather from a lack of knowledge of pronunciation rules for plural and possessive forms. However, articulation test scoring would reflect a substitution of /s/ for /z/ in the final position. Clinicians might conclude, inaccurately, that the client is unable to produce /z/ in the final position.

Results of the five most frequently used standardized articulation tests at state institutions for the deaf—Fisher-Logemann Test of Articulation Competence (Fisher and Logemann 1971), Photo Articulaton Test (Pendergast et al. undated), the Templin-Darley Tests of Articulation (Templin and Darley 1960), Arizona Articulation Proficiency Scale (Fudala and Reynolds 1986), and Goldman-Fristoe Test of Articulation (Goldman and Fristoe 1969)—were further examined (Bally and Allen 1991) to determine the extent to which pronunciation deficits affect speech intelligibility in deaf and hard of hearing populations. All five tests were noted to have selected stimuli that would require knowledge of pronunciation rules to produce appropriate responses. In addition to the example previously cited ("toes"), other words that occurred on common articulation tests included such stimuli as "wagon" ("g" has alternate pronunciations), "knife" (silent letters include "k" and "e"), and "scissors" ("sc" usually pronounced as /sk/, "ss" usually pronounced as /s/, and final "s" pronounced as /z/). Responses to more than one third of the stimulus items on each of the analyzed tests could reflect either pronunciation *or* articulation errors or both. As a result of such ambiguous stimulus items, deficits in pronunciation skills would be recorded as errors in articulation.

Similarly, articulation tests are not designed to measure the ability to syllabify words. Although clients with only minimal residual hearing are often able to produce the correct number of syllables in articulating a spoken word, the Bally and Marasco study (1991) showed that they were often unable to identify the number of syllables in a written word. They would also unlikely be able to demonstrate a knowledge of where syllables should be separated. No tests that measured the ability to syllabify accurately were found in the literature.

The ability to use appropriate stress on syllables (and words) may be included in test batteries for speech and voice. The Phonologic Level Speech Evaluation (Ling 1976) and the NTID Voice and Speech Examination (1975) are both used to measure stress production. Both are designed for work with hard of hearing and deaf populations. The Ling evaluation differentiates use of stress as "faulty" or "normal" (160), but does not include an error analysis. The NTID examination response form allows clinicians to indicate the presence or absence of stress as a prosodic feature. Neither tool examines the conceptual understanding and ability to use word structure and semantics as a predictor of stress.

Measuring Pronunciation

The tests described above may be adapted for use with deaf and hard of hearing populations. The clinician may integrate informal test procedures while administering articulation tests to determine if some of the errors are related to pronunciation. Articulation errors may be differentiated from pronunciation errors by providing additional stimuli in which there are similar orthographic constructs, such as additional words ending with /s/ and /z/, to see if responses are consistent. Stimuli with direct grapheme-phoneme equivalents for the target sound (such as "jazz" or "buzz") may then be introduced to see if the target sound may be articulated in the final position. If the subject is successful, articulation error may be ruled out. However, if the subject is not successful, the error still may not be classified as either an articulation or pronunciation error. More information may be gained from additional tasks. The clinician may require the subject to say words that are differentiated only by the final (target) phonemes (such as "bus" and "buzz") to see if the subject attempts to differentiate the sounds. Any effort to differentiate or modify the production of the final phonemes may suggest that the error may be related to articulation. Finally, the clinician may make an inquiry of the client, asking if she thinks the final sounds of the two words are pronounced the same or differently. If the client responds that the words are pronounced differently, there may be some reason to believe the error is in articulation.

Errors in pronunciation reflect a lack of knowledge of the inherent principles of English that dictate the correct pronunciation of familiar as well as unfamiliar words. Individuals with hearing loss are primarily dependent on orthographic information for vocabulary acquisition but are sometimes unable to effect a successful conversion from a graphemic base to a phonemic base for the purpose of oral productions.

The clinician may also make an informal assessment of syllabification using articulation test results. The production of polysyllabic words may be examined with respect to the rules for syllabification (Fry, Fountoukidis, and Polk 1985) listed later in this chapter. However, in most tests, representatives of all the rules may not be included, nor is the nomenclature of this area examined.

The use of stress is more functionally assessed in the Ling and NTID evaluations mentioned above. The only missing element is that a functional nomenclature for work with stress cannot be assessed.

Having established a need to assess pronunciation skills as an entity separate from articulation skills, Bally and Marasco (1991) undertook a review of other standardized tests. This review did not reveal any tests that inventory a client's overall knowledge or application of pronunciation rules in English. Only the Word Attack subtest of the Woodcock Reading Mastery Test (Woodcock 1987) probes graphemic structures using nonsense words as stimuli. Although this subtest examines an individual's ability to pronounce specific graphemic structures, it does not provide a comprehensive picture of a subject's acquisition, knowledge, and application of such principles. Further, it does not examine a client's ability to understand nomenclature commonly associated with pronunciation skills, syllabification, and stress, or the client's abilities to use a dictionary as a resource for independently improving these skills.

The absence of normative data and effective tools that can measure pronunciation skills and differentiate pronunciation and articulation ability has led to the development of an assessment procedure for effectively measuring pronunciations skills, including defining specific skills, designing a tool to evaluate these skills, establishing norms for normal hearing populations, and comparing the skills of deaf adults/adolescents to these norms.

The Pronunciation Skills Inventory (PSI)

The Pronunciation Skills Inventory (PSI) (appendix A) is an assessment tool designed primarily for use with prelingually deaf adults. The purposes of this tool are to inventory a subject's acquisition, understanding, and use of rules and principles that govern the pronunciation of words for spoken English, as well as to determine her understanding of related nomenclature. Additionally, the PSI assesses the client's abilities to use a dictionary as an independent tool for effecting correct pronunciation of words.

To create such an inventory the orthographically based graphemic system and the orally based phonemic system were explored, compared, and contrasted to define their inherent rules and principles. A listing of the nomenclature commonly used to describe these principles was compiled (i.e., consonant, silent letter, syllable, stress, etc.). From this information eighteen probe areas were identified and test items designed.

The PSI includes eighteen probe items (appendix A), a Clinician's Response Form, a Client Stimulation Form, and a Profile Form for scoring and interpretation. A Clinician's Guide includes normative data for the target population, normative data for normal hearing grade school children, an in-depth explanation of each respective test item and its objectives, and notes that suggest possible errant responses as well as clinical applications.

Scoring is based on a five-point differential with a 1 being 85–100 percent correct, reflecting an understanding and ability to complete the task, and a 5 being 0–20 percent correct, indicating a "lack of understanding of the question." A 3 rating (a score of 21–84 percent) reflects an understanding of the question or principles. A 2 or 4 reflect a lack of understanding of the question or terminology used and, when stimulated with examples, equal scores of 85–100 percent and 21–84 percent respectively.

This scoring facilitates intervention planning by differentiating a subject's skill abilities from her understanding of commonly used nomenclature. For example, on item 10, a client is required to identify the number of sounds and letters in respective words. The test trials for the PSI showed that many subjects substituted the number of syllables for the number of sounds. Such observations should be noted on the Clinician Response Form after the PSI score for each item as indicated.

The PSI was used on two test populations to establish normative data on hearing children regarding instruction and acquisition of targeted pronunciation skills. The first population was a group (N=116) of normal hearing elementary school children, kindergarten through the fourth grade in Fairport, New York. In addition, a group of teachers (N=30) of elementary school children was surveyed to determine their perception of pronunciation skill acquisition and the source of the tested skills to see how closely they matched the actual skills of the children. A high correlation (over 90 percent) between teacher perception and actual skills was noted for all probed items. The second test population was a group of prelingually deaf university-level adults (N=85). The PSI was administered as part of a test battery given to the adults prior to their entrance into an elective program of aural rehabilitation. Test results were averaged for both populations. The results of this comparison (appendix B) demonstrated a dramatic contrast between populations. The deaf adults had significantly fewer pronunciation skills and a more limited understanding of related nomenclature. Appendix B shows normative data that contrasts the mean grade levels for acquisition of pronunciation skills of normal hearing children with those of the deaf adult group.

Based on results of their study with the PSI, Bally and Marasco (1991) made the following recommendations:

1. Results of standardized tests of articulation should be viewed with respect to pronunciation rules inherent in the English language.

2. The impact of a client's understanding and use of pronunciation skills should be assessed for all prelingually deaf clients when it affects speech intelligibility.

3. Pronunciation skills and articulation skills should be co-examined.

4. An understanding of rules and principles related to pronunciation of English words should be an integral part of clinical intervention for clients whose speech intelligibility is affected.

Pronunciation Skills Training

An effective starting point for the introduction of pronunciation skills is to work from the client's assessed knowledge. Most clients will know the alphabet. Many will have had some experience with producing sounds in the context of articulation therapy. Therefore, it may be effective to establish the parallel systems of letters, (graphemes or the orthographic system) sounds (phonemes or the phonemic system).

The phonemic system of American English contains forty-three phonemes—including twenty-four consonants, fourteen vowels, and five diphthongs (Singh and Singh 1976)—recognized in the International Phonetic Alphabet (IPA) (Kenyon and Knott 1953). Phonemes are classes of sounds that, when combined in particular sequences make words unique. For example, /v/ and /f/ are considered to be separate phonemes because they differentiate the words "fan" and "van" or "fine" and "vine." Graphemes are represented here in quotes such as "fine," and phonemes are identified in slashes, such as /fīn/. The Thorndike Barnhart system is used throughout this chapter, unless otherwise noted. (See figure 10.1.) It should be noted that speech production (articulation) of particular phonemes may vary depending on their context or how they are co-articulated. These may be referred to as allophones, which are slightly different sounds classified as the same phoneme. Neither hearing speakers nor those with hearing loss are generally aware of these differentiations, but development of awareness and accurate production within context falls within the purview of articulation therapy as necessary.

The orthographic system of English employs only twenty-six written characters to represent the forty-three Thorndike phonemes. Consequently many letters have more than one corresponding sound. For example, the grapheme "c" may represent the phonemes /s/ as in "acid," /k/ as in "acrid," or /sh/ as in "ocean." Some vowels represent even a greater number of sounds. Some consonants may also be silent, such as the "c" and one "l" in the word "kickball." The contexts in which one produces these sounds vary and are sometimes inconsistent: "gave, slave, wave, and shave" have a "long a," but "have" has a "short a". In addition, specific combinations of two graphemes unique to a single phoneme are called *digraphs*. For example, "sh" is pronounced /sh/, not as a sequence of /s/ followed by /h/ ("shy," "brash"). Finally, words spelled the same way may have different pronunciations depending on their syntactic function ("record," "read").

The orthographic system employs five characters to represent fourteen vowels and five dipthongs. Persons with hearing loss are statistically more apt to hear the low-frequency vowel sounds than high-frequency consonant sounds (Katz 1994). From this one might assume that an individual would utilize this auditory information and more consistently produce vowel sounds correctly. However, therapists report that it is more difficult to stimulate the less visible vowel sounds than the more visible consonants. This difficulty may become more understandable when one considers that there are only five vowel graphemes that represent and must be translated, depending on the context, into sixteen (Thorndike) or more different phonemes. Therapists traditionally stimulate practice with such phonemes in articulation therapy by giving clients practice lists with words that have a specific target sound. For example, listings for "long a" would include "gave, slave, wave, brave," etc. However, when the individual encounters the word "have," she is likely to generalize the "long a" and mispronounce the word.

Selecting a Functional Pronunciation System

To help clients develop independent skills, it may be necessary to identify a user-friendly pronunciation system. Such a system allows an individual to effect an easy transition from graphemes to phonemes for the purpose of pronouncing words. It should be learned easily or be accessible on a day-to-day basis. Functional and readily accessible systems include dictionary pronunciation systems and phonic systems used to teach reading.

When the habilitation process is one-on-one, the dictionary pronunciation system used should be the one the client prefers. If an individual has experience using a particular dictionary system that is comfortable and/or familiar, it may be desirable to continue with that system. The approaches described in this chapter can be easily adapted for use with any given system. The objective for the professional is to introduce a system that the client can use quickly and efficiently for pronunciation success.

A comparison of dictionary systems designed for children and adolescents by speech-language pathologists at the Model Secondary School for the Deaf in a 1978–1979 survey (MSSD 1979) resulted in the endorsement of the Thorndike/Barnhart system as shown in the Student Dictionary Series (1978) for use with deaf and hard of hearing students in institutional settings. (See table 10.1.) This selection was made because

1. the system used symbols to represent phonemes that more nearly resembled their graphemic counterparts;

2. the symbols were easily translated into fingerspelling (the IPA symbols for /ng/ or /ae/, for example, could not be readily achieved with handshapes);

3. the symbols used to represent phonemes could easily be elicited on typewriters and word processors making the development of worksheets more easily managed;

4. the series was graded to learning levels (beginning, intermediate, advanced);

Table 10.1   Thorndike Pronunciation Key

						Foreign Sounds
a	hat, cap	j	jam, enjoy	u	cup, butter	
ā	age, face	k	kind, seek	u̇	full, put	
ä	father, far	l	land, coal			Y as in French *du*.
		m	me, am			Pronounce (ē) with the lips rounded as for (ü).
b	bad, rob	n	no, in	ü	rule, move	
ch	child, much	ng	long, bring	v	very, save	
d	did, red			w	will, woman	à as in French *ami*.
		o	hot, rock	y	young, yet	Pronounce (ä) with the lips spread and held tense.
e	let, best	ō	open, go	z	zero, breeze	
ē	equal, be	ô	order, all	zh	measure, seizure	œ as in French *peu*.
ėr	term, learn	oi	oil, voice			Pronounce (ā) with the lips rounded as for (ō).
		ou	house, out	ə	represents:	
f	fat, if				a in about	N as in French *bon*.
g	go, bag	p	paper, cup		e in taken	The N is not pronounced, but shows that the vowel before it is nasal.
h	he, how	r	run, try		i in pencil	
		s	say, yes		o in lemon	
i	it, pin	sh	she, rush		u in circus	
ī	ice, five	t	tell, it			H as in German *ach*.
		th	thin, both			Pronounce (k) without closing the breath passage.
		ŦH	then, smooth			

Note: The pronunciation of each word is shown just after the word, in this way: ab bre vi ate (ə brē′vē āt). The letters and signs used are pronounced as in the words below. The mark ′ is placed after a syllable with primary or heavy accent, as in the example above. The mark ′ after a syllable shows a secondary or lighter accent, as in ab bre vi a tion (ə brē′vē ā′shən).

Some words, taken from foreign languages, are spoken with sounds that do not otherwise occur in English. Symbols for these sounds are given in the key as "foreign sounds."
Source: Thorndike and Barnhart 1988.

5.   it provided training in dictionary function and use for students on appropriate levels.

Contrasting the Systems

Clinicians may find that contrasting the graphemic with the phonemic system may be effective in helping clients to distinguish between the two systems. Because most clients know the alphabet, the graphemic system may be more easily established. The use of fingerspelling or writing may be employed to help teach or reinforce knowledge of all twenty-six component letters and ordering them correctly. The ability to pronounce the names of the letters (/bē/, /sē/, /dē/, etc.) may be taught later as a separate objective once clients have learned the phonemic counterparts.

Phoneme/grapheme Relationships

The letters "b, d, h, k, l, m, n, p, r, v, w, and z," with rare exceptions, have one-on-one grapheme-to-phoneme relationships and may be established easily with a client. For example, when a "b" is seen in a written word, it generally makes the /b/ sound, unless it is a silent letter. This principle holds true for the other graphemes in the group. Clients who can successfully identify the components of the alphabet in written or nonverbal form and the sounds that the letters make are demonstrating an understanding of the two systems and the ability to decode, map, and recode.

Other phoneme/grapheme concepts may also be taught. The letters "f" and "j" are also consistent, but may have alternate spellings—for example, "ph" has the same phoneme as "f" (/f/) and "dg" has the same phoneme as "j" (/j/). "S" may represent both /s/ and /z/ phonemes, such as in the initial and medial positions in "scissors." "T" may represent the phonemes /t/ as in "fortress," /ch/ as in "picture," or /sh/ as in "nation." "G" may represent both /g/ and /j/ phonemes, as in "regard" or "margin." The letter "c" may be produced as /s/, /k/, or /sh/ depending on its context or derivation. The letter "x" can be produced as /z/ in the initial position ("xerox") or as the phoneme blends /ks/ or /gz/ in medial or final positions ("toxic" or "exact") depending on the context.

Teaching which phonemes are to be produced in which contexts may be a more complex task. Some, such as "x," consistently become /z/ at the beginning of words (except in "x-ray") and /ks/ or /gz/ (depending on voicing) in the medial and final positions. "C" is less consistent in specific contexts in which it translates to the /s/, /sh/ or /k/ phonemes, a result of the inherent pronunciation rules of the parent language from which it was assimilated into English.

Digraphs

Clients may not understand that digraphs have a unique function in grapheme/phoneme relationships. Digraphs are combinations of two graphemes that, in tandem, represent a single phoneme. The phoneme is unique to this graphic representation and is *not* produced as the sequential combination of the two counterparts. "Th" is pronounced /th/ or /TH/, not as a sequential combination of /t/ followed by /h/.

To effect the accurate production of the phonemes, articulation therapy may be integrated at this point of pronunciation training. The concept of voicing may be highlighted as phonemes are established. The presence of articulation errors need not deter continued teaching of the rules and principles of pronunciation.

Silent Letter Rules

Students in the Bally and Marasco (1991) study demonstrated confusion in identifying silent letters. Some students did not know the rules, some did not know there were silent letters, and some confused the concept with "unvoiced sounds."

Table 10.2   Silent Letter Rules

Primary Rules

1. If there is a double, eliminate one (except "cc" when the c's occur in separate syllables).

2. If there is a "ck," eliminate the "c" (same as previous rule if one assumes that "c" represents /k/) (e.g., "duck" =/duk/).

3. If "e" appears in the final position and the word has one or more additional vowels, eliminate the final "e" (e.g., "choke" = /chōk/).

4. If "t," "c," and "h" appear together ("tch"), eliminate the "t" (e.g., "match" = /mach/).

5. If "g," "h," and "t" appear together ("ght"), eliminate the "gh" (e.g., bright = /brīt/).

6. If "w" and "r" appear together ("wr"), eliminate "w" (e.g., "wrap" = /rap/).

7. If "k" and "n" or "g" and "n" appear together ("kn" or "gn") in the same syllable, eliminate the "k" or "g" respectively (e.g., "knot" = /not/ or "gnat" = /nat/).

Secondary Rules

8. If "mb" appears in the same syllable, eliminate the "b" (e.g., "comb" = /kōm/).

9. If "alk" appears in the same syllable, eliminate the "l" (e.g., "chalk" = /chôk/).

10. If "ould" appears in a word, eliminate the "l" (e.g., "should" = /shůd/).

11. If "alm" appears in a word in the same syllable, eliminate the "l" (e.g., "palm" = /päm/).

12. If "ps" appears in a word in the same syllable, eliminate the "p" (e.g., "psalm" = /säm/).

Silent letters may be introduced as those letters for which a grapheme, in specific contexts, is not interpreted or produced as a phoneme. In English, rules relative to specific combinations are applied with varying degrees of frequency. These include the primary and secondary rules shown in table 10.2.

In addition to the examples shown in table 10.1, dozens of unique or minor instances of silent letters can be found in English, such as the "s" in "island" or the "b" in "debt" or "doubt." Such instances should be explained to a client when vocabulary containing them is introduced.

It may be useful to review phonics programs for the content related to phoneme-grapheme relationships and format or present them in ways that are more accessible to deaf and hard of hearing individuals. A visual presentation using an orthographic base, for example, may be more desirable as the primary source of pronunciation information.

Syllabification

The concept of the vowel as the basis of the syllable, the relationship of syllabification to syntactic structures, and the role of syllabification in pronunciation may all be established with clients with hearing loss. Syllables sometimes are part of phonics lessons because syllabification affects vowel sounds (for example, an open vowel rule), and sometimes they are part of spelling or English lessons. There is no close agreement on various lists of syllabification rules, and some of the rules have numerous exceptions (Costigan 1985). Although there is some disagreement among professionals, the rules for syllabification shown in table 10.3 based on Fry, Fountoukidis, and Polk (1985) may serve as guidelines for the professional.

Stress

The concept of stress may be explained as emphasis on a particular syllable: "Stress is related to syllable nucleus and is used to denote differing degrees of prominence in words containing more than one syllable" (Singh and Singh 1976, 170). It is achieved by giving more intensity with an increase in the breath force on the stressed syllable in a word. Longer duration or higher pitch may also be

Table 10.3   Rules for Syllabification

Rule 1. VCV +	A consonant between two vowels tends to go with the second vowel unless the first vowel is accented and short. Examples: *bo-nus, kitch-en*
Rule 2. VCCV	Divide two consonants between vowels unless they are a blend or digraph. Examples: *lec-ture, moth-er*
Rule 3. VCCCV	When there are three consonants between two vowels, divide them between the blend or the digraph and the other consonant. Example: *en-trance, wran-gler*
Rule 4. Affixes	Prefixes always form separate syllables, (*re-union*), and suffixes form separate syllables only in the following cases:

Table 10.3 *Continued*

	a. The suffix *y* tends to pick up the preceding consonant. Example: *for-ty*
	b. The suffix *-ed* tends to form a separate syllable only when it follows a root that ends in *d* or *t*. Example: *parad-ed, jaunt-ed*
	c. The suffix *-s* never forms a syllable except when it follows an e. Example: *trucks, bus-es*
Rule 5. Compounds	Always divide compound words. Example: *cow-boy*
Rule 6. Final *le*	Final *le* picks up the preceding consonant to form a syllable. Example: *gar-gle*
Rule 7. Vowel Clusters	Do not split common vowel clusters, such as:
	a. *r*-controlled vowels (*ar, er, ir, or,* and *ur*). Example: *ar-ter-y, mirr-or*
	b. Long vowel digraphs (*ea, ee, ai, oa,* and *ow*). Example: *crea-ture, sai-lor*
	c. Broad *o* clusters (*au, aw,* and *al*). Example: *au-di-ence*
	d. Dipthongs (*oi, oy, ou,* and *ow*). Example: *cow-ard, roy-al*
	e. Double *o*: Example: *school*
Rule 8. Vowel Problems	Every syllable must have one and only one vowel sound. a. The letter *e* at the end of a word is silent. Example: *June* b. The letter *y* in the middle or at the end of a word operates as a vowel. Example: *E-gypt, cy-clone* c. Two vowels together with separate sounds form separate syllables. Example: *ar-e-a*

used to place stress on words. In polysyllabic words, stress may be given to a syllable based on the specific vowel sound, the syntactic and grammatical structure of a written word, and the type of sentence. For example, suffixes do not receive stress; each half of a compound word receives equal stress; a word such as "conflict" may receive different stress when it is a verb or a noun; and an important word in a sentence may receive stress. Although stress is governed by a general set of rules in English, at times the rules may not be consistent.

Training for the use of stress may be studied in both word and sentence contexts. It may include components of auditory training for identification of stressed syllables and voice therapy for changes in pitch and intensity, which generate appropriate stress.

Integrated Therapy Approaches

The introduction of the rules and principles as well as the nomenclature of pronunciation may occur at any time there is a phonetic component being considered from other therapy perspectives. When clients are learning to articulate sounds, it is logical for them to understand the orthographic contexts that should elicit the target phonemes. The lipreading component of therapy should be based on an understanding that a person is focusing on the mouth movements of phoneme sequences as opposed to the orthographic sequences of letters for the same word. In auditory training, the same phoneme/grapheme relationships may also be used as a basis for developing word and sound level listening skills. To present the information outside of such integrated contexts may be less meaningful and therefore less effective.

Teaching Approaches

In teaching pronunciation rules, it may be effective to encourage the client to use analytic thinking skills. In doing so, the professional may present several examples of words governed by a single rule. For example, "knit, knot" and "knock" may be presented representing words with a silent /k/ in the "kn" context. First, the clinician may ask a directed question such as, "Which letter does *not* make a sound in the following words?" Then the stimulus words may be presented both in writing and by modeling them orally so that the client may lipread them. The clinician may then identify correct responses and direct the client to generalize a rule that describes the contexts in which the /k/ is not produced (e.g., when "kn" appears in the same syllable, the "k" is eliminated). Additional stimulus words such as "know, knife, kitten," and "kite" may help the client to identify the context(s) in which the rule is applied. These activities may be integrated with work on auditory training, speechreading, or articulation goals, as described in the previous section.

Cultural Considerations

When working with individuals who identify themselves as culturally Deaf, the client's motivation for improving pronunciation skills may be examined. Such factors may be used to design or select activities or to encourage and reinforce accurate pronunciation in contexts relevant to the client's perceived needs. For example, if a client wishes to develop pronunciation skills for the workplace, activities may be developed that focus on the pronunciation of relevant terminology.

The Communication Scale for Deaf Adults (CSDA) (Kaplan, Bally, and Brandt 1991) may provide the professional with information related to the client's motivation and objectives for improving pronunciation skills. An interview format is recommended to determine the extent of and the reasons for motivation to work in this area. Individuals who have established speech skllls may wish to use a knowledge of pronunciation rules and principles for maintaining, improving, or retrieving any waning skills. Individuals who may have grown up in manually based programs may perceive oral English as a "second language" and thus need a carefully integrated program design that uses the principles of pronunciation as a basis for correctly determining which phonemes should be articulated.

Psychosocial Aspects

When teaching pronunciation skills, many clients find the discovery of an unknown rule or principle of pronunciation to be interesting or puzzling elements of a previously unexplored system or systems. However, the professional may anticipate instances wherein a culturally Deaf individual, in learning such information often considered common knowledge for a hearing person, may express surprise, anger, or frustration that "no one told me that before." The absence of such "common knowledge" among some Deaf clients may be attributed to the absence of oral approaches in some institutions for reasons described earlier. Others may learn this kind of information incidentally through audition or because it is generalized within "hearing" or mainstreamed curricula. The professional may wish to address these concerns candidly or, when a client's responses seem extreme or may detract from the therapy process, the professional may wish to refer the client for counseling.

Resources

Many of the resources mentioned earlier in this chapter may be adapted for use with deaf and hard of hearing populations. An orthographic base may be most expeditious for teaching pronunciation skills. Also, skills may be reinforced using auditory or visual (lipreading) input as appropriate for each individual's needs and preferences.

A review of the literature revealed only two programs designed for teaching pronunciation skills to deaf and hard of hearing individuals are currently in use. Both are directed at university-level students and were designed for use in specific pronunciation skills courses. These include the two-part program *Key Picture/ Word Strategy to Facilitate the Learning of Merriam-Webster Pronunciation Symbols* (Pshirrer 1981), *Pronunciation II: NGEC175* (Nutter and Subtelny undated), used at the National Technical Institute for the Deaf (NTID), and *The Pronunciations Skills Guide for Deaf and Hard of Hearing Adults* (Bally and Marasco 1991). Two versions of the latter, using the Webster and Thorndike systems, were used as course texts at NTID and Gallaudet University respectively. Both have limited availability through their respective institutions.

The teaching and remedial phonics materials and programs described earlier may also be useful to the clinician. Many are organized with a focus on specific consonant or vowel groups. Others provide labeled pictures or flash cards that may be incorporated into a teaching approach that uses the written word as the primary stimulus. Clinician modeling is successful as a reinforcing technique, and the tapes may be used when clients have enough residual hearing and need secondary auditory training activities.

Summary

This chapter has discussed the assessment and teaching of pronunciation skills. It described the challenges facing deaf and hard of hearing persons in developing effective pronunciation skills as well as the challenges facing professionals who do training in this area. It described how assessment tools might be used, introduced the Pronunciation Skills Inventory, designed to be used in conjunction with standardized articulation tests to assess client skills, enumerated some of the principles and rules that may be included in pronunciation skills training, and described some of the intervention programs and materials that the professional might use.

References

Allen, A. S., and S. J. Bally. 1991. *The applicability of five standardized articulation tests to deaf and hearing populations: A comparative study.* Unpublished study. Washington, D.C.: Gallaudet University, Department of Audiology and Speech-Language Pathology.

Bally, S. J. 1994. *Pronunciation Skills Inventory (PSI).* Washington, D.C.: Gallaudet University, Department of Audiology and Speech-Language Pathology.

Bally, S. J., and K. L. Marasco. 1991. Assessing pronunciation skills of prelingually deafened adults and children. Presentation to American Speech-Language Hearing Association, Atlanta, Georgia.

Bowen, J. D. 1975. *Patterns of English pronunciation.* Rowley, Mass.: Newbury House, Inc.

Byrne, J. 1984. On teaching articulatory phonetics via an orthography. *Memory and Cognition* 12 :181–189.

Cartier, F. A., and T. T. Martin. *The phonetic alphabet,* 2d ed. 1971. Dubuque, Iowa: William C. Brown Company.

Catran, J. 1986. *How to speak English without a foreign accent.* Sherman Oaks, Calif.: Jade Publications.

Context Phonetic Clues. 1984. North Billerica, Mass.: Curriculum Associates, Inc.

Compton, A. J. 1983. *Compton phonological assessment of foreign accent.* San Francisco: Carousel House.

———. 1987. *Compton P-ESL Program: Pronouncing English as a second language.* San Francisco: Carousel House.

Costigan, P. 1977. A validation of the Fry syllabification generalization. Unpublished master's thesis, Rutgers University, New Brunswick, N.J. Available from ERIC.

———. 1985. In *The NEW reading teacher's book of lists,* ed. E. Fry, D. Fountoukidis, and J. Polk. Englewood Cliffs, N.J.: Prentice Hall.

EPIC (Emphasizing Phonics in Context). 1978 New York: McCormick-Mathers Publishing Co.

Fisher, H. B., and J. A. Logemann. 1971. *The Fisher-Logeman Test of Articulation Competence.* Boston: Houghton Mifflin.

Fox, B., and D. K. Routh. 1976. Phonemic analysis and synthesis as word attack skills. *Journal of Educational Psychology* 68:70–74.

Fry, E., D. Fountoukidis, and J. Polk. 1985. *The NEW reading teacher's book of lists.* Englewood Cliffs, N.J.: Prentice Hall.

Fudala, J. B., and W. M. Reynolds. 1986. *Arizona Articulation Proficiency Scale.* Los Angeles: Western Psychological Services.

Goldman, R., and M. Fristoe. 1986. *Goldman-Fristoe Test of Articulation.* Circle Pines, Minn.: American Guidance Service.

Hall, M. A. 1981. *Teaching reading as a language experience,* 3rd ed. Columbus, Ohio: Charles E. Merrill.

Heilman, A. W. 1993. *Phonics in proper perspective,* 7th ed. New York: Maxwell Macmillan International.

Hooked on phonics 1993. Orange, Calif.: Hooked on Phonics, Inc.

Kaplan, H., S. J. Bally, and F. D. Brandt. 1991. Communication Self-Assessment Scale for Deaf Adults. *Journal of the American Academy of Rehabilitative Audiology* 2(3): 164–182.

Katz, J. 1994. *Handbook of clinical audiology,* 3rd ed. Baltimore: Williams & Wilkins.

Kenyon, J. S., and T. A. Knott. 1953. *A Pronouncing dictionary of American English*. Springfield, Mass.: G. & C. Merriam.

Ling, D. 1976. *Speech and the hearing impaired child: Theory and practice*. Washington, D.C.: Alexander Graham Bell Association for the Deaf.

———. 1989. *Early intervention for hearing-impaired children: Total communication options*. Boston: College Hill Press.

Ling, D., and A. H. Ling. 1978. *Aural rehabilitation: The foundations of verbal learning in hearing impaired children*. Washington, D.C.: Alexander Graham Bell Association for the Deaf.

Listen and do: Consonants. 1963. Boston: Houghton Mifflin.

National Technical Institute for the Deaf (NTID) Voice and Speech Examination. 1975. Rochester, N.Y.: National Technical Institute for the Deaf.

Nutter, M. M., and J. D. Subtelny. n.d. *Pronunciation II: NGEC 1975*. Rochester, N.Y.: National Technical Institute for the Deaf Communication Center.

Paul, P. V., and S. P. Quigley. 1994. *Language and deafness*. San Diego, Calif.: Singular Publishing Group, Inc.

Pendergast, K., S. Dickey, J. Selmar, and A. Soder. n.d. *Photo Articulation Test*. Danville, Ill.: Interstate Printers & Publishers, Inc.

Phonics in context. 1993. Baldwin, N.Y.: Educational Activities, Inc.

Pickafit. 1967. Boston: Houghton Mifflin.

Picture cards. 1986. Boston: Houghton Mifflin.

Pshirrer, L. 1981. *Key picture/word strategy to facilitate the learning of Merriam-Webster pronunciation symbols*. Rochester, N.Y.: National Technical Institute for the Deaf.

Rice, G. V. 1980a. *Focus on phonics IIb: Student workbook*. Syracuse, N.Y.: New Reader's Press.

———. 1980b. *Focus on phonics IIb: Teacher's edition*. Syracuse, N.Y.: New Reader's Press.

———. 1982a. *Focus on phonics IIa: Student workbook*. Syracuse, N.Y.: New Reader's Press.

———. 1982b. *Focus on phonics IIa: Teacher's edition*. Syracuse, N.Y.: New Reader's Press.

———. 1982c. *Focus on phonics III: Student workbook*. Syracuse, N.Y.: New Reader's Press.

———. 1982d. *Focus on phonics III: Teacher's edition*. Syracuse, N.Y.: New Reader's Press.

———. 1983a. *Focus on phonics I: Student workbook*. Syracuse, N.Y.: New Reader's Press.

————. 1983b. *Focus on phonics I: Teacher's edition.* Syracuse, N.Y.: New Reader's Press.

————. 1985a. *Focus on phonics IV: Student workbook.* Syracuse, N.Y.: New Reader's Press.

————. 1985b. *Focus on phonics IV: Teacher's edition.* Syracuse, N.Y.: New Reader's Press.

Scott, L. B. 1982. *Developing phonics skills: Listening, speaking, reading, and writing.* New York: Teacher's College, Columbia University.

Singh, S., and K. S. Singh. 1976. *Phonetics: Principles and practices.* Baltimore: University Park Press.

Stern, D. A. 1992. *The sound and style of American English.* Lyndonville, Vt.: Dialect Accent Specialists, Inc.

Templin, M. C., and F. L. Darley. 1960. *The Templin-Darley Tests of Articulation.* Iowa City, Iowa: State University of Iowa, Bureau of Educational Research and Service Extension Division.

Thorndike, E. L., and C. L. Barnhardt. 1979. *Scott, Foresman advanced dictionary.* Glenview, Ill.: Scott Foresman & Co.

Thorndike, E. L., and C. L. Barnhardt. 1988. *Thorndike-Barnhart student dictionary.* Glenview, Ill.: Scott, Foresman & Co.

Woodcock, R. W. 1987. *Woodcock Reading Mastery Tests* (revised). American Guidance Service.

Word analysis cards. 1984. North Billerica, Mass.: Curriculum Associates, Inc.

Appendix 10A
Pronunciation Skills Inventory
Clinician's Guide

OVERVIEW

The Pronunciation Skills Inventory (PSI) is a clinical tool for assessing the knowledge and skills of deaf and hard of hearing children, adolescents, and adults related to the pronunciation of English words. It examines a client's understanding of how orthographics (graphemes) may be used as a guide to an accurate pronunciation of spoken vocabulary. The PSI should be used *in conjunction with* a standardized test of articulation.

TEST ADMINISTRATION

It is *important* that the clinician review the Clinician's Guide, read test instructions, and administer the PSI as directed. Deviance from the instructions may be considered "stimulation" and affect test scoring. For example, in item 1, the clinician directs the client to "say the alphabet." If the client does not understand the term "alphabet" and the clinician re-directs with "say the ABCs," the item should be considered as stimulated and scored as a 2, 4, or 5. The PSI uses the "stimulability" ratings to provide useful clinical information to the clinician. In the case of item 1, the clinician will know if the client is familiar with the common nomenclature "alphabet" for the task.

SCORING

Scoring procedure is clearly identified on the PSI in boxes at the end of each item. Scores should include:

1. a "raw score"—the number of correct responses out of the total number targeted

2. a "percent score" computed from the raw score

3. a "stimulability" evaluation (circling "yes" or "no" indicates if the responses were stimulated by examples or use of explanation of nomenclature)

4. a "PSI Score": the percent score and the stimulability evaluation are interpreted and assigned to a five point differential:

    1 Understands task, scores 85–100%

    2 Stimulated by example, scores 85–100%

    3 Understands task, scores 21–84%

    4 Stimulated by example, scores 21–84%

    5 Does not understand task and/or not stimulable by example, scores 0–20%

PSI scores may then be transferred to the Pronunciation Skills Profile for review and analysis.

INVENTORY OF CONTENT

The following is a discussion of each item of the test. It includes clarification of directions as well as objectives, possible responses, scoring suggestions, norms, therapy implications, and other insights gained from experience using this inventory.

1. *The alphabet:*
a. The client is instructed to "say the alphabet." The primary objective is to see if the client is able to identify the letters of the English alphabet. If the client does not respond to the task (i.e., understand the term "alphabet") the clinician may stimulate by instructing the client to "say the ABCs." If the client is still unable to respond, the clinician may write or fingerspell the alphabet until she understands *or* the clinician feels that the client is not able to complete this task. The primary objective is for the client to be able to identify the graphemes of the English alphabet.

If the client's speech is not intelligible, the clinician may direct the client to fingerspell or write the alphabet. It was noted in the test population that some students who omit letters when reciting or fingerspelling are able to complete the written task without omissions. A high percentage of the test population completed the test without error. Clients who transpose two or more sequences of letters should be tested further in sequencing tasks to explore the possibility of specific learning disabilities.

Elementary Test Population (hearing): PSI __1__ at grade __K__
Adult Test Population (deaf): PSI <u>1.05</u>

b. The objective of this item is to record phonetically the clients' production of the grapheme names: /bē, sē, dē/ etc. A moderate percentage (46 percent) of the test population routinely used graphemes and phonemes interchangeably. This may indicate that a client does not know the function or appropriate use of the two (grapheme and phoneme) systems. The clinician may also gain some preliminary insights as to the client's articulation skills. This can be used as a pretest for a clinical objective directed at these skills. Clinical trials have shown that deaf clients who are generally unintelligible for connected speech are often successful in learning to spell words intelligibly.

Note: 85 percent of the adult deaf test population substituted phonemes for graphemes at least some of the time. The clinician can stimulate correct responses by using the letter "w" as an example, noting that the name of the letter is "double u" but the sound it makes in words is /w/. Successful work in the area of pronunciation skills should be based on a client's clear understanding of the difference between graphemes and phonemes.

2. *Vowel identification:* The client is instructed to "identify the vowels." The word "vowel" may be spelled orally or written without being considered as stimulation. After a reasonable amount of time, if the client is unable to identify the vowels, the clinician may stimulate by identifying "a" as a vowel. If so, this should be reflected as a 2, 4, or 5 stimulated score. The clinician should record responses by assigning numbers that indicate the order in which the vowels are presented. For example, if the client says "o" as the first vowel s/he can identify, place a number 1 in the box below the "o." A "sometimes y" response should be noted under "Comments" but not included in scoring.

Elementary Test Population (hearing): PSI _1.0_ at grade _4_
Adult Test Population (deaf): PSI 1.21

3. *Diacritically marked vowels:* The client is instructed to explain the difference between long and short vowels. Acceptable responses may take a variety of forms:
a. Client may give examples. Only accurate examples should be considered as "1" responses. A "3" score should indicate that the client understands that the diacritical markings influence or dictate the phoneme that the vowel produces (such as /a/ in "ate").

Elementary Test Population (hearing): PSI _2.6_ at grade _4_
Adult Test Population (deaf): PSI 4.05

b. The client may give examples of words that include long or short vowels and should then be directed to isolate the vowel sounds.
Discussion: _____% of the adult test population equated long and short vowels with the duration of vowel production.

Adult Test Population (deaf): PSI ____

c. Client may describe that long vowels are the same as the name of the letter (grapheme), whereas short vowels take a different sound.
Parts 3b and 3c should not be considered stimulated responses, unless the clinician gives examples of correct responses. However, they should be scored separately and considered as different skill levels.

Adult Test Population (deaf): PSI ____

4. *Vowel production:* The client is instructed to look at the "nonsense" words on the Client Stimulus Form and say each one. The stimulus words were selected to represent vowel combinations common to English. This item probes the client's ability to generalize inherent rules for vowel production. Vowel production should be phonetically recorded. The clinician may wish to record the entire word production for further analysis.

Part 4b requires the client to use speech decoding abilities to determine word equivalents for the test words. These equivalent words are common English words with their traditional spellings. Clinicians should be cautioned to use care in determining if these responses are correct. Clients may either sign the word, give its correct (traditional) spelling, define the word, or use it in context to demonstrate accuracy of choice.

Elementary Test Population (hearing): PSI __1__ at grade __1__
Adult Test Population (deaf): PSI 1.21

5. *Consonant identification:* The client is instructed to designate the name given to letters that are not vowels: *consonants.* The client should be asked to spell this word and the clinician should record his response. The word "constants" or something similar is frequently offered and should be considered as a level 3 response as it reflects some understanding of the concept that consonants generally are consistent whereas vowels change their sounds. This task may be stimulated by saying "'A, E, I, O, and U' are the vowels. What are the other letters called?"

Elementary Test Population (hearing): PSI 1.56 at grade __4__
Adult Test Population (deaf): PSI 3.20

6. *Consonants versus vowels:* The client is asked to differentiate between vowels and consonants. Correct responses should reflect a basic understanding that vowels are the core or main structure of words (perhaps adding that there must be a vowel in every word, although the same cannot be said for consonants). Stimulate by saying, "You know what the vowels are and you know the other letters are called consonants. Why do we separate them into the two groups?"

Elementary Test Population (hearing): PSI 2.68 at grade __4__
Adult Test Population (deaf): PSI 4.29

7. *Consonant production:* The client is instructed to produce the words indicated on the Client Stimulus Form. These "nonsense" words include consonants that have alternative phonemes within the English language. Responses should be directed toward the underlined parts of words as indicated on the Clinician's Response Form and recorded phonetically. The clinician may also wish to transcribe the entire client response for further analysis. Correct responses:

1. cend
2. bigh*t*
3. *p*hat
4. brix
5. *w*rat
6. ham*b*
7. *g*eans
8. *g*nap
9. *dj*ello
10. *j*as

Part 7b instructs the client to identify the "real word" that is pronounced the same as the nonsense word. The client must use speech decoding to determine a common English word with the same phonemic structure. Correct responses should be verified by having the client fingerspell, spell, define, or use the word in a sentence. Correct responses:

1. *c*end = (send)   6. ham*b* = (ham)
2. bi*ght* = (bite)   7. *g*eans = (jeans)
3. *ph*at = (fat)   8. *g*nap = (nap)
4. brix = (bricks)   9. *d*jello = (jello)
5. *w*rat = (rat)   10. jas = (jazz)

8. *Plurals, past tenses, and contractions:*

a. The client is instructed to pronounce the words indicated on the Client Stimulus Form. The clinician should listen to the production of plural and possessive endings to determine if correct voicing and syllabification are assigned and used for each item. Responses should be recorded phonetically. Correct responses:

1. lips(s) _____   2. beds(z) _____   3. buses(əz) _____
4. buzz*es*(əz) _____   5. Beth's(s) _____   6. Bill's(z) _____

b. The client is instructed to pronounce the words indicated in part 8b of the Client Stimulus Form. The clinician should listen to the production of contractions, specifically to determine if the correct pronunciation and syllabification are used for each item. Responses should be recorded phonetically. Correct responses:

1. didn't /didənt/   3. it's /its/
2. isn't /izənt/   4. won't /wunt/

c. The client is instructed to pronounce the words indicated in part 8c of the Client Response Form. The clinician should listen to the past tense verb endings to determine if the correct voicing and syllabification are assigned to and used for each item. Responses should be recorded phonetically. Correct responses:

1. begg*ed*(d) _____   2. dipp*ed*(t) _____
3. fad*ed*(_d) _____   4. wait*ed*(_d) _____

9. *Phoneme production:* The client is asked to produce the sound (phoneme) that each letter (grapheme) makes. This may be stimulated as directed on the Clinician Response Form, using "w" and explaining that the name of the letter is /dubləlyü/ whereas the sound is /w/. Alternate productions should be solicited for "c" and "g" as directed.

Responses should be recorded phonetically. Responses to this item should be compared to results from item 1. Note any grapheme for phoneme substitutions. Compare results with standardized articulation test results. Correct responses:

b ( )	k ( )	s ( )
c ( )( )( )	l ( )	*t ( )( )
d ( )	m ( )	v ( )
f ( )	n ( )	w ( )
*g ( )( )	p ( )	x ( )
h ( )	q ( )	y ( )
j ( )	r ( )	z ( )

* items have alternate sounds ("c"=/s/k/sh/, "g"=/g/j/, "t"=/t/sh/ch/)

Elementary Test Population (hearing): PSI <u>2.23</u> at grade <u>2</u>
Adult Test Population (deaf): PSI <u>3.23</u>

10. *Grapheme/phoneme differentiation:* The client is instructed to look at the test items for item 10 on the Client Stimulus Form and indicate the number of letters and sounds in each respective word. If the client gives the correct answer to the first five stimuli on the letters column, a score of 1 may be assigned. If the client says there is "one" sound in each of the first five items, he is probably indicating the number of syllables. If so, it should be clarified that the clinician wants "sounds" not "syllables." Scoring would then be 4 or 5, noted as stimulated.

This item probes the ability to differentiate phoneme/grapheme differences in words. It further explores the client's ability to identify digraphs (diphones) such as "th" and "sh," equivalencies for letters such as "x" and "q," and silent letter rules. These are tested in greater depth in subsequent items.

Elementary Test Population (hearing): PSI __1__ at grade __4__
Adult Test Population (deaf): PSI 1.20

11a. *Digraphs (consonants) (a.k.a. diphones):* The client is instructed to identify sounds in which two consonant letters equal one sound (digraphs). Correct responses may include "sh," "ch," "th," "TH," "wh," "ph," and "ng." An additional correct response may be "gh" for /f/, which occurs inconsistently and therefore should be noted under "comments" and may need to be "deep tested." Responses may also include blends (such as "fl" or "br") as well as letter combinations that include silent letters (such as "kn" or "ght"), which should not be given scoring credit.

Elementary Test Population (hearing): PSI 3.04 at grade __4__
Adult Test Population (deaf): PSI 3.63

11b. *Digraph production (consonants):* The client is instructed to say the nonsense words, which include five digraphs. The clinician only needs to transcribe the production of the digraph. The results should be examined and compared with articulation test results. The clinician should note if there is an effort to produce the two component graphemes as separate phonemes. No normative data is available on this item.

11c. *Digraphs (vowels):* The client is instructed to identify sounds in which two vowel letters equal one sound (digraphs). Correct responses may include "ai, au, ay, ea, ee, ei, ey, oa, oe, oi, oo, ou, oy, and uy". These responses may include the diphthongs.

11d. *Digraph production (vowels):* The client is instructed to say the nonsense words, which include fourteen vowel digraphs. The clinician needs to transcribe only the production of the digraph. The results should be examined along with articulation test results. The clinician should note if there is an effort to produce the two component graphemes as separate phonemes. No normative data is available on this item.

12. *Silent letters:* The client is instructed to identify the silent letters in the words listed in item 12 of the Client Stimulus Form. Some words do not have silent letters. Correct responses are indicated on the Clinician's Response Form.

1. bell (1) _____	6. night (gh) _____	11. debt (b) _____
2. time (e) _____	7. knot (k) _____	12. watch (t) _____
3. flop (-) _____	8. comb (b) _____	13. walk (l) _____
4. tree (e) _____	9. duck (c or k) _____	14. feed (e) _____
5. wrap (w) _____	10. tax (-) _____	15. island (s) _____

Elementary Test Population (hearing): PSI 2.52 at grade 3
Adult Test Population (deaf): PSI 3.31

Client is instructed to pronounce the words on item 12b of the Client Stimulus Form. Clinician should transcribe response phonetically and determine if silent letters (or equivalents as reflected on articulation tests) are being produced.

13. and 14. *Syllabification (grapheme/phoneme base):* The client is instructed to indicate the number of syllables for each of the words of item 13 on the Client Stimulus Form. The client is given the same instructions for item 14 but the clinician says each of the words on the Clinician's Response Form. The clinician should record the client's responses and compare them to correct responses indicated on the Clinician's Response Form.

13. *Elementary Test Population (hearing):* PSI 1.24 at grade 4
Adult Test Population (deaf): PSI 2.17

14. *Elementary Test Population (hearing):* PSI 1.16 at grade 4
Adult Test Population (deaf): PSI 1.98

15. and 16. *Stress (grapheme/phoneme base):* The client is instructed to indicate the syllable that is stressed in each of the words of item 15 on the Client Stimulus Form. The client is given the same instructions for item 16 but the clinician says each of the words on the Clinician's Response Form. Responses should be compared to correct responses indicated on the Clinician's Response Form.

15. *Elementary Test Population (hearing):* PSI 2.52 at grade 4
Adult Test Population (deaf): PSI 3.10

16. *Elementary Test Population (hearing):* PSI 2.60 at grade 4
Adult Test Population (deaf): PSI 3.20

17. and 18. *Syllable/stress and dictionary skills:* The client is directed to locate the stimulus words for both items. For item 17 the client is asked to identify the number of syllables and the stressed syllables and then apply this information to pronouncing the stimulus words. Locating skills are assessed through observation. For item 18 the client is directed to locate, pronounce, and use unfamiliar words found on the Client Stimulus Form.

17a. *Elementary Test Population (hearing):* PSI 1.0 at grade 4
Adult Test Population (deaf): PSI 1.80

17e. *Elementary Test Population (hearing):* PSI 1.72 at grade 4
Adult Test Population (deaf): PSI 2.33

17f. *Elementary Test Population (hearing):* PSI 2.20 at grade 4
Adult Test Population (deaf): PSI 1.60

18b. *Elementary Test Population (hearing):* PSI 3.0 at grade 4
Adult Test Population (deaf): PSI 2.89

Appendix 10A (continued)
Pronunciation Skills Inventory

Directions:

Each item should receive a raw score (RS) indicating number of items correct, a percent score (number right out of total possible) as well as an inventory score (PSI) based on the following scale:

1 = Understands task, scores 85–100%

2 = Stimulated by example(s), scores 85–100%

3 = Understands task, scores 21–84%

4 = Stimulated by example(s), scores 21–84%

5 = Does not understand task and/or not stimulable by example, scores 0–20%

Use Client Response Form for items with asterisks (*).

Clinician Note: The clinician should review the Clinician's Guide prior to administering the Pronunciation Skills Inventory. The Guide includes correct responses, protocols for administration, and normative data as well as rehabilitation directives. The Client Stimulus Form should be used to cue responses. The Client Profile Form should be used for clarification of test results.

PRONUNCIATION SKILLS INVENTORY

Clinician's Response Form

Client name: _____ ID/SSN: _____

Clinician name: _____ Date: _____

1. ALPHABET: Instruct client to "say the alphabet." Transcribe responses phonetically.

a /e/	( )	j /dze/	( )	s /es/	( )		
b /bi/	( )	k /ke/	( )	t /ti/	( )		
c /si/	( )	l /el/	( )	u /yu/	( )		
d /di/	( )	m /em/	( )	v /vi/	( )		
e /i/	( )	n /en/	( )	w /dub l yu/	( )		
f /ef/	( )	o /o/	( )	x /eks/	( )		
g /dzi/	( )	p /pi/	( )	y /wai/	( )		
h /ets/	( )	q /kyu/	( )	z /zi/	( )		
i /ai/	( )	r /ar/	( )				

1a. RS: /26 % _____	Stim.? Y N	PSI: 1 2 3 4 5
b. RS: /26 % _____	Stim.? Y N	PSI: 1 2 3 4 5

Comments:

2. VOWELS: Instruct the client to "tell me which letters are vowels." Check, if correct. Number responses in order given.

a   e   i   o   u

| 2. RS: /5 % _____ | Stim.? Y N | PSI: 1 | 3 | 5 |

Comments:

*3. a. VOWEL DESIGNATIONS: Ask the client to "explain the difference between long and short vowels."
Response:

   b. If unable to explain 3a: Indicate number 3 on the Client Stimulus Form. Ask the client to "pronounce each vowel."

       1. a_____   6. ā_____
       2. e_____   7. ē_____
       3. i_____   8. ī_____
       4. o_____   9. ō_____
       5. u_____   10. ü_____

   c. If unable to produce correct resonses to item 3b: Give client a dictionary and ask client to "use the dictionary to help you tell me how to pronounce the vowels on this list." (Client Stimulus Form Number 3)

       1. a_____   6. ā_____
       2. e_____   7. ē_____
       3. i_____   8. ī_____
       4. o_____   9. ō_____
       5. u_____   10. ū_____

3a. RS: /1	% _____	Stim.? Y N	PSI: 1	2	3	4	5
b. RS: /10	% _____	Stim.? Y N	PSI: 1	2	3	4	5
c. RS: /10	% _____	Stim.? Y N	PSI: 1	2	3	4	5

Comments:

4. VOWEL FUNCTION

   a. *Vowel production:* Indicate number 4 on Client Stimulus Form. Instruct the client to "Say the following 'words'." Score based on the accuracy of vowel production.

   b. *Speech decoding:* Ask the client to "tell me the real (or equivalent) word by spelling or signing it" (example: "shue" = "shoe").

	Correct vowel production	ID of "real word"
1. mee (me)	_____	_____
2. boan (bone)	_____	_____
3. rume (room)	_____	_____
4. nou (now)	_____	_____
5. nead (need)	_____	_____
6. shie (shy)	_____	_____
7. lain (lane)	_____	_____
8. tew (to, too, two)	_____	_____
9. tyde (tide, tied)	_____	_____
10. poynt (point)	_____	_____

| 4a. RS: /10 % _____ Stim.? Y N PSI: 1 2 3 4 5 |
| b. RS: /10 % _____ Stim.? Y N PSI: 1 2 3 4 5 |

Comments:

5. CONSONANT IDENTIFICATION: Ask the client, "What are letters that are not vowels called?" (Consonants)

| 5. RS: /1 % _____ Stim.? Y N PSI: 1 3 5 |

Comments:

6. CONSONANT/VOWELS: Ask the client to "explain the difference between vowels and consonants." Response:

| 6. RS: /1 % _____ Stim.? Y N PSI: 1 3 5 |

Comments:

7. CONSONANT FUNCTION: Indicate the following "words" on Client Stimulus Form Number 7.

   a. *Consonant function:* Tell the client to "Say the 'words'." (Score based on the accuracy of production of underlined consonants).

   b. *Speech decoding:* Ask the client to "Tell me the real (or equivalent) word" by spelling it or signing it. (Example: rase = race)

	Correct consonant production	ID of "real word"
1. cend (send)	_____	_____
2. bight (bite)	_____	_____
3. phat (fat)	_____	_____
4. brix (bricks)	_____	_____
5. wrat (rat)	_____	_____
6. hamb (ham)	_____	_____
7. geans (jeans)	_____	_____
8. gnap (nap)	_____	_____
9. djello (jello)	_____	_____
10. jas (jazz)	_____	_____

7a. RS: /10	% _____	Stim.? Y N	PSI: 1 2 3 4 5
b. RS: /10	% _____	Stim.? Y N	PSI: 1 2 3 4 5

Comments:

8. GRAMMATICAL CONSTRUCTS: Indicate the words for part 8 of the Client Stimulus Form. Tell the client to "say the words."

   a. *Possessives/Plurals:* (Note production of word endings)

      1. lips(s) _____   2. beds(z) _____
      3. buses(əz) _____   4. buzzes(əz) _____
      5. Beth's(s) _____   6. Bill's(z) _____

8a. RS: /6	% _____	Stim.? Y N	PSI: 1 2 3 4 5

Comments:

   b. *Contractions:* (Note production of second syllable)

      1. didn't   3. it's
      2. isn't   4. won't

8b. RS: /4	% _____	Stim.? Y N	PSI: 1 2 3 4 5

Comments:

   c. *Past tense:* (Note production of word endings)

      1. begged(d) _____   2. dipped(t) _____
      3. faded(əd) _____   4. waited(əd) _____

8c. RS: /4	% _____	Stim.? Y N	PSI: 1 2 3 4 5

Comments:

9. PHONEME PRODUCTION: Instruct the client to "tell me what sounds (specific) letters make in words." Transcribe responses. This task may be stimulated with the grapheme "w" by contrasting the grapheme "double u" with the phoneme /w/. Use a blackboard or fingerspelling.

   ```
   b ( )              k ( )        s ( )
   *c ( ) ( ) ( )     l ( )       *t ( ) ( )
   d ( )              m ( )        v ( )
   f ( )              n ( )        w ( )
   *g ( ) ( )         p ( )        x ( )
   h ( )              q ( )        y ( )
   j ( )              r ( )        z ( )
   ```

   * items have alternate sounds ("c"=/s/k/sh/, "g"=/g/j/, "t"=/t/ch/)

9. RS: /24	% _____	Stim.? Y N	PSI: 1 2 3 4 5

Comments:

10. GRAPHEME/PHONEME: Instruct the client to "look at each of the words" on the Client Response Form, part 10. "Say them aloud, and tell me: (a) the number of

letters in each, and (b) the number of sounds in each." If the response to 1b (sounds) is "one" the number of sounds may be *stimulated* by saying to client, "That's the number of syllables. How many sounds does it have?"

		Number of letters	Number of sounds
1)	tub	(3)_____	(3)_____
2)	wine	(4)_____	(3)_____
3)	shop	(4)_____	(3)_____
4)	box	(3)_____	(4)_____
5)	step	(4)_____	(4)_____

| 10a. RS: /5 % _____ Stim.? Y N PSI: 1 2 3 4 5 |
| b. RS: /5 % _____ Stim.? Y N PSI: 1 2 3 4 5 |

Comments:

11a.   DIGRAPH IDENTIFICATION: (Consonants): Ask the client to "tell me the sounds in which two letters equal one sound." (If client correctly indicates that the "sh" was a single sound in the previous exercise, use it as a stimulus and ask client to generate others.)

Responses: _____ _____ _____ _____ _____ _____ _____ _____
              (sh)   (ch)   (th)   (*TH*)   (zh)   (ng)   (ph)   (wh)

Comments:

| 11a. RS: /6 % _____ Stim.? Y N PSI: 1 2 3 4 5 |

11b.   DIGRAPH PRODUCTION (Consonants): Instruct the client to say the following five "words" on the Client Stimulus Form:

1. shim /_____/   3. chup /_____/   5. phop /_____/
2. lang /_____/   4. thull /_____/

| 11b. RS: /5 % _____ Stim.? Y N PSI: 1 2 3 4 5 |

Comments:

11c.   DIGRAPH IDENTIFICATION (Vowels): Instruct client, "Now tell me the vowel sounds in which two letters equal one sound."

Responses: _____ _____ _____ _____ _____ _____ _____ _____ _____ _____
              ai   au   ay   ea   ee   ei   ey   oa   oe   oi

              _____ _____ _____ _____
              oo   ou   oy   uy

| 11c. RS: /5 % _____ Stim.? Y N PSI: 1 2 3 4 5 |

Comments:

11d. DIGRAPH PRODUCTION (Vowels): Instruct the client to "say the following fourteen words" on the Client Stimulus Form:

1. dail /_____/   6. beil /_____/   11. moop /_____/

2. saud /_____/   7. mey /_____/   12. hout /_____/

3. tay /_____/   8. board /_____/   13. doy /_____/

4. sead /_____/   9. loe /_____/   14. shuy /_____/

5. reen /_____/   10. poin /_____/

11d. RS: /14 % _____ Stim.? Y N PSI: 1 2 3 4 5

Comments:

12. SILENT LETTERS: Indicate the following words on the Client Stimulus Form, and
    a. Instruct the client to "say each word"
    b. Instruct the client to "tell me which letters are 'silent letters'"

1. bell (l) _____   6. night (gh) _____   11. debt (b) _____

2. time (e) _____   7. knot (k) _____   12. watch (t) _____

3. flop (-) _____   8. comb (b) _____   13. walk (l) _____

4. tree (e) _____   9. duck (c or k) _____   14. feed (e) _____

5. wrap (w) _____   10. tax (-) _____   15. island(s) _____

12a. RS: /15 % _____ Stim.? Y N PSI: 1 2 3 4 5
b. RS: /15 % _____ Stim.? Y N PSI: 1 2 3 4 5

Comments:

*13. SYLLABIFICATION (Grapheme): Indicate the following words on the Client Stimulus Form. Ask the client to "tell me the number of syllables in each word."

Number of syllables

1. rousemicker   (3)_____

2. audishoble   (4)_____

3. treys   (1)_____

4. coufraine   (2)_____

5. hyphus   (2)_____

13. RS: /5 % _____ Stim.? Y N PSI: 1 2 3 4 5

Comments:

14. SYLLABIFICATION (Auditory/Visual): Say the following words twice. Ask the client to "tell me the number of syllables in each word."

	Number of syllables
1. cheeroid	(2)_____
2. omnifutile	(4)_____
3. kwatz	(1)_____
4. sergid	(2)_____
5. reductive	(3)_____

14. RS: /10 % _____ Stim.? Y N PSI: 1 2 3 4 5

Comments:

*15. STRESS (Grapheme): Indicate the following words on the Client Stimulus Form. Explain, "The words are divided into syllables." Instruct the client to "tell me the syllable of each word that gets the most emphasis or stress.

1. choc tive
2. mer i ca
3. ex train
4. lip lock
5. re dib a ble

15. RS: /10 % _____ Stim.? Y N PSI: 1 2 3 4 5

Comments:

16. STRESS (Auditory/Visual): Say the following words twice. Instruct the client to "tell me which syllable has the stress or emphasis."

1. un pip less
2. a rout
3. cob i tant
4. grump ing
5. a clop tic

16. RS: /10 % _____ Stim.? Y N PSI: 1 2 3 4 5

Comments:

*17. SYLLABLE/STRESS: Instruct the client to "look up each of following words; (a) tell me how many syllables are in the word, (b) tell me the syllable that gets the stress, and (c) pronounce the word."

1. pneumonia (   )
2. revenue (   )

17a. locating (dictionary) RS: /2	% _____	Stim.?	Y N	PSI: 1 2 3 4 5
b. locating (pron. guide) RS: /2	% _____	Stim.?	Y N	PSI: 1 2 3 4 5
c. I.D. number of syllables RS: /2	% _____	Stim.?	Y N	PSI: 1 2 3 4 5
d. I.D. stress RS: /2	% _____	Stim.?	Y N	PSI: 1 2 3 4 5
e. pron. syllables RS: /2	% _____	Stim.?	Y N	PSI: 1 2 3 4 5
f. pron. stress RS: /2	% _____	Stim.?	Y N	PSI: 1 2 3 4 5

Comments:

18. DICTIONARY SKILLS: Instruct the client to indicate which of the following words are not familiar. When you have found two with which client is unfamiliar, instruct the client to "find the selected words in the dictionary." Then instruct the client to "pronounce the word, tell me the part of speech, define the word, and use the word correctly in a sentence."

1. rhyme ( )		4. gnu ( )		
2. quiche ( )		5. aisle ( )		
3. svelte ( )		6. fatigue( )		

18a. pronounc. RS: /2	% _____	Stim.?	Y N	PSI: 1 2 3 4 5
b. part/speech RS: /2	% _____	Stim.?	Y N	PSI: 1 2 3 4 5
c. define RS: /2	% _____	Stim.?	Y N	PSI: 1 2 3 4 5
d. use RS: /2	% _____	Stim.?	Y N	PSI: 1 2 3 4 5

Comments:

Source: Bally 1994.

PRONUNCIATION SKILLS INVENTORY

Client Stimulus Form
(*Note:* Numbers correspond to numbered items on the Clinician's Response Form.)

3. Say each of the following sounds:

    1. a   6. ā
    2. e   7. ē
    3. i   8. ī
    4. o   9. ō
    5. u   10. ū

4. Study each word. Say it the best you can. Tell the real word that is pronounced the same. (Example "shue = shoe")

    1. mee   6. shie

    2. boan   7. lain

    3. rume   8. tew

    4. nou   9. tyde

    5. nead   10. poynt

7. Look at each word. Say it the best you can. Tell me the real word that is pronounced the same (Example: "knaime" = "name").

    1. cend   6. hamb

    2. bight   7. geans

    3. phat   8. gnap

    4. brix   9. dgello

    5. wrat   10. jas

8. Look at each word. Say it the best you can.

    a.   1. lips   4. buzzes
         2. beds   5. Beth's
         3. buses   6. Bill's

    b.   1. didn't   3. it's
         2. isn't   4. won't

    c.   1. begged   3. faded
         2. dipped   4. waited

10. Look at each word and say it to yourself. For each word, tell me: (a) how many letters it has and (b) how many sounds it has.

    1. tub

    2. wine

    3. shop

    4. step

    5. box

11b. Say the following five words:

    1. shim

    2. lang

    3. chup

    4. thull

    5. phop

11d. Say the following fourteen words:

1. dail		2. saud	
3. tay		4. sead	
5. reen		6. beil	
7. mey		8. boad	
9. loe		10. foin	
11. moop		12. hout	
13. doy		14. shuy	

12. Look at each word. Tell me which letters are the silent letters. Say each word.

1. bell	6. night	11. debt
2. time	7. knot	12. watch
3. flop	8. comb	13. walk
4. tree	9. duck	14. feed
5. wrap	10. tax	15. island

13. Look at each word and say it aloud. Tell me how many syllables are in each word.

    1. rousemicker

    2. audishoble

    3. treys

    4. coufraine

    5. hyphus

15. Look at each word and say it aloud. They are separated into syllables. Tell me which syllable gets the most emphasis or stress.

    1. choc tive

    2. mer i ca

    3. ex train

    4. lip lock

    5. re dib a ble

17. Look up these words in the dictionary. Tell me which syllable gets the most emphasis or stress. Pronounce the word.

    a) pneumonia   b) revenue

18. Here are some words. Choose two that you don't know. Find each one in the dictionary. Say each one. Tell me what part of speech it is. Explain its meaning in your own words. Use the word in a sentence.

    1. rhyme   4. gnu

    2. quiche   5. aisle

    3. svelte   6. fatigue

Appendix 10B
Preliminary Comparative Data:
Mean PSI Scores for Grade Schoolers/Prelingually Deaf Adults

Item (#)	Skill	Grade K (n = 25)	Grade 1 (n = 22)	Grade 2 (n = 22)	Grade 3 (n = 22)	Grade 4 (n = 25)	Deaf Adults (n is denoted by ( ) after mean)
1	Recite ABC's	1–	1–	1–	1–	1–	1.05 (78)
2	Identify vowel	5–	2.14–	1.18=	1.18=	1=	1.21 (78)
3 a,b,c	Long vs. Short Vowels	5–	4.54–	3.73=	3+	2.6+	4.05(a) (52) 3.30(b) (23) 3.5 (c) (8)
4,7,8	Pronounce Words	5–	4.84–	3.38+	3.27+	2.2+	4.03(a) (65)
5	Consonants	5–	5–	3.14=	2+	1.56+	3.20 (62)
6	Vowels vs. Consonants	5–	5–	4.73=	4+	2.68+	4.29 (69)
9	Phonemes	5–	3.30=	2.23+	2.82=	2.44+	3.23 (72)
10a	Number of letters	5–	1.45=	1=	1=	1=	1.20 (77)
10b	Number of sounds	5–	3.27+	3.82=	3.09+	2.84+	3.83 (77)
11	Digraphs	5–	4.72–	4.18–	4.27–	3.04+	3.63 (77)
12	Silent letters	5–	4.18–	3=	2.55+	2.52+	3.31 (71)
13	Number of syllables/ written word	5–	5–	2.82–	1.36+	1.24+	2.17 (68)
14	Number of syllables/ spoken word	5–	5–	2.05–	1.73=	1.16+	1.98 (70)
15	Stress– written word	5–	5–	3.64–	2.82=	2.52+	3.10 (68)
16	Stress– spoken word	5–	5–	3.95–	2.64–	2.6+	3.2 (52)
17a	Word find	5–	5–	3.86–	4.64–	1+	1.8 (51)
17b	Stress	5–	5–	4.14–	4–	1.72+	2.33 (33)
17c	Pronunciation	5–	5–	4.33–	3–	2.2–	1.6 (23)
18a	Locate	5–	5–	5–	1.36=	1+	1.40 (56)
18b	Pronunciation	5–	5–	3.95–	2.55=	3.0=	2.89 (56)

Source: Bally and Marasco 1991.

Note: Numbers under each grade indicate mean score for each probe area; "–" after number indicates score worse than deaf population; "+" indicates score better than deaf population; "=" indicates score within .5 of deaf population.

11

Language Skills

Maureen Nichols and Mary June Moseley

■ ■ ■ ■

This chapter will discuss needs of deaf and hard of hearing individuals in the development and refinement of language. "Language" will be defined, specific areas of focus will be described, and techniques for language therapy will be discussed within the framework of an integrated model.

Language is defined as "a socially shared code or conventional system for representing concepts through the use of arbitrary symbols and rule-governed combinations of those symbols" (Owens 1992, 4). This socially shared code allows the exchange of information between two individuals, which is a part of the larger process of communication—"the process of exchanging information and ideas between participants" (Owens 1992, 7). Communication includes a linguistic code that may be received and expressed through several modes: (1) listening (and/or speechreading) and speaking, (2) signing, and (3) reading and writing. In addition, communication may include suprasegmental devices (e.g., rising intonation signalling a question form); nonlinguistic cues (body posture, facial expression, etc.); and metalinguistic cues (the ability to analyze and judge language as an entity separate from its content, a skill required in reading and writing) (Owens 1992).

American Sign Language (ASL), as described in chapter 1 is an example of visual-gestural communication. Communication is said to occur, regardless of the language used, when information is exchanged between two people (Kretschmer and Kretschmer 1978). Thus, this chapter will explore ways to develop language skills leading to effective verbal, signed, or written communicative exchange, depending on the needs and desires of the individual. For example, comprehension of new word meanings may be taught to Deaf students although their expression of those words will be in their own preferred mode and may be either oral or signed.

Language Characteristics of Individuals with Hearing Loss

The language learner must have knowledge of and expertise in several different areas of language (Lund and Duchan 1993; Owens 1992). These areas include: semantics (meaning); syntax and morphology (word order/grammatical information); phonology (sounds); and pragmatics (appropriate use of language—the ability to express one's intentions, the knowledge of how to carry on a conversation, and the ability to take the receiver's perspective in order to provide sufficient information to a conversational partner to ensure understanding of the message). The following paragraphs will review the literature in the areas of semantics, syntax, and pragmatics. Phonology (the sound system) is discussed at length in chapter 9.

Semantics

Two major aspects of semantics, *vocabulary* and *figurative language*, appear problematic for adolescents and some adults with hearing loss (McAnally, Rose, and Quigley 1994).

Studies in the deaf population have found that vocabulary development of deaf children is similar to that of hearing children with comparable characteristics but occurring at a slower pace (Quigley and Paul 1984). The first words of young deaf children (whether signed or spoken) appear to be similar to those of their hearing peers (McAnally, Rose, and Quigley 1994). However, vocabularies of young deaf children may contain fewer lexical items than those of hearing peers. They tend to have difficulty with English function words and less knowledge of common content words (McAnally, Rose, and Quigley 1994). These difficulties appear to persist into adolescence.

In studies that measure educational achievement of school-age children (i.e., administration of the Stanford Achievement Test), a typical profile has been found within deaf students. Their lowest performance usually is on the vocabulary subtest with higher scores attained on other areas of the test. Scores on subtests that involve less language, such as Arithmetic Computation and Spelling, are higher than scores on subtests that involve meaningful language, such as Arithmetic Reasoning and Paragraph Meaning (Quigley and Paul 1984).

In addition, studies have shown that deaf students of all ages are typically unable to comprehend as many words from standard English text as hearing children (Quigley and Paul 1984). In a recent survey, the median-scaled score for

SAT-8 reading comprehension for seventeen-year-old deaf and hard of hearing students was the grade equivalent of 4.5 (Holt 1993).

Figurative language is crucial to communication in English, both in speech and in writing. Estimates suggest that figurative language may constitute as much as two-thirds of spoken and written materials (Boatner and Gates 1969). The most common forms of figurative language are metaphors, similes, and idioms, most requiring the ability to determine similarities and differences between various attributes (McAnally, Rose, and Quigley 1994). Difficulty in the development of metaphors, similes and idioms has been demonstrated in the deaf population (Giorcelli 1982). Educators of deaf and hard of hearing individuals believe that difficulty with figurative language contributes to the major problems students evidence in language development, including reading (Quigley and Paul 1984). In addition, clinical evidence indicates difficulties with figurative language in adolescent deaf and hard of hearing children, particularly in the use of idioms (Hughes, Brigham, and Kuerbis 1986; McAnally, Rose, and Quigley 1994).

Syntax

In the area of development of English syntax, research indicates that deaf and hard of hearing children appear to develop similarly to hearing children, although at a slower rate (Kretschmer and Kretschmer 1978; Quigley and Paul 1984). Much of the research in the area of English syntax has been with written language. Quigley and his associates (Quigley, Power, and Steinkamp 1977; Quigley and Paul 1984) have extensively studied written syntax with deaf and hard of hearing children, ages ten to eighteen years. They have identified specific problematic syntactic structures: the verb system, negation, conjunction, complementation (problems with infinitives), relativization, and question formation. Students appear to use a subject-verb-object sentence pattern for all types of sentences. Difficulty in writing sentences may translate into difficulty in producing clear written discourse.

Yoshinaga-Itano (1986), summarizing studies on written language compositions, indicated that, in comparison to hearing children, children with severe to profound hearing loss show: (1) less productivity with respect to clause, sentence length, and composition length: (2) lack of complexity; and (3) more grammatical errors of additions, substitutions, omissions, and inappropriate word order. The studies described above primarily look at problems with the product rather than describe the process used. A more functional approach to instruction might focus on written language as a process of connected discourse and thus might have the potential for increasing literacy (McAnally, Rose, and Quigley 1994).

Pragmatics

Little research describes the comprehension and use of communicative intentions by deaf and hard of hearing individuals. Clinical observations suggest that most deaf adolescents and adults are able to express their intentions in such a way as to ensure that their needs are met.

Again, there is limited research on the use of discourse rules by children with hearing loss. However, this area is perceived by experienced teachers as problematic for Deaf individuals (e.g., Brackett 1983). Specific areas cited as difficult are topic maintenance, appropriate topic choice, and repair of conversational breakdown.

In addition, there is little research showing how individuals with hearing loss take the perspective of the receiver, a perspective demonstrated by providing clear and concise information in a timely manner. This area is important to evaluate in individuals with hearing loss, particularly the use of cohesive devices in English (DeVilliers 1988; Kretschmer 1989). Cohesive devices are the words that tie sentences together in discourse. They include syntactic forms such as pronominalization, conjunction, relativization, as well as temporal adverbs (e.g., before, now, then), ellipsis (e.g., a partial sentence such as "on the table" typically used in response to a question), articles, and synonyms (Kretschmer 1989; Lund and Duchan 1993).

Pronominalization, conjunction, and relativization—syntactic forms mentioned in the discussion of written syntax as problematic for adolescents with hearing loss—are necessary to provide sufficient information in discourse for understanding. There is some indication that this area may also be problematic in oral English discourse. Hughes and Moseley (1988) found that five college-age students seeking language therapy demonstrated problems with ellipsis, relativization, and use of articles.

Students who experience difficulty in this area have described their problem in the following terms: "I just can't seem to get my point across no matter if I write, sign, or talk!"; "My friends tell me to 'get to the point!'"; "when I leave a message on my brother's answering machine, I have to call back because I can't get it across the first time" (Hughes and Moseley 1988).

Vocabulary and figurative language as well as written language and pragmatics difficulties will be discussed below in more detail. These areas comprise the *language* part of the integrated therapy model and are particularly appropriate for high school aged adolescents working on communication skills. Therefore, the remainder of this chapter will provide recommendations for developing a therapy program in the context of working with a group of adolescents in a classroom setting. Adaptations for individual therapy settings and suggestions for late-deafened adults will be discussed briefly throughout this chapter.

Vocabulary

Vocabulary is an important aspect of literacy. Knowledge of vocabulary is correlated with successful reading comprehension (Quigley and Paul 1984). As stated previously, it has been documented that the vocabulary levels of Deaf children are below those of their hearing peers (McAnally, Rose, and Quigley 1994). The average English vocabulary level of a Deaf eighteen-year-old individual is comparable to that of a nine-year-old hearing child (Cooper and Rosenstein 1986).

Quigley and Paul (1984) state that the difficulty Deaf students have with English vocabulary is demonstrated by their consistently low scores on the SAT Word Meaning Subtest. The problem appears to extend beyond understanding word meanings. Students appear not to see relationships between words or appreciate words as parts of larger categories (Kretschmer and Kretschmer 1978).

A whole language approach to teaching reading and writing does not advocate teaching words in isolation but rather teaching them in context through literature and integrating all aspects of language in meaningful situations (Nagy 1988; Schleper 1992; Westby 1990). The focus is on *how* the individual uses language and what strategies are needed to increase not only vocabulary, but the entire spectrum of language—signed, spoken, written, or read. Vocabulary is taught as a way of enabling students to understand and express concepts and ideas (Nagy 1988). Two important principles of whole language literacy instruction are: (1) students need to be actively involved in purposeful reading and writing tasks, and (2) students need to learn and apply strategies for decoding meaning (Blachowicz 1991).

Vocabulary Assessment

Standardized tests used to evaluate the expressive and receptive vocabularies of students may include published instruments such as the Peabody Picture Vocabulary Test (Dunn and Dunn 1981), Expressive One-word Picture Vocabulary Test (Gardner 1979), and the Comprehension Subtest of the Stanford Achievement Test (1989). These tests are not standardized for Deaf students, but may be used to provide diagnostic information about known and unknown word meaning.

In addition to the information provided by these tests, informal assessment procedures may be included to determine the facility with which the students use their vocabulary across the continuum of signed or spoken language and in reading and writing. Receiving input from the student's academic teachers regarding vocabulary facility and weaknesses and asking the students to reflect on their own vocabulary growth help determine how well the student applies vocabulary knowledge in everyday communication situations.

A full vocabulary assessment should include observation of the student in the classroom and reading a cross section of student writing samples, including journal writing. Close monitoring of what books the student is reading and understanding gives the teacher information regarding the level of text difficulty the student may be able to comprehend.

In addition, students can assess themselves on the correct use of new vocabulary. They can determine how consistently and how well they remember new words (e.g., using charts and journals) and how willing they are to try out newly learned concepts.

Teaching Strategies for Vocabulary

The literature on programming describes many vocabulary teaching and enrichment programs (e.g., Crais 1990; Johnson and Pearson 1984). Characteristics of the most successful vocabulary teaching programs include the following (Nagy 1988):

1. Exposure in meaningful contexts

2. Connections between the words and the student's own life experiences and prior knowledge

3. Varied information about each word

4. Multiple exposures to new words

5. An active role taken by the student in the word learning process

Each of these areas will be discussed below.

1. *Exposure in meaningful contexts* (Nagy 1988; Stahl 1986). The most important way of promoting vocabulary growth is to increase the amount of information that the student reads. Students are exposed to words in a variety of contexts, including student selected materials such as text books, contemporary fiction, poetry, newspapers, magazine articles (including those written by/about Deaf persons), journals, letters, student- and teacher-written essays and short stories. Focus is primarily on the meaning of what is read, and individual words are seen as a part of the whole passage.

Reading provides exposure to words and concepts in a variety of contexts. Many new words are learned incidentally, but wide reading does not automatically ensure that all new vocabulary will be learned. It is not always possible for even the most skilled reader to figure out the word meanings from context. The informal measures described above may help ascertain how the students are deriving meaning from what they read and if direct vocabulary instruction may be needed. Teachers and clinicians must find the correct balance for each student of incidental vocabulary learning and direct vocabulary instruction.

Specific strategies for figuring out word meaning during reading may help students become better readers. One strategy, which has a strong visual component, gives the students a series of choices for figuring out the meaning of an unknown word when it is encountered in a text (see figure 11.1). This "five finger" method suggests the following choices:

1. Recognize the word

2. Guess what the word means from the context and keep reading

3. Figure out what the word means from root, prefix, or suffix

4. Ask a friend or teacher what the word means; and

5. Look it up in the dictionary (MSSD English Department 1993).

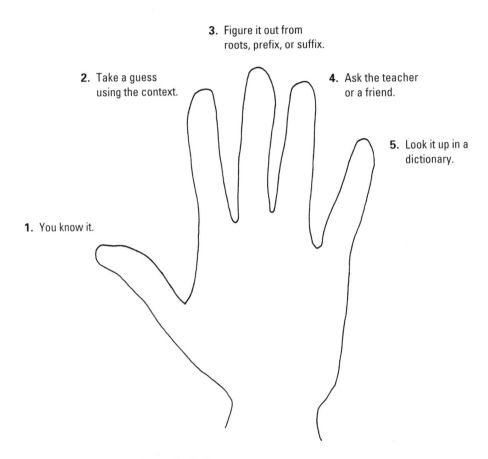

3. Figure it out from roots, prefix, or suffix.

2. Take a guess using the context.

4. Ask the teacher or a friend.

5. Look it up in a dictionary.

1. You know it.

Figure 11.1. Word Attack skills
Source: Adapted from Welsh-Charrier 1995.

A picture of a hand with five fingers (figure 11.1) may serve as a visual reminder for the student.

A second strategy for figuring out word meaning is for the teacher to model the process of guessing and predicting word meanings. The teacher can test to see if the guesses are correct by doing a "think aloud" activity with the class. For example, a transparency of the text may be projected on a screen so that all participants can read along as the teacher makes predictions, guesses at word meanings, tests the hypotheses to see if they make sense, and generally thinks out loud about what the passage means. Students then take turns doing the think aloud activity so that a variety of approaches and techniques can be shared and the students can learn from each other (Cummins 1991).

A third strategy, "dialogue journaling" (a written conversation with the teacher), helps the students learn new vocabulary words related to their own experiences, needs, and interests (Bailes, Searls, Slobodzian, and Staton 1986). (Journaling is discussed in more detail in the section entitled "Writing.") During this journaling process students might ask the teacher about the meaning of a specific word or might write about how they figure out what a new word means. Writing about word meaning is a metacognitive activity that allows both teacher and student to better understand the vocabulary learning process.

2. *Connections between words and the student's prior knowledge.* Students learn more quickly and retain the knowledge when they can make it a part of an already existing schema (Johnson, Pittleman, and Heimlick 1986). Therefore, it is important to make a connection between new words and concepts to information that the student already knows. Johnson, Pittleman, and Heimlick (1986) describe three instructional strategies for vocabulary development that involve activating prior knowledge: semantic associations, semantic mapping, and semantic feature analysis.

The use of *semantic associations* encourages students to discuss words that share common features. The words can be chosen from novels, a textbook, or an article about current events. For example, students can brainstorm all the words related to the word "hearing aid." The list of generated words (written on the board or on a piece of paper to be kept in students' notebooks) could include "expensive, fragile, distortion, beneficial, intolerable, costly, outrageously expensive, and feedback." Students would expand the associations through discussion. For example, one student might know the word "feedback" as part of the communication process, but can learn, through semantic associations, that it also means the annoying "eeeeee" sound a hearing aid makes under certain conditions. Generating English sentences with the words and sharing them with the class is an additional reinforcing activity.

Semantic mapping or *webbing* is organizing information in graphic form. This technique may be used as a prereading or prewriting activity (Johnson and Pearson 1984). The main idea or topic is written in the center of a sheet of paper and the students brainstorm and generate related words and concepts to place in separate and appropriate categories surrounding the topic. If, for example, the topic is "Dormitory Life," one category labeled "roommates" might contain the ideas of friendship, arguments, and negotiation. Another category entitled "rules" might contain the words "strict, too numerous, prison, get you ready for life, help you learn what to do," etc. To encourage higher order thinking skills, the students should be responsible for deciding in which category each word and concept should be placed. As with semantic association, discussion is an important part of this process. Students likely will disagree about the appropriate placement of the words in the web and will need to do some explaining and compromising.

Through semantic mapping students learn new words and concepts and see new applications and relationships among words. They can also think about "old" words in a new way and become more flexible with meaning. This activity is similar to the speechreading constellations described in chapter 8, but with a focus on vocabulary.

Semantic feature analysis taps a reader's prior organization of knowledge

Things that happen in school

Feelings about school activities	winning a soccer championship	losing the soccer championship	listening to a debate on handgun control	deciding where to take the last field trip	having a new chair in teacher's lounge	hearing about a new science discovery			
excited	+	−	+	+	−	+			
agog	+	−	−	−	−	+			
proud	+	−	−	−	−	+			
ambivalent	−	−	+	+	−	−			
apathetic	−	−	−	−	+	−			
lackadaisical	−	+	−	−	−	−			
provocative	−	−	+	−	−	+			

Figure 11.2. Semantic feature analysis
Source: Johnson and Pearson 1984.

and has potential for greatly increasing vocabulary in a systematic way. Students use higher order thinking skills such as comparing, contrasting, and categorizing to learn within specific categories of words. Students are asked to generate a list of words that have features in common. The words are placed in a list and a matrix is constructed with possible features of the words across the top (Johnson and Pearson 1984). A visual representation such as this matrix enables students to see similarities and differences between words and between concepts (see figure 11.2.).

3. *Varied information about each word.* Students benefit from learning that many words have multiple meanings and various grammatical forms and may be used correctly in some contexts but not in others. For example, the word *cozy* can be used to describe a small room, but it would not be appropriate to use it to describe a person's small nose. There are shades of meaning and clusters or groups of words with similar, but discretely different meanings. Blachowicz

(1991) discusses semantic gradients in which students are required to rank order a group of words such as "cool, hot, lukewarm, boiling, freezing, super cooled, and tepid."

Learning antonyms and synonyms for words encourages students to increase their knowledge of the word and become more flexible with language. Many students are interested in studying word derivations and word sources from other countries and cultures. If, for example, a student is reading Shakespeare, it could be pointed out that Shakespeare was responsible for introducing or popularizing almost two thousand words that are used in the English language today.

In addition, vocabulary can be expanded by learning adjective strings or groups of words that can be used interchangeably. It may build an individual's confidence to learn that a sunset can be described not only as beautiful, but as gorgeous, magnificent, breathtaking, incredible, etc.

Learning about analogies is a way of increasing vocabulary and developing analogous reasoning at the same time. It increases the students' ability to see relationships between words and concepts. Analogy work requires students to use the higher order thinking skills of comparing and contrasting and to see part/ whole relationships. Students can write analogies themselves, leaving out one part and asking other students to complete them.

Students can learn the different grammatical forms and meanings of specific words by constructing "word families" on charts that are displayed in the classroom or therapy room and copied into the students' notebooks for further reference (Tompkins 1993). The notebooks may serve as a referral source during writing tasks when the student wants to figure out the correct word form independently from the teacher. Instead of just learning how to use one new vocabulary word, the student can learn how to use the grammatical variations of a word: for example *boredom, bore, boring, boringly*. (See table 11.1.)

Student-created dictionaries and thesauruses can be made containing often-used words or words that are interesting and important to the student. These books can be shared with friends or class members to spark discussion and further increase students' interest in words.

4. *Multiple exposure to new words*. More than one exposure to a new vocabulary word is needed before it becomes part of the students' reading, writing, and signing (speaking) language repertoire. Reinforcement in a variety of experiences with new words is related to effective learning (Blachowicz 1991; Routman 1991). Many different activities can be used to provide this practice. For example, the teacher can generate sentences, poems, and stories that include the new vocabulary words. The students can participate in cooperative learning group activities in which they give each other feedback as to whether the words have been used correctly, or they can make necessary corrections.

In addition, new vocabulary words can be presented daily in written context, in a "word of the day" format related to daily news or announcements. For example, the teacher can write on the blackboard, "All afternoon classes will be canceled this afternoon. I assume that most of you will be ECSTATIC." Students

Table 11.1 Word Families

Noun	Verb	Adjective	Adverb	Notes
teacher	teach	teachable	—	I notice that *er* means person
boredom	bores	boring	boringly	Many adverbs end in *ly*. I wonder if all adverbs end that way.
competition	competed	competitive	competitively	

Model Sentences

1. My *teacher* was born in Ghana.   (noun)

2. Please *teach* us to read Spanish.   (verb)

3. I was so stubborn in elementary school, that the faculty did not think I was *teachable*!   (adjective)

4. I often suffer from *boredom* on Sundays.   (noun)

5. That class really *bores* me!   (verb)

6. What a *boring* movie that was.   (adjective)

7. He explained the directions very *boringly*.   (adverb)

8. The sports *competition* will be tomorrow.   (noun)

9. John *competed* in the race.   (verb)

10. My brother and I are very *competitive*.   (adjective)

11. The twins ran *competitively*.   (adverb)

can guess what the word means and explain to other students why they made that guess. The teacher can use the target vocabulary words when writing in dialogue journals with students (see section entitled "Writing").

The students share with class members and/or with the teacher when and where they read recently learned vocabulary words—in textbooks, literature, newspapers, captioned movies, and/or TV. Vocabulary lists can be posted in the classroom or listed in notebooks and journals for further reinforcement.

5. *An active role taken by the student in the word learning process.* Students can make their own decisions about the kind of words they choose to learn and

can evaluate how often they use newly learned words in their writing, signing, and/or speaking. For example, a student seen by one of the authors wanted to learn vocabulary related to religion; words that would be immediately applicable to a church she was attending. Vocabulary work in this area accompanied work on speechreading and the use of strategies for communication, thus fitting into the integrated therapy model.

Figurative Language

Student use of figurative language is difficult to assess because of the many linguistic, metalinguistic, and nonlinguistic factors involved (Nippold 1985). Therefore, assessment of a student's proficiency with figurative language should be an ongoing process that can include both formal and informal measures.

Formal assessment tools include the Gouchnour Idiom Screening Test (Gouchnour 1977) and the Test of Language Competence-Understanding Metaphoric Expressions subtest (Wiig and Secord 1985). These tests provide information regarding a student's ability to choose the correct meaning of a specific figurative language expression within a multiple choice format. Such tests provide information on idioms and metaphoric expressions common to English, but may not provide information on individual needs.

Informal analysis may involve monitoring what the students are reading, how well they are understanding the text, and what strategies they currently use for deriving meaning from figurative and idiomatic expressions in context. Informal analysis is likely to yield more specific information on individual student needs.

Journal writing with a student is a way to assess what figurative language the teacher uses that the student comprehends. The student might ask the teacher for clarification as part of their written dialogue. Careful reading of the student's written work may reveal that a student is already adept at developing similes and metaphors and using idiomatic expressions. Students can be responsible for evaluating their own progress in writing figurative language by reading through their written narratives over a period of time.

Nippold and Martin (1989) found that a group of hearing students' understanding of idioms increased significantly when the idioms were tested in two-sentence story contexts instead of in isolation. Prinz (1983) reported that it is more difficult for a student to explain the meaning of a word on a multiple choice test. These findings suggest that contextual information will yield more information about a student's knowledge of idioms and is important to consider when developing an original test or interpreting the results of formal tests.

Teaching Strategies for Figurative Language

Initially, students need to develop an awareness that figurative expressions in the English language are difficult to learn for many second language learners, not only for Deaf people. This awareness that the language itself is difficult and that the students are not impaired learners, can motivate them to attempt to attach meaning to different forms of figurative language when they are encountered during reading.

Students fluent in ASL may compare figurative and idiomatic aspects of ASL with those of English and discuss how difficult it often is for people learning ASL to understand these idiomatic expressions. Students can make lists or posters depicting ASL idiomatic expressions to further develop the concept that all languages have idiomatic expressions. During these discussions it is also possible to introduce idiomatic and figurative expressions from the native languages of international students in the class.

It is important that Deaf students engage in a wide variety of reading tasks that will expose them to numerous forms of figurative language in context. Students need to develop and use the strategies of skilled readers such as utilizing prior knowledge, using contextual clues, predicting, guessing the meaning, testing out the proposed meaning to see if it makes sense, and skipping over a part of the text that is not understood and coming back to it later to determine the meaning after more information has been obtained. Teachers can teach students these strategies and demonstrate their use by doing a think-aloud activity as described by Farr (1992) and Cummins (1991). In this activity, the teacher explains her thought processes and describes her strategies as she is using them to derive meaning from the particular passage. Later, students themselves can demonstrate the think-aloud activity while reading and can thus do peer teaching of figurative language.

Some researchers (e.g., Nippold and Martin 1989) advocate the learning of figurative language in context, but also realize the need for some direct teaching, especially the skills of seeing likenesses and differences or learning to compare two objects. These skills are basic to many forms of figurative language, especially similes and metaphors. One concrete strategy to help the student appreciate likenesses and differences is the following: the teacher may show the students two objects and then lead them through a process of filling out a grid that compares various features of the objects, such as size, shape, color, texture, use, etc. By practicing comparison and contrast activities with the teacher, students may show an increased ability to use higher order thinking skills independently when reading and writing. A list of features such as size, color, texture, and placement can also be used as prompts to promote more critical thinking in future tasks. With practice, the students can automatically make comparisons utilizing many parameters.

Various forms of humor such as jokes, puns, riddles, hyperbole, and slang can be taught in a similar manner as idioms, metaphors, and similes. These forms of figurative language can be discussed and analyzed as they appear in the context of what the student is reading. Direct instruction can start with a discussion that these elements occur frequently in the English language.

A comparison of the visual nature of Deaf humor and the humorous auditory play on words that abounds in spoken languages can help students realize that both languages, ASL and English, have specific characteristics related to humor, and that they both can be valued. Students should understand that what is humorous to one person may not be funny to another person. Instructional materials for direct teaching may include teacher-generated multiple choice activities for students to choose the correct meanings of riddles, puns, or jokes. Students can make a notebook with examples of various categories of humor. Transparencies of good examples can be made, and class discussion activities can be conducted to reinforce learning.

Goldstein (1986) suggests using cartoons and comic strips to teach vocabulary and figurative language. Newspapers and magazines are inexpensive, readily available, and current, and they often generate a high degree of interest. She suggests that students identify new words within the humorous context, discuss the meaning of the word or words, and then write the newly acquired words or expressions in a notebook. This activity will give the student repeated opportunities to practice the new concepts and provide a record of that new information.

Newspaper headlines, especially articles on the sports pages, are good sources for examples of slang and figurative language. Bulletin boards or journals and notebooks can be made featuring a wide variety of newspaper headlines for students to discuss.

The activities described above have been presented in the context of a group setting. Most activities are equally appropriate for an individual setting and may be adapted (e.g., using paper instead of chalkboards, discussion between the clinician and client only, or perhaps bringing a third party into the therapy room). Specific vocabulary and/or idioms may be integrated easily with other aspects of the integrated therapy model—speechreading activities, pronunciation skills, communication strategies, etc. In addition, the emphasis on functional vocabulary and figurative language involves the participation of the student in making decisions about the types of skills he or she needs and is consistent with the Integrated Therapy Model as described in chapter 2.

In addition, these activities have emphasized the refinement of written, spoken, or signed language and have been appropriate for the adolescent or adult who was congenitally deafened. Adults who are deafened later in life may have different needs in the areas of semantics because a language base has already been established. Some of the specific needs in this area may center around working on new vocabulary or idiomatic expressions. For example, the client may learn the names of current politicians and countries, or new slang and vocabulary from current events (i.e., "Whitewater," "information superhighway," "roller blading") and from the changing social, political, and educational environment. In addition, words and figurative expressions related to the person's work setting may be explored and utilized during communication therapy sessions.

Written Language

Deaf individuals have the need to perform a variety of writing tasks in everyday life at school or work and in social situations. As described earlier in this chapter, considerable research has documented and described the problems of Deaf writers (Kretschmer and Kretschmer 1978). Students have related to one author of this chapter their many negative experiences with writing, especially with teachers handing back their writing covered with red marks.

One approach is to perceive a Deaf student as a developing writer who needs more experience with the English language, often a second language, not as a disabled writer who needs to be fixed. Thus, the student may feel more free to experiment with a wide variety of writing tasks (journal writing, biography, poetry, and essays). Deaf students have many interesting experiences and ideas to put down on paper (Ewoldt 1993–1994). With this approach, students may be more willing to share their work with others, to ask for constructive criticism, and to use feedback from others to revise and improve what they are writing.

Assessment of Writing

Assessment of a Deaf student's writing can include using a standardized test such as the Test of Written Language (TOWL) (Hammill and Larsen 1985). This test is not standardized on Deaf students; however, it may provide diagnostic information regarding sequencing, grammatical structure, spelling, and the mechanics of writing, such as punctuation and capitalization.

Proponents of the whole language philosophy (e.g., Baskwill and Whitman 1988) recommend that informal writing evaluation should occur on a daily basis using observation, recording, and interpretation of what students are saying and doing during the writing process.

Areas that can be evaluated are the students' ability to use written communication when performing the following writing tasks:

1. Writing an emergency message

2. Using the TTY

3. Writing in a journal

4. Writing through interactive computers

5. Personal letter writing

In assessing all five areas it is necessary to determine: (a) the intent or purpose of the communication, (b) the intended audience or receiver of the message, (c) the effectiveness of the communication, (d) how well the writer determines if the written communication was effective, and (e) what repair strategies the student uses to improve the written message (Horn et al. 1983).

Emergency Message The emergency message should state the problem and describe what kind of help is needed. It needs to be specific and to include all important information, but not unnecessary details. The grammar and spelling need to be clear enough for the reader to understand the message, but do not need to be perfect. If the first written emergency message is not clear enough, the writer must be able to identify problems that interfere with communication and correct them quickly.

TTY Conversation The student should know TTY protocol, abbreviations, rules of turn taking, and appropriate greetings and closing of conversations (Deyo 1984). The student should focus on sending a clear message and on not becoming overly concerned with minor typographical errors or spelling errors that do not interfere with the message. Specific questions to be asked are: Can the student formulate and answer questions clearly? What clarification and repair strategies does the student use when the message is not understood by the receiver or when the student does not understand what has been typed? Can the student use a relay service effectively? Using a TTY that has a printer will enable hard copies of conversations to be saved and evaluated over time.

Journal writing Depending on the type of journal being used (see the section on journal writing in this chapter), changes and improvements in vocabulary and the mechanics of writing can be assessed. More importantly, expression of more critical thinking skills can be noted by both teacher and student.

Interactive Computer Writing Students can receive feedback and suggestions from other writers involved in this form of collaborative writing regarding specific ways their writing can be improved (O'Connor, Peyton, and Bloomquist 1990). Saving and evaluating hard copies of the writing will aid the teacher in evaluating growth and improvement. (See the description of Computer Networks for Writing later in this chapter.)

Personal and Business Letter Writing A variety of letters can be evaluated, depending upon a student's experiences and need: cover letters for résumés, requests for information, or thank you and sympathy notes are just a few examples.

Teaching Strategies for Writing

The whole language approach to teaching writing has many applications for developing writers. Writing is taught as a process rather than just focusing on the end product. Rather than have the student write a piece and submit it to the teacher who does all the editing and correcting, the student goes through many steps in the writing process.

The Writing Process The main stages of the process include prewriting, writing, revision, editing, and postwriting (Goodman 1986). The prewriting process includes rehearsal activities such as group discussion or using graphic organizers such as webs, as a way of coming up with ideas related to a specific topic. This gives the students the opportunity to use their prior knowledge about a topic and to think critically about the topic without having to worry at this stage about grammar or mechanics.

During the writing stage of the process, the student writes a rough draft, then shares it with several classmates (peers) who give feedback regarding content but not grammar, spelling, or punctuation at this point. For example, if a student wrote a sketchy story about his former school, feedback from peers might include what they liked and didn't like about the story or questions such as, "What did your school look like? What did your teacher look like? Was your teacher mean or nice? Did your teacher remind you of anyone else that you know? Can you compare that teacher with any other teacher?"

Students use the feedback for the next stage of the process—revision of their writing. They may write drafts as necessary until they are satisfied with the organization and content of their writing piece. It is helpful to remind students at this stage that most writers write many drafts before they are satisfied. Teachers can share their own writing drafts and final pieces as examples. Students enjoy reading their teachers' writing and listening to them describe their writing process. Powers (1994) describes how one teacher shared a term paper on which she received a disappointing grade of C and let the class read the professor's red ink comments. The teacher then led the class in a discussion of how her paper could have been improved.

If direct teaching of grammar or punctuation is necessary, it is done at this point in the writing process within the context of the student's own work. Class mini-lessons, such as in subject-verb agreement, or individual instruction can be conducted at this time. The student may keep a list of all grammar and punctuation skills that have been taught and should be expected to apply these skills in all future writing. Students are taught editing skills and are responsible for self-editing all work before it is turned into the teacher for teacher editing. Some students may prefer to add a step to the writing process and ask a friend or classmate to edit a piece of writing after self-editing and before teacher editing.

After the student has already completed the revision or self-editing process, the teacher may edit the writing. Instead of correcting a grammatical or punctuation error directly on the student's work, the teacher may make comments on yellow sticky notes. For example, if the student has grammatical errors, the teacher may advise the student to review his lesson on plurals. Thus, the student becomes responsible for correcting the error and producing a completed product.

Journal Writing Journal writing is a way for Deaf students to practice, expand, and refine their writing skills. Many different kinds of journals have been used successfully with elementary- through college-age Deaf students (Bailes et al. 1986; Staton 1990).

A *dialogue journal* is a written conversation between student and teacher about a student-selected topic. Bailes et al. (1986) describe how teacher and student take turns writing back and forth, sharing thoughts, experiences, reactions and insights. The student's grammar and spelling are not corrected, nor is any grade given for the student's work. Instead, the teacher models correct English grammar, syntax, and spelling; and over time, changes in the student's written English occur (Bailes et al. 1986).

A student/client may write in a dialogue journal about how he or she reacted in difficult communication situations. This may provide a way of analyzing responses and discussing more effective and assertive ways to handle future situations. Keeping a daily communication journal can be an especially beneficial way for a late-deafened adult to keep track of progress and to note change over time.

Staton (1985) studied dialogue journals of elementary, secondary, and postsecondary Deaf students and found that writing competence and grammatical fluency increased over time. Also evident were improvements in reading comprehension, including better understanding of idioms and inferences. In addition to improving language skills, students using dialogue journals showed refined thinking skills (Mettler and Conway 1991). Deaf college students demonstrated greater ability to express and to elaborate their ideas in English, as well as to demonstrate a greater understanding of the subject matter of courses in which dialogue journals were used (Staton 1990).

Literature journals are described by Welsh-Charrier (1991) as a place where students and teachers discuss, through writing, books, chapters, and stories the student is reading. Dialogue journals and literature journals have several similar characteristics, focusing on student interests and not emphasizing grammatical or spelling errors. Literature journals are content oriented and provide a way for the teacher to gain insight into what the student understands about the text being read and into what the student needs in terms of instruction. Based on needs observed by the teacher when writing journal dialogues with a student, individual lessons on grammar or spelling, or direct teaching of reading strategies, can be conducted.

Schleper (1993) used children's picture books to teach literary elements such as foreshadowing, symbolism, and onomatopoeia to Deaf adolescents. He found that the students demonstrated improved ability to understand the above literary devices and that they incorporated these elements in their written compositions.

Hartman and Kretschmer (1992) found that Deaf students who discussed what they were reading using ASL, and then wrote about what they were reading using English, increased their understanding of what they were reading. The literature journal was a place where the students were able to bridge the gap between the two language forms of written English and signed ASL.

Peer reading journals are another form of literature journals (Mettler and Conway 1991). Students have a written conversation with peers about books they have selected to read. The teacher reads the entries, responds in writing, and develops a three-way reading journal. The teacher can also suggest kinds of questions the students might ask each other. Students may also write back and forth about topics of mutual interest. The teacher may periodically join the written conversation to encourage deeper thinking about a topic or lead the conversation in a different direction.

In two separate studies, the use of interactive conversational writing and writing about experiences with no correction of syntax were shown to result in improvement in the use of syntactic skills (Harrison, Simpson, and Stuart 1991; Staton 1985). Staton (1985) described the use of a dialogue journal and hypothesized that functional interactive conversation can be created through writing rather than face-to-face conversations. She further hypothesizes that correct grammar emerges through the communication experience. Harrison, et al. (1991) indicated similar findings using noncorrective writing.

Computer Networks for Writing   Collaborative writing on computer networks is being used with a wide age range of Deaf students (Bruce, Peyton, and Batson 1993). The ENFI (Electronics Networks for Interaction) approach was developed at Gallaudet University in Washington, D.C., in 1985. The purpose of this program was to give Deaf students opportunities to use written English in different ways.

ENFI uses a computer network within classes for collaborative "real-time" written interaction. Messages are composed by all participating individuals and transmitted to all other screens involved in the network. As individuals type and send messages, the written message scrolls up the screen, with the name of the sender attached, forming a script similar to that of a play. Individuals may compose on a private window at the bottom of their screen as other messages from participants continue to scroll up the screen. Participants can thus read previous messages as well as continue composing new ones. The computer stores the entire conversation so that it may be reviewed at any time (Bruce, Peyton, and Batson 1993).

The ability to create natural conversation and dialogue is emphasized in network-based programs. Students may discuss, role play, respond to one another, collaborate in writing text, play language games such as Twenty Questions, and participate in a variety of other language activities involving print (Bruce, Peyton, and Batson 1993). In addition, there is potential for working with many aspects of language: developing narratives; using syntax and semantics; practicing pragmatic abilities such as the expression of different intentions; using cohesive devices; and learning rules for conducting discourse. O'Conner, Peyton, and Bloomquist (1990) found that students enrolled in the ENFI program scored better on the English Language Proficiency Test than students not enrolled in the program. Gains were noted in language acquisition and in the reading and writing processes. The authors described ENFI as an "opportunity to interact in print about print" (17).

Story Narratives   Mozzer-Mather (1990) described a strategy for writing story narratives. Deaf students were videotaped signing narratives of remembered experiences in ASL. Next, the students watched the videotape and wrote the same stories in English. Because the written drafts were not as complex and detailed as the signed stories, using the video, Mozzer-Mather made lists of English glosses as memory prompts and gave them to the students. (Glosses are English words written entirely in capital letters to indicate that they are to be regarded as symbols of signs. The meanings of the glosses roughly parallel the meanings of the English words used.) Using the list of glosses, the students wrote another draft of the story that was longer and more detailed and that contained fewer grammatical errors than the first draft. This technique used ASL to help refine English. Mozzer-Mather proposed investigating the strategy of asking older Deaf students to watch their signed narratives on video and then to create their own list of glosses before writing the stories in English.

Pragmatics

Knowledge of how to participate in discourse and take the receiver's perspective are necessary for clear communication. These two areas will be discussed in the following section.

Discourse

Assessment Observation of an individual's discourse skills is one of the major ways of obtaining information about his or her ability to participate in a conversation and keep the conversation moving (Roth and Spekman 1984b). Information gathering usually includes such elements of discourse as social versus nonsocial speech; turn-taking and talking time; conversational and topic initiation; maintenance and termination; on-topic exchanges (contingency); and/or conversational repairs (Roth and Spekman 1984a).

Task-oriented group activities are valuable for permitting an analysis of turn-taking skills. Fabricating situations in which breakdown of the conversation occurs may provide information about needs in this area (see also the discussion of repair strategies in chapter 3). Greeting and farewell rituals may be observed in the natural process in which they occur: coming to and leaving a communication therapy situation.

Role playing may provide a way to observe the adolescent or adult in conversational interaction. A check sheet can be used to indicate whether such behaviors exist regularly, part of the time, or not at all. Published checksheets exist that can help objectify needs in this area (for example, Deyo and Hallau 1983; Prutting and Kirchner 1987; Wiig and Bray 1984). In addition, a written transcript of the utterances used during a specific activity may provide valuable information about discourse skills, including the specific amount of on-topic utterances and contingent utterances (Hughes and Moseley 1988).

Programming Some published programs exist for teaching individuals the rules of discourse (for example, Deyo and Hallau 1983; Wiig and Bray 1984). Deyo and

Hallau's (1983) program, *Communicate with Me: Conversation Strategies for Deaf Students,* is specifically designed for adolescents with hearing loss. The purpose of this program, which focuses on student-to-adult interactions, is to help deaf and hard of hearing students improve their conversation skills. It includes seven units covering the following areas: (1) selecting appropriate topics and communication methods, (2) gaining attention, (3) turn-taking, (4) ending conversations, (5) repair strategies, (6) maintaining and changing topics, and (7) combined practice areas from all units.

The *Communicate with Me* program was designed for students seven to fifteen years old. The program uses role-play activities, visuals in the form of pictures, cards, and books, as well as checklists for rating self or others through videotape analysis. The stories in the books and the pictures represent everyday life situations encountered specifically by deaf and hard of hearing students. For example, one of the role-play activities describes a situation in which the student must approach a Deaf principal, begin a conversation about selling copies of the school newspaper, and then end the conversation (Deyo and Hallau 1983).

This program addresses a specific area of language within a conversational format. In addition, it provides pictorial representation of the activities as well as discussion. The use of visual/pictorial design in instructional materials for children with hearing loss is desirable (Diebold and Waldron 1988). The stories and pictures are relevant to experiences of Deaf individuals. The flexibility of this program provides the potential for integrating other areas of language (e.g., semantics, pragmatic intentions, etc.) into the existing lessons.

No written evaluation of the *Communicate with Me* program is identified. However, a similar program, using role-playing and video analysis was tried for eighteen weeks with twelve- to thirteen-year-old Deaf children in Queensland (Murphy and Hill 1989). The focus of this program was on communicative function, and the program included general functions such as how to initiate and maintain conversations, as well as specific functions such as how to ask a favor, how to cope with being teased, how to make polite queries, etc. Analysis of this program indicated student improvement and awareness of the skill being facilitated as well as generalization to other spontaneous interactions.

The activities described above are appropriate for use in a group, but may be adapted to an individual client-clinician relationship. In addition to such activities, a direct discussion approach may prove beneficial; for example, talking with the client about conversational routines (greeting, ending conversations, etc.). This may be especially helpful for the late-deafened adult, who may need some specific knowledge/discussion of the aspects of discourse that make conversation possible.

Taking the Receiver's Perspective

This area focuses on the informativeness of a message and the ease with which that message can be conveyed. Table 11.2 presents an example of a message that

Table 11.2 Partial Transcript of Conversation between Bob (B) and a Clinician (C)

Conversational Turn		Utterance
1	B:	We just got that for a vacation house.
2	C:	Do you go there every year?
3	B:	Uh we bought it this year or last year. But uh It's a uh, we have a um, pool so we can play sometimes.
4	C:	Oh that's great!
5	B:	They're very competitive inside You like ping-pong?
6	C:	Uh-huh Yeah
7	B:	He plays ping-pong a lot because they like to be very competitive.
8	C:	Who's that? Your brothers you mean?
9	B:	They still try to compete and they say I'm better than you. [clinician laughs] And all that stuff And uh . . .

Source: Hughes and Moseley 1988.

is difficult to understand and requires clarification in order for communication to occur. For example, in turn 3 Bob does not respond directly and appropriately to the preceding question: the conversation is not contingent. In turns 5 and 7, Bob uses pronouns in two different ways: without a preceding referent and with unclear number (*he* and *they* are used with no indication of number of people involved).

Such communication is an example of the problem with taking the receiver's perspective, also described in the literature as presupposition or role taking (Roth and Spekman 1984a and 1984b). Hughes and Moseley (1988) report deaf and hard of hearing students who, when they seek communication therapy, claim, "I just can't seem to get my point across no matter if I write, sign or talk!"

The process of providing clear information is based on the premise that some information in a message is "old" and some is "new." The sender and the receiver must differentiate between the two areas, inferring information about their partner and the context in order to choose appropriate words (or signs) to express meaning. Shared information or knowledge can be established in several ways: (1) by mutually monitoring aspects of the physical setting; (2) by sharing some general knowledge of the communication situation itself or of the communicative partner (for example, age, status, past experiences); and (3) by mutually monitoring the preceding discourse (Roth and Spekman 1984a).

In English, written and verbal discourse use linguistic cohesive devices to assure that information is exchanged clearly (Halliday and Hasan 1976). Examples of cohesive devices are the use of relative clauses (describing a person or object); of pronominalization (pronouns specify a previously used referent); of direct and indirect references (*a* refers to "new" information; *the* to "old" information); and of ellipsis, substitution, and conjunction. In addition, the use of adjectives and specific nouns (identifying objects by name, rather than calling an object "that thing") help to provide information.

Assessment Assessing the informativeness of a message may be done through the use of the referential communication task or barrier game (Hughes and Moseley 1988; Roth and Spekman 1984b). One version of this task is to erect a barrier between two participants and present each person with a set of pictures (photographs or designs) that are exactly alike. One of the individuals must describe a specific picture or design in such a way that it is easily identifiable by the person on the opposite side of the barrier who may ask for feedback as needed. The degree of feedback necessary to complete the task may vary from consistent feedback to none and will help delineate the need for clarification to convey a message. In addition, a transcript of such an activity may indicate what kinds of cohesive devices the individual used to help convey information.

The barrier game activity may be varied in several ways. For example, the complexity of the activity itself may be varied by using photographs, line drawings, modern designs, or real objects. The role and age of the receiver may be varied by using different individuals to see how the client responds to cognitive level, status, and familiarity.

Assessment may also include evaluating the client's informativeness in such discourse activities as describing an event or favorite TV show or movie, retelling a story, describing an activity such as purchasing a car or taking a vacation, or conversing spontaneously. A written transcript of such discourse will provide a clear account of contingency, timing, need for clarification during a verbal interaction, and cohesive devices used.

Programming The following section will discuss several possible ways to approach programming in the area of providing adequate information to a receiver. These approaches may be selected depending on their usefulness with either English or with ASL.

Hughes and Moseley (1988) describe two teaching approaches. The first they refer to as a linguistic orientation, appropriate for teaching written or spoken English skills. This approach involves direct instruction specifically on each of the syntactic/linguistic devices found to be indicators of the ability to take the receiver's perspective.

For example, the purpose and use of relative clauses may be discussed and practiced (identifying or nonidentifying relative clauses) (Swan 1984). Different types of adjective classes (size, color, shape, texture, etc.) and how they are used in relation to nouns, may be consciously discussed. Pronoun reference may be directly practiced. Such a direct instructional approach may later become more interactive, through journal or computer writing, so that the practice on these specific structures becomes more communicative in nature. For example, adjective types may be applied to the description of a new dress bought to wear to homecoming events. Practical application to writing and providing information is the goal of any direct instruction.

The second approach described by Hughes and Moseley (1988) is a visual/conceptual approach and is appropriate for either English or ASL. This approach has appeared clinically effective with clients who seem to have overall sign and spoken receptive and expressive language difficulties. These students may also have difficulty formulating their thoughts into sign or onto paper, respond inappropriately to questions, have a limited vocabulary, and seem to have no strategies to repair communication breakdowns.

The visual/conceptual approach is based on systematically identifying similarities and differences in two like pictures. Distinguishing features are discussed and analyzed. The following are examples of the types of features that are relevant for such a discussion:

1. *Similarities*—identification of the main idea/topic of each picture, such as similar people, objects, space, color, etc.

2. *Differences*—identification of emotions, body characteristics (hair color, hair length, overall height of individuals, positioning of arms/legs), clothing descriptors, location of the picture (inside, outside), texture of objects, angle of the camera (aerial, lateral), etc.

In conjunction with both of these approaches, anticipatory strategies (those strategies used to prepare for a communication event, thus reducing the possibilities of communication breakdown) and repair strategies (such as rephrasing, changing mode of communication, etc.) are taught.

Clients may evaluate themselves by watching videotapes or by using check sheets to indicate use of cohesive devices or identification of similarities and differences. A checklist can also be used to review any written work the students do, whether describing a picture or writing an essay.

Hughes (Hughes and Moseley 1988) reports clinical success with this methodology within a three- to six-month period. In addition, clients report a noticeable difference in their own daily communication: "My parents seem to understand me better, I don't have to repeat as much"; "I was able to leave a message on my brother's answering machine with one call—instead of being cut off by the beep and having to call back"; "I used the checksheet while proofing this letter I'm writing to you."

Wallach and Miller (1988) suggest helping students develop an appreciation for the use of cohesion in English by analyzing their own textbooks. For example, pronouns can be identified and circled in a text, then others substituted to vary meaning and complexity. Charts can be made to help categorize vocabulary and pronouns specific to a particular narrative or text. For example, "In this story, Steven is referred to as: a child, the boy, he, his, the baby, etc." Other writers (e.g., Lund and Duchan 1993) suggest similar activities.

Summary

This chapter has discussed areas of language important for communication therapy with adolescents and adults. The term "language" was defined, and characteristics of deaf and hard of hearing individuals were described. The focus of this chapter has been on strategies for assessing and programming for several aspects of language including vocabulary, figurative language, written language, and pragmatics. The aspects of pragmatics discussed were the use of discourse rules and the ability to take the receiver's perspective.

References

Bailes, C., S. Searls, J. Slobodzian, and J. Staton. 1986. *It's your turn now!: Using dialogue journals with deaf students*. Washington, D.C.: Gallaudet University, Pre-College Programs.

Baskwill, J., and P. Whitman. 1988. *Evaluation: Whole language, whole child*. New York: Scholastic Inc.

Blachowicz, C. 1991. Making connections: Alternatives to the vocabulary notebook. *Reading Teacher*. 45:643–649.

Boatner, M. T., and J. E. Gates. 1969. *A dictionary of idioms for the deaf*. Washington, D.C.: National Association of the Deaf.

Brackett, D. 1983. Group communication strategies for the hearing impaired. *Volta Review* 85:116–128.

Bruce, B., J. K. Peyton, and T. Batson. 1993. *Network-based classrooms: Promises and realities*. New York: Cambridge University Press.

Cooper, R., and J. Rosenstein. 1986. Language acquisition of deaf children. *Volta Review* 68:57–58.

Crais, E. 1990. World knowledge to word knowledge. *Topics in Language Disorders* 10: 45–62.

Cummins, A. 1991. A thinking skills strategy. *Learning '91* 19:53.

DeVilliers, P. A. 1988. Assessing English syntax in hearing-impaired children: Eliciting production in pragmatically-motivated situations. *JARA Monograph Supplement* 2: 41–71.

Deyo, D. 1984. *Ring/flash: Telephone skills for deaf and hard of hearing students.* Washington, D.C.: Gallaudet University, Pre-College Programs.

Deyo, D., and M. Hallau. 1983. *Communicate with me: Conversation strategies for Deaf students.* Washington, D.C.: Gallaudet University, Pre-College Programs.

Dunn, L., and L. Dunn. 1981. *Peabody Picture Vocabulary Test, rev. ed.* Circle Pines, Minn.: American Guidance Service.

Diebold, T. J., and M. B. Waldron. 1988. Designing instructional formats: The effects of verbal and pictorial components on hearing-impaired students' comprehension of science concepts. *American Annals of the Deaf* March: 30–35.

Ewoldt, C. 1993-94. Language and literacy from a deaf perspective. *The Whole Language Newsletter* 13:2–5.

Farr, R. 1992. Implementing a whole language approach: conceptual and practical issues. Paper presented at ASCD Mini-Conference on Whole Language Instruction, Alexandria, Virginia.

Gardner, M. 1979. *Expressive One-Word Picture Vocabulary Test.* Novato, Calif.: Academic Therapy Publications.

Giorcelli, L. 1982. *The comprehension of some aspects of figurative language by deaf and hearing subjects.* Doctoral dissertation, University of Illinois, Urbana.

Goodman, K. 1986. *What's whole in whole language.* Portsmouth, New Hamp.: Heinemann.

Goldstein, B. 1986. Looking at cartoons and comics in a new way. *Journal of Reading* 29: 657–661.

Gouchnour, E. 1977. *Gouchnour Idiom Screening Test.* Danville, Ill.: Interstate Printers & Publishers.

Halliday, M. A. K., and R. Hasan. 1976. *Cohesion in English.* London: Longman.

Hammill, D. D., and S. C. Larsen. 1985. *Test of Written Language.* Austin, Tex.: Pro-Ed.

Harrison, D. R., P. A. Simpson, and A. Stuart. 1991. The development of written language in a population of hearing-impaired children. *Journal of the British Association of Teachers of the Deaf* 15:76–85.

Hartman, M., and R. Kretschmer. 1992. Talking and writing: Deaf teenagers reading *Sarah, plain and tall. Journal of Reading* 36:174–180.

Holt, J. A. 1993. Stanford Achievement Test, 8th ed.: Reading comprehension subgroup results. *American Annals of the Deaf* 138:172–175.

Horn, R., J. Mahshie, M. Wilson, and S. Bally. 1983. Audiologic habilitation with the hearing impaired adolescent/adult: An integrative approach. Miniseminar presented at American Speech-Language-Hearing Convention, Cincinnati, Ohio.

Hughes, M. C., and M. J. Moseley. 1988. A descriptive pragmatic inventory for deaf adolescents: Implications for intervention. Miniseminar presented at American Speech-Language-Hearing Association, Boston, Massachusetts.

Hughes, M. C., E. Brigham, and T. Kuerbis. 1986. Approaches to teaching figurative language to hearing-impaired adolescents/adults. Miniseminar presented at the ASHA Convention, Detroit, Michigan.

Johnson, D., and P. Pearson. 1984. *Teaching reading vocabulary.* New York: Holt, Rinehart and Winston.

Johnson, D., S. Pittleman, and E. Heimlick. 1986. Semantic mapping. *The Reading Teacher* 39:778–783.

Kretschmer, R. E. 1989. Pragmatics, reading and writing: Implications for hearing-impaired individuals. *Topics in Language Disorders* 9:17–32.

Kretschmer, R. R., and L. W. Kretschmer. 1978. *Language development and intervention with the hearing impaired.* Baltimore: University Park Press.

Lund, N. J., and J. F. Duchan. 1993. *Assessing children's language in naturalistic contexts,* 3rd ed. Englewood Cliffs: Prentice Hall.

McAnally, P. L., S. Rose, and S. P. Quigley. 1994. *Language learning practices with deaf children,* 2d ed. Austin, Tex.: Pro-Ed, Inc.

Mettler, R., and D. Conway. 1991. Peer reading journals: A student to student application of dialogue journals. In *Perspectives in Education and Deafness,* ed. M. Abrams. Washington, D.C.: Gallaudet University, Pre-College Programs.

Mozzer-Mather, S. 1990. *A strategy to improve deaf students' writing through the uses of glosses of signed narratives.* Washington, D.C.: Gallaudet University Research Institute Publication #WP90-4.

Murphy, J., and J. Hill. 1989. Training communication functions in hearing-impaired adolescents. *Australian Teacher of the Deaf* 30:26–32.

Nagy, W. 1988. *Teaching vocabulary to improve reading comprehension.* Urbana, Ill.: National Council of Teachers of English.

Nippold, M., 1985. Comprehension of figurative language in youth. *Topics in Language Disorders* 5:1–20.

Nippold., M., and S. Martin. 1989. Idiom interpretation in isolation versus context: A developmental study with adolescents. *Journal of Speech and Hearing Research* 32: 59–66.

O'Connor, D., J. Peyton, and C. Bloomquist. 1990. The performance of ENFI and non-ENFI students on Gallaudet University's English Placement Test, 1989–1990. *Teaching English to Deaf and Second Language Students* 8(2):10–17.

Owens, R. E., Jr. 1992. *Language development: An introduction,* 3rd ed. New York: Merrill.

Powers, R. 1995. Personal communication. Model Secondary School for the Deaf, Washington, D.C.

Prinz, P. 1983. The development of idiomatic meaning in children. *Language and Speech* 26:263–272.

Prutting, C. A., and D. M. Kirchner. 1987. A clinical appraisal of the pragmatic aspects of language. *Journal of Speech and Hearing Disorders* 52:105–119.

Quigley, S., and P. Paul. 1984. *Language and deafness.* San Diego, Calif.: College Hill Press.

Quigley, S. P., D. J. Power, and M. W. Steinkamp. 1977. The language structure of Deaf children. *Volta Review* 79:73–83.

Roth, F. P., and N. J. Spekman. 1984a. Assessing the pragmatic abilities of children, part 1: Organizational framework and assessment parameters. *Journal of Speech and Hearing Disorders* 49:2–11.

————. 1984b. Assessing the pragmatic abilities of children, part 2: Guidelines, considerations, and specific evaluation procedures. *Journal of Speech and Hearing Disorders* 49:12–17.

Routman, R. 1991. *Invitations: Changing as teachers and learners.* Portsmouth, N. H.: Heinemann.

Schleper, D. 1992. *Prereading strategies.* Washington, D.C.: Gallaudet University.

————. 1993. *Using picture books to introduce literary devices to deaf adolescents.* Washington, D.C.: Gallaudet Research Institute.

Stahl, S. 1986. Three principles of effective vocabulary instruction. *Journal of Reading* 29: 662–668.

Stanford Achievement Test. 1989. New York: Psychological Corporation.

Staton, J. 1985. Using dialogue journals for developing thinking, reading, and writing with hearing-impaired students. *Volta Review* 87:127–154.

————. 1990. *Conversations in writing: A guide for using dialogue journals with deaf secondary and post secondary students.* Washington, D.C.: Gallaudet University Research Institute.

Swan, M. 1984. *Basic English usage.* Oxford: Oxford University Press.

Tompkins, L., 1993. Personal communication: Washington, D.C. Gallaudet University.

Wallach, G., and L. Miller. 1988. *Language intervention and academic success.* Boston: College Hill Press.

Welsh-Charrier, C. 1991. *The literature journal.* Washington, D.C.: Gallaudet University, Pre-College Programs.

————. 1995. Word attack skills figure (adapted). Washington, D.C.: Gallaudet University, Model Secondary School for the Deaf.

Westby, C. E. 1990. The role of the speech-language pathologist in whole language. *Language, Speech, and Hearing in Schools* 21:228–237.

Wiig, E. H., and C. M. Bray. 1984. *Let's talk: Intermediate level.* Columbus, Ohio: Merrill.

Wiig, E., and W. Secord. 1985. *Test of Language Competence.* Columbus, Ohio: Merrill.

Yoshinaga-Itano, C. 1986. Beyond the sentence level: What's in a hearing-impaired child's story? *Topics in Language Disorders* 6:71–84.

Communication Therapy Case Studies

Introduction

The last section of this book will emphasize the application of the integrated communication therapy model. In chapter 12, Wilson and Scott show varying skills that may be integrated, with specific emphasis on telephone training. Chapter 13 provides three detailed therapy plans for clients with differing needs and aspirations. Each of the case studies follows a client through the assessment and therapy process and discusses the outcomes of the application of this model.

12

Telephone Communication Training

Mary Pat Wilson and Susanne M. Scott

■ ■ ■ ■

Many deaf and hard of hearing clients who seek aural rehabilitative services indicate a desire to develop or enhance telephone skills in order to meet communicative needs in their workplace and personal lives. In the past, telephone training was limited primarily to use of the voice telephone for the hard of hearing client and incorporated traditional auditory training with use of communication strategies and codes. However, recent advancements in technology and the passage of the Americans with Disabilities Act (ADA) have led to "communication access" for all deaf and hard of hearing people, resulting in an increase in the variety of telecommunication options available. Due to these technological advancements and their legal implications, the role of the aural rehabilitationist in the area of telephone training is evolving. This expanded role now includes familiarity with the variety of options available to the deaf and hard of hearing client to maximize his access to the outside world through many forms of telecommunication. This chapter will present an overview of some of the recent options for telecommunication use and provide an approach to telephone training that integrates both receptive and expressive skill areas.

Developments in Telecommunication Use for the Deaf

In today's world, the telephone has become such an integral part of our lives that it is difficult to imagine living without it. Yet, prior to 1964, the majority of deaf and hard of hearing people had virtually no access to the telephone and had to depend upon hearing friends and relatives to make their telephone calls. In 1964 Robert Weitbrecht, a deaf engineer at the Stafford Research Institute, developed a modem that interfaced a Teletype Corporation Model 32ASR with the telephone network and called it a Teletypewriter (TTY) (Harkins 1991). Although this development was a major breakthrough in telephone access for the deaf, the use of TTYs was not widespread until the production of smaller, modern day telecommunication devices for the deaf (TDDs). Many more deaf and hard of hearing people purchased TDDs as the prices lowered and more models were produced (Conlon-Mentkowski 1988).

The term TDD did not gain wide acceptance, however, because it implied that the device could only be used by a deaf individual. The Federal Communications Commission (FCC) has proposed the term Text Telephone (TT) to replace the old terms TTY and TDD. The FCC defines a TT as a device that employs graphic communication in the transmission of coded signals through a wire or radio communication system. The term TT is currently being used by the Telecommunications Relay Service (TRS), described in the next paragraph, as well as being used regularly in Europe (Boone 1992). However, the term TT is not acceptable to members of the deaf community in the United States (Telecommunications 1994). Telecommunications for the Deaf, Inc. (TDI), a consumer support organization for visual telecommunication users, endorses a return to the use of the acronym TTY to represent all Text Telephones. (The acronym TTY will be used throughout the remainder of this chapter to represent all types of text telephones, except when referring specifically to the TRS.)

Although TTYs are connected to the general telephone network, the fact that few hearing people have TTYs has precluded deaf and hard of hearing users from unassisted telephone conversations with the general public (Taylor 1988). However, a recent solution to this problem has been developed in the form of the TRS. This service involves having a communications assistant (CA) who "relays" telephone conversations between a voice telephone user and a text telephone (TT) user. The CA has two telephone lines: one line is connected to the TT user and the other to the voice telephone user. During the relay process, the CA speaks on the line what is read from the TT and, in turn, types on the TT the spoken words to be read by the deaf or hard of hearing person (Taylor 1988). A deaf or hard of hearing person who has intelligible speech can access a part of the relay service called Voice Carry Over (VCO). VCO is a form of TRS in which the deaf or hard of hearing person speaks directly to the other user. The CA does not voice in this conversation but types back the hearing person's response to the deaf or hard of hearing person. This process can save time by reducing the typing to one way, instead of back and forth (Boone 1992). As a result of the ADA (Title IV), twenty-four hour relay services have been mandated nationwide. These services are required of all common carrier telephone companies, without restrictions on type, length, or number of calls made by the relay user (Compton and Flexer 1992).

Title III of the ADA, dealing with Public Accommodations, also impacts upon telephone access for the deaf and hard of hearing person. This title mandates that auxiliary aids and services must be provided to individuals with vision or hearing impairments or other individuals with disabilities, unless undue burden would result. Some auxiliary aids and services for telephone reception include: telephone handset amplifiers, hearing aid compatible telephones, TTYs, computers as TTYs, electronic mail, facsimile transmission (FAX), video telephone, speech to text, and cellular vibratory numeric and alpha numeric pagers (Compton and Flexer 1992). Many of these telecommunication systems and auxiliary aids are discussed in greater detail in chapter 6.

Aural Rehabilitationist's Role

As advancements in technology have created change in the variety of telecommunication options available to the deaf and hard of hearing person, they have also brought about evolution in the role of the aural rehabilitationist in providing the service of telephone training. In addition to providing training in receptive and expressive skill areas, the aural rehabilitationist may also provide information and training in the use of the various telecommunication options and auxiliary aids, as well as information about the ADA as it pertains to access in the workplace and other public places. In short, the aural rehabilitationist serves as an advocate for the deaf and hard of hearing consumer, while at the same time encouraging the individual to acquire the knowledge and confidence to request equal access for himself.

Assessing Needs and Skills

With the new developments and options now available to deaf and hard of hearing consumers, telephone training can mean a variety of things to any given consumer depending upon the number of different situations in which he uses some form of telecommunication. The first step for the aural rehabilitationist in providing this service is to determine telephone communication use and needs at home, in the workplace, and in social situations. This can be accomplished through the interview process, as described in chapter 2, and through the use of questionnaires (Castle 1980, 1984; Erber 1982, 1985). These questionnaires provide information about frequency of telephone use, types of calls placed, familiarity with the persons called, use of telecoil or other coupling arrangements, and perceived difficulty in receptive and expressive communication on the voice telephone. Previous telecommunication experiences should also be discussed, as well as familiarity with the use of telephone directories, operator assistance, long distance calling, and communication software (for using a personal computer as a TTY).

Following needs assessment, the aural rehabilitationist should evaluate the client's current telephone skills using formal and informal assessment tools. (A framework for assessment is provided in chapter 2.) For voice telephone use, skills to be evaluated would include: reception and expression of numbers, letters (including a coded alphabet), proper names, closed-set sentences, and open-set sentences. During the assessment of voice telephone skills, the clinician and client can also evaluate the effectiveness of various coupling arrangements, such as use of a hearing aid on the telecoil compared to the microphone setting (Wallber, MacKenzie, and Clymer 1987), use of portable telephone amplifiers, and use of an amplified handset with and without the hearing aid. (For a detailed discussion of the various telephone devices, see chapter 6.) For TTY use, skills to be evaluated include the ability to formulate and type a clear and understandable message, use of a keyboard (typing ability), knowledge of TTY abbreviations, and reading comprehension. For both the conventional telephone and the TTY, the client's knowledge of telephone protocols and etiquette should also be evaluated. As one component of informal assessment, role play provides an effective tool for determining the client's "functional" telephone abilities. Through role play, the client and clinician can "act out" a variety of telephone conversations (e.g., making an appointment, ordering on the phone, making a social call, etc.) in order to evaluate the client's communicative effectiveness and use of receptive and expressive strategies.

Establishing Goals

Following the process of needs assessment and skill assessment, the client and clinician must negotiate to arrive at goals for telephone training. If the client has developed a more realistic perception of his communication skills through the assessment process, he will know the skills that are in his inventory. Through discussion with the clinician of the variety of uses for the telephone, the client may come to a better understanding of what skills are necessary to be successful in a given situation and may be able to determine if the skills possessed match the skills required. As a result, the client and clinician may need to establish separate sets of goals for different types of telephone calls, especially if the client uses a variety of telecommunication options for making these calls. For example, a client may choose to use the TTY only when communicating with deaf friends, the relay service when making certain business calls, and the voice telephone for setting up appointments and communicating with family and hearing friends. Although each of these options requires specific skills, some skills are applicable to all types of telephone communication, such as using appropriate strategies, formulating specific questions, and shortening utterances to include the most salient information. The process of telephone training should include education and training in those areas that can be generalized to all telephone communication, as well as practice, through role play and structured phone calls, in each of the specific methods that the client uses.

Although an occasional client, such as a late-deafened adult, will request training in use of the TTY, it is the authors' experience that the majority of deaf or hard of hearing clients who seek telephone training services are interested in use of the *voice* telephone, at least in some situations. In face-to-face communication, the deaf or hard of hearing individual has relied on visual feedback, or paralinguistic information, to be understood and to understand others. Due to the absence of this visual feedback use of the voice telephone creates a unique challenge both receptively and expressively. The individual must now derive meaning by voice alone for comprehension on the telephone. As a result, "listening comprehension, sound patterns, stress and intonation, fluency of speech, use of social register and attention to context become very crucial skills for effective telephone communication" (Feuille-LeChevallier 1983, xi).

The deaf or hard of hearing individual, who may have experienced little difficulty sending and receiving information with a TTY, may now experience restrictions with the voice telephone due to limited residual hearing or limited speech intelligibility over the telephone. Although he may still be able to communicate freely with family members in an open-set format, he may need to structure other calls and limit the amount of information being conveyed. In certain situations, special code systems might be needed to communicate effectively.

Options for Telephone Communication

The following section presents available options for training of telephone conversation skills based on the client's auditory reception ability, speech intelligibility, and use of communication strategies. Although these skills and abilities do not fully determine the degree of freedom (e.g., open set or limited set) in a given telephone conversation, they do suggest a starting point for the process of telephone training. With additional practice, persistent use of strategies, and the development of confidence on the telephone, many clients are able to use the voice telephone for those situations that they have deemed important. For those situations in which the TTY or TRS is the client's method of choice or is most appropriate based on assessment results, suggestions will be made for incorporating these methods into the telephone training process as well.

Open-Set Telephone Communication

In this chapter, open-set voice telephone communication is defined as fluent conversation between two talkers/listeners in which the topic may be unknown or frequently changing and be low in predictability and/or redundancy. Examples of open-set voice telephone communication are: (1) a social conversation between two old friends who have not spoken in a long time, and (2) a business-related conversation between a customer and a representative from a complaint department of a large department store. In the first example, the participants are familiar with one another and may have some known and predictable topics to discuss. However, the topic may frequently change and may include new names, places, or events that are unfamiliar to the listener. In the second example, the participants are strangers, and the topic (or nature of the specific complaint) may be entirely unknown to the business representative receiving the call. In addition, the responses of the business representative and the course of action recommended to the caller are not highly predictable.

The deaf or hard of hearing client who is able to participate successfully in open-set telephone communication must be able to communicate fluently, both expressively and receptively, without the aid of visual cues. Expressively, this requires speech that is highly intelligible with minimal voice and/or articulation errors and a limited need for repetition or other communication strategies. Receptively, this requires demonstrated auditory recognition for open-set word and sentence materials and a limited need to request repetition or other clarification from the speaker. Open-set communication on the telephone can also include modes other than voice-to-voice communication: for example, two individuals using the TTY and fluently communicating about a variety of topics, or an individual who has highly intelligible speech but is unable to use the voice telephone receptively using the VCO with the relay service.

Limited-Set Telephone Communication

Limited-set voice telephone communication is defined here as a conversation between two talkers/receivers in which the topic is clearly known or defined and there is a high degree of predictability in the questions and responses that constitute the conversation. Examples of limited-set voice telephone communication are: (1) making appointments or ordering items by telephone (e.g., pizza, mail-order clothing, etc.), and (2) two familiar people conversing about a specified topic (e.g., discussing details about a trip home from college). In the first example, the participants are strangers, but the topic is circumscribed, and the caller can plan most of the dialogue prior to making the call. In addition, the responses and subsequent questions of the listener have a high degree of predictability. In the second example, the participants are familiar with one another, and the topic can be clearly limited to the specific details that are important to convey (e.g., the name of the airline, flight number, and time of arrival). Again, the caller can plan much of the dialogue prior to making the call.

The deaf or hard of hearing client who is able to participate successfully in limited-set voice telephone communication must have some ability to communicate without the aid of visual cues. Expressively, this requires speech that is intelligible when the topic is known or when the speaker has practiced producing preplanned utterances and vocabulary words. Receptively, this requires demonstrated auditory discrimination for closed-set word and sentence materials, as well as familiarity with a variety of communication strategies.

Telephone Communication with Special Code Systems

Voice telephone communication with special code systems is defined as the use of speech and nonspeech codes that employ special words, numbers, sounds, or letters for giving and receiving information over the telephone (Castle 1984). An example of a telephone conversation using a code system is a short conversation about one subject or idea in which the caller controls the conversation by structuring successive thoughts as yes/no questions, and the receiver answers in one of three ways: "no" (one syllable), "yes-yes" or "o-k" (two syllables), or "please repeat" (three syllables). The response may be sent by speaking or by tapping the pattern into the mouthpiece of the telephone (Erber 1982).

The deaf or hard of hearing client who is able to participate successfully in a telephone conversation using a special code must have speech that can be understood on the telephone by the listener, but may have limited reception ability and be unable to understand conversation on the telephone. In addition, the caller must be familiar with the code used and be able to explain it well to the listener. For this reason, special codes are usually reserved for use with family and close friends. There are also codes that do not require the use of speech at all, similar to Morse code, which can be used by individuals with limited speech and hearing ability. However, the limitations of this method preclude its widespread use. Furthermore, the availability of the relay service nationwide has facilitated telephone communication for all deaf and hard of hearing individuals. This advancement has virtually eliminated the need for using some of these tedious code systems, except in rare circumstances.

An Integrated Approach to Telephone Communication Training

The preceding descriptions of the different types of voice telephone communication emphasize the need for a client to possess a variety of receptive and expressive communication skills for successful use of the telephone. In addition, he needs a limited knowledge of conversational protocol and a basic understanding of equipment as well. In the process of acquiring and refining these skills through telephone training, role play, and actual use, the client must integrate many as-

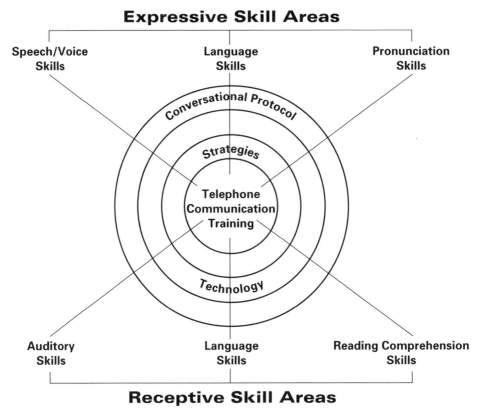

Figure 12.1. Telephone Communication Training Model

pects of communication in a given telephone conversation for its successful completion.

In chapter 2, the process of integrated therapy was described as "an approach in which all aspects of communication are integrated in a given session into a meaningful, situationally based context" (p. 29). Similarly, telephone communication can be described as a process in which many aspects of communication are integrated into a purposeful, conversationally based exchange. Communicative effectiveness is enhanced through skill development and the use of appropriate strategies and conversational protocol.

A visual representation of the process of telephone communication training is shown in figure 12.1. (See chapter 2 for a comparison to the Integrated Therapy Model.) This model depicts three concentric circles surrounding Telephone Communication Training: Communication Strategies, Technology, and Conversational Protocol. These represent global areas involved with both receptive and expressive aspects of skill development and incorporated into the therapy process as well. The areas of Communication Strategies and Technology were introduced and previously discussed in depth in chapters 3 and 6. The outermost concentric circle in this model represents Conversational Protocol, defined as the etiquette or conventions that govern telephone conversations. For voice telephone calls, conversational protocol includes initiating the call, using appropriate greetings, turn taking, formulating questions, providing appropriate responses, and politely concluding the call. For a TTY call, conversational protocol also includes using the appropriate abbreviations.

In addition to the concentric circles, the model also depicts spokes that represent the specific skill areas. These are the same skill areas as described in chapter 2, with the obvious omission of Speechreading Skills. (When video technology becomes a commonplace component of everyday telephone communication in the not too distant future, then speechreading skills can be added to the model.) The expressive areas in this model consist of Speech/Voice Skills and Pronunciation Skills, and the receptive areas include Auditory Skills and Reading Comprehension Skills. The Language Skills area encompasses both expressive and receptive modalities. The only addition to this model in the skill areas is Reading Comprehension Skills, which become a factor in telephone communication when the client uses the TTY.

The focus of telephone communication training is to provide information about telecommunication usage, options, protocol, technology, and strategies and to develop or enhance communication skills necessary to complete calls successfully using the mode(s) selected as most appropriate by the client and clinician. This process may involve some work in all of the skill areas listed in the model, depending upon the needs of the client. Using the integrated therapy approach, these receptive and expressive skills and abilities are identified, enhanced, and applied to the process of successful telephone communication. The following sample cases will demonstrate the application of an integrated therapy approach to the process of telephone communication training as previously described in this chapter. In addition, these cases will serve as a vehicle for the introduction and discussion of a variety of therapy procedures and techniques for telephone communication training.

Sample Case One: Using Open-Set Telephone Communication

A twenty-five-year-old hard of hearing woman enrolled in aural rehabilitation to prepare for telephone communication on the job. She had just been hired to work in an advertising firm as a member of an advertising team.

The client presented with a bilateral, moderately severe to severe, sensorineural hearing loss. Her open-set word recognition scores were 80 percent for the right ear and 60 percent for the left ear. The client was aided binaurally with behind-the-ear (BTE) hearing aids with a powerful telecoil, and she demonstrated significant benefit from amplification. Aided thresholds were consistent with a mild to moderate hearing loss range and open-set word recognition in sound field (in quiet) was 80 percent.

At the start of aural rehabilitation therapy, an information gathering interview was used to determine the client's current telephone use and anticipated use on the job. Based on the client's report, she currently was using the voice telephone on a regular basis, but primarily for social and personal calls. She anticipated using the telephone frequently at work for conducting business with both clients and colleagues. She was pursuing telephone communication training at this time to increase her overall confidence on the telephone and to learn appropriate telephone strategies and conversational protocol for business calls.

Following the interview process, the client's communication skills were evaluated to determine appropriate goals for telephone communication training. To evaluate receptive skills on the telephone, the CID Everyday Sentences (Davis and Silverman 1978) were presented over the telephone while the client used her hearing aid on telecoil and an amplified handset on the telephone. She received a score of 92 percent, indicating that she was able to understand the content of the message without difficulty. This was followed by a tracking procedure (DeFilippo and Scott 1978) used over the telephone (Erber 1982) to assess the client's use of receptive communication strategies. When the client missed information, she relied heavily on repetition, suggesting a limited repertoire of repair strategies.

To evaluate expressive skills, the client read a passage while the clinician judged speech intelligibility using a modification of the Gallaudet Speech Intelligibility Rating Scale (Frisina and Bernero 1958). The client received a rating of 1.5 on the scale, indicating that she is easily understood by the general public, but has minor articulation and/or pronunciation errors. Voice characteristics were judged to be within normal limits. Assessment of articulation skills, using the Fisher-Logemann Sentence Articulation Test (Fisher and Logemann 1971), indicated inconsistent, mild distortion of /s,z/ in some words. Assessment of pronunciation skills, using the Pronunciation Skills Inventory (Bally 1984), indicated knowledge of most of the pronunciation rules of English, with the exception of rules for production of plural, possessive, and past tense word endings, as well as rules for stress in words. To assess the client's use of expressive communication strategies over the telephone, a modification of the tracking procedure was employed in which the client was the sender of the information and the clinician was the receiver. When the clinician did not understand, the client had to use expressive strategies to make herself understood. As with receptive strategies, the client demonstrated use of a limited repertoire of expressive repair strategies when the listener had difficulty understanding.

Following assessment, the client and clinician discussed results and negotiated preliminary goals. Agreement was reached to focus on the following areas in therapy: use of appropriate expressive and receptive communication strategies in nonface-to-face situations, use of appropriate conversational protocol for business calls, and refinement of speech intelligibility through improved pronunciation and articulation. Based on the client's expressive and receptive skills and current telephone use, the format chosen for training was *open-set* telephone communication.

Prior to actual telephone practice, the client and clinician discussed anticipatory and repair communication strategies, as well as the use of an assertive approach to communication. The client listed the different types of business calls that she would be making on the job and then used anticipatory strategies to predict possible vocabulary and sequence of dialogue that would occur during those telephone calls. She also anticipated potential places in the conversation where a communication breakdown might occur, such as while conveying or receiving lists of numbers, names, or addresses over the telephone. To avoid these breakdowns, the clinician provided lists of repair strategies developed for use on the telephone (Castle 1980, 1984), and the client practiced using the strategies in a variety of situations.

Conversational protocol for business telephone calls was introduced and practiced through the use of "dialog" exercises (Feuille-LeChevallier 1983). These "dialogs" were used to present common business situations on the telephone and served as a device for introducing vocabulary and for practicing appropriate language for some of the most frequent communicative situations occurring in the context of business telephone calls—beginning a call, placing a call on hold, giving and taking a message, handling a wrong number, transferring a call, returning a call, and terminating a call.

Through the process of anticipating vocabulary and practicing dialogues related to business telephone calls, the client and clinician were able to identify core vocabulary words that the client had difficulty pronouncing. By analyzing these errors, the clinician could determine if the mispronunciations were the result of inappropriate stress or syllabification; of inappropriate use of plural, possessive, and/or past tense endings; or of lack of awareness of specific silent letter rules. Following analysis of the errors, specific pronunciation rules were taught as well as advanced dictionary skills, as appropriate. In preparation for role play of telephone conversations, the client then practiced correct pronunciation of all of the identified core vocabulary words. Additional work on expressive skills included practice with expressive communication strategies. The client and clinician used the same list of repair strategies that was previously presented for receptive practice, but the client modified these strategies to use them expressively in order to increase her own intelligibility when she was not understood. For example, she would rephrase a sentence or spell a word that the listener had misunderstood.

Following preliminary expressive and receptive skill training, the client was ready to practice integration of the acquired skills. To accomplish this, the client and clinician engaged in role play telephone conversations of the various types of previously planned business calls. After each call, they evaluated the effectiveness of the strategies used and reviewed any mispronunciations of vocabulary words. With continual refinement of skills during role play conversations, the client developed the confidence to begin making actual business calls. She then placed calls to various businesses to obtain information, while the clinician monitored the calls. The types of telephone conversations practiced in therapy included the following: responding to a classified advertisement to inquire about a job, apartment, or product for sale; calling specialty stores to determine if they sell a particular product; and calling a museum to obtain information about an exhibit.

Although open-set voice telephone use was the client's mode of choice for most situations, the clinician recommended that the client consider the use of the Voice Carry Over (VCO) with the Telecommunications Relay Service (TRS) in the following situations: when there is a bad telephone connection or a very noisy environment, when calling a foreign speaker, or when time is very limited and the information is critical. In order to prepare the client for VCO use, general information about the TRS was presented, and the protocol for using the VCO was discussed. The client then made several actual telephone calls through the relay service to become accustomed to the procedures and to feel comfortable enough to use the service on her own.

Over the course of the time that the client was enrolled in aural rehabilitation, she had begun her new job and was using the voice telephone at work on a regular basis. This provided her with the opportunity to practice her new skills in real-life situations and integrate the use of appropriate communication strategies for successful telecommunication use. In addition, the client kept a log of her telephone calls, including strategies used and their effectiveness. Through the process of analysis and discussion in therapy, she was able to modify those strategies that were not effective and to improve her success rate in future calls. By the completion of the aural rehabilitative process, the client had gained the skills and confidence to feel independent in her use of telecommunication options.

Sample Case Two: Using Limited-Set Telephone Communication

A twenty-three-year-old deaf college senior enrolled in aural rehabilitation to develop and enhance voice telephone skills for specific situations. His current use of the voice telephone was limited to communication with hearing family members. In most other situations he relied on the TTY. His reason for requesting services was to develop the skills to enable him to use the voice telephone for making appointments, for ordering food and products, and for handling emergency situations.

The client presented with a severe to profound, sensorineural hearing loss in the left ear and a moderate to profound, rising to severe, sensorineural hearing loss in the right ear. Open-set word recognition scores were 0 percent for both ears; however, closed-set discrimination testing, using a Modified Rhyme Test (MRT) (Kreul et al. 1968), revealed scores of 36 percent for the left ear and 72 percent for the right ear. The client was aided monaurally, on the right ear, with a behind-the-ear (BTE) hearing aid with a powerful telecoil, and his aided thresholds were in the mild to moderate hearing loss range. Aided closed-set discrimination testing with the MRT in sound field (in quiet) yielded a score of 78 percent.

At the start of aural rehabilitation therapy, an information gathering interview was used to determine the client's current telephone use and his goals for future use. In addition to the interview, the client completed a telephone communication questionnaire (Castle 1984) to provide additional information about telephone usage. Based on the information gathered, the client was currently using the voice telephone to communicate with hearing family members and close friends, but using the TTY in all other situations. He stopped using the voice telephone with strangers after several frustrating calls. He was pursuing telephone communication training, before he graduated, to develop the skills and confidence to use the voice telephone in structured situations, such as in ordering and setting up appointments by phone. He also wanted to develop the confidence to feel capable of using the voice telephone in emergency situations.

Following the interview process, the client's communication skills were evaluated to determine appropriate goals for telephone communication training. To evaluate receptive skills, the Test of Auditory Comprehension (Trammell et al. 1976) was administered to the client. He passed all subtests through subtest eight, a task involving discrimination, memory, and sequencing of details in context. He was unable to complete tasks involving competing messages at a 0 dB signal-to-noise ratio. The client's ability to obtain information over the telephone in quiet was assessed using a variety of formal and informal measures. During this assessment, the client used his hearing aid on the telecoil setting and an amplified handset on the telephone. Tasks included: closed-set word discrimination (76 percent); closed-set sentence discrimination (100 percent); identification of letters of the alphabet (19 out of 26 correct); identification of numbers embedded in sentences (90 percent); and identification of proper names embedded in sentences (65 percent without spelling and 90 percent following spelling). During this evaluation, the client used only the strategies of asking for repetition and requesting spelling when he did not understand.

To evaluate expressive skills, the client read a passage while the clinician judged speech intelligibility using a modification of the Gallaudet Speech Intelligibility Rating Scale (Frisina and Bernero 1958). The client received a rating of 2.5 on the scale, indicating that he has obvious voice and/or articulation errors, but his speech can be understood if the topic is known and/or the listener has time to adjust to his speech. Suprasegmentals and voice were informally assessed and found to be within normal limits, with the exception of excessive nasal resonance, during production of some vowels, and of slightly monotone pitch. Assessment of articulation skills, using the Fisher-Logemann Sentence Articulation Test (Fisher and Logemann 1971), indicated distortion of sibilants and affricates in all positions of words, as well as substitution of w/r in the initial position of words. Assessment of pronunciation skills, using the Pronunciation Skills Inventory (Bally 1984), indicated knowledge of most of the pronunciation rules of English, but difficulty in using the dictionary for pronunciation of unfamiliar, multisyllabic words. Use of expressive communication strategies, when the listener had difficulty understanding, was limited to repetition and writing in face-to-face situations and to repetition only over the telephone.

Following assessment, the client and clinician discussed results and negotiated preliminary goals. Based on the client's expressive and receptive skills and his expectations for telephone use, the most appropriate format for training was *limited-set* telephone communication. Agreement was reached on the format of therapy and on the following areas of focus for therapy: use of anticipatory communication strategies to structure telephone calls; use of expressive and receptive communication strategies during telephone communication; improved intelligibility of core vocabulary words through articulation and pronunciation practice; and knowledge of appropriate procedures for emergency telephone calls.

Before actual telephone practice could begin, the client and clinician worked on predicting vocabulary and dialogue for a variety of possible telephone calls (e.g., ordering pizza or making appointments). This was accomplished by listing vocabulary, possible questions that the caller would ask, possible questions that the caller would be asked, and the sequence of this dialogue for each type of telephone call. The creation of language constellations was one technique used for this predictive activity (Kaplan, Bally, and Garretson 1987, 53). The constellations created were then used for receptive practice through role playing the telephone call and for expressive practice through articulation and pronunciation work on the identified core vocabulary for that telephone call. In addition to predicting dialogue, the client worked on structuring questions more specifically to limit the responses of the other person during the telephone conversation. Through these activities the client recognized that highly predictable dialogue and vocabulary can be associated with many situations and that communication can be more successful when planned ahead.

Following work on these anticipatory strategies, the client and clinician practiced using repair strategies for situations when communication breakdown occurred. Repair strategies were listed, defined, and used in the context of face-to-face situations and then on the telephone during role-play situations. Particular emphasis was placed on number and letter strategies most appropriate for telephone usage, such as digits, counting, and coded alphabet strategies (Castle 1980, 1984). (See chapter 3 for examples and lists of the various types of anticipatory and repair strategies.)

Through the process of creating language constellations for a variety of telephone conversations, the client and clinician identified core vocabulary words related to each situation. Work on expressive skills was then initiated to improve intelligibility of the identified vocabulary words: teaching dictionary skills and the modification of phoneme production, as appropriate. The goal of this practice was to increase the likelihood that the listener on the telephone would understand the speaker's speech within the context of a highly predictable conversation.

Procedures for handling emergency situations were introduced by first discussing the various types of emergency resources (e.g., rescue squad, ambulance, fire department, police department, etc.), the types of services they provide, and the way to access them via the telephone. Following this discussion, different types of emergencies were identified (e.g., a fire, a car accident, a serious injury, etc.), and language constellations were created for each situation. As core vocabulary words were identified for each situation, pronunciation and articulation practice was introduced as needed.

At this point in the therapy process, the client was ready to integrate the acquired skills through role-play telephone conversations with the clinician. The various types of calls that had been previously planned—ordering pizza, setting up an appointment, or reporting an emergency—were role played and then analyzed by the client and clinician. As problems such as the need to restructure questions to be less open-ended were identified, possible solutions were generated prior to role playing that situation again. When the client had gained the confidence to place an actual call, he used the therapy setting to make an appointment with his dentist. Following that successful call, he began to use the telephone outside of therapy for ordering pizza from his dorm and for other limited-set phone conversations. He continued to rely on the TTY in an open-set format for most telephone use, but felt that he had developed the skills and confidence to use the voice telephone in some situations.

Summary

In this chapter, an overview of the available options for telecommunication use for the deaf and hard of hearing individual was presented. In addition, an approach to telephone training that integrates both receptive and expressive skill areas was described and schematically represented. Sample cases were presented to illustrate the application of an integrated approach to telephone communication training and to provide suggestions for therapy procedures and techniques.

References

Bally, S. J. 1984. *Pronunciation Skills Inventory.* Unpublished assessment tool, Gallaudet University, Washington, D.C.

Boone, M. 1992. This news is for you. *SHHH Journal* 13(1):37–39.

Castle, D. L. 1980. *Telephone training for the deaf.* Rochester, N. Y.: National Technical Institute for the Deaf.

———. 1984. *Telephone training for hearing impaired persons,* 2d ed. Rochester, N. Y.: National Technical Institute for the Deaf.

Compton, C. L., and C. Flexer. 1992. The Americans with Disabilities Act: Implications for the profession of audiology. Paper presented at the American Academy of Audiology Annual Convention, Nashville, Tennessee.

Conlon-Mentkowski, S. 1988. Overview of state regulated relay services. *Gallaudet Research Institute Monographs,* series B:2.

Davis, H., and S. R. Silverman. 1978. *Hearing and deafness,* 4th ed. New York: Holt, Rinehart, and Winston.

DeFilippo, C. L., and B. L. Scott. 1978. A method for training and evaluating the reception of ongoing speech. *Journal of the Acoustical Society of America* 63:1186–1192.

Erber, N. P. 1982. *Auditory training.* Washington, D.C.: Alexander Graham Bell Association for the Deaf.

———. 1985. *Telephone communication and hearing impairment.* San Diego, Calif.: College-Hill Press.

———. 1988. *Communication therapy for hearing-impaired adults.* Abbotsford, Victoria, Australia: Clavis Publishing.

Feuille-LeChevallier, C. 1983. *Tele-Vesl business telephone skills.* Haywood, Calif.: The Alemany Press.

Fisher, H. B., and J. A. Logemann. 1971. *Fisher-Logemann Test of Articulation Competence.* Boston: Houghton Mifflin.

Frisina, D. R., and R. J. Bernero. 1958. A profile of the hearing and speech of Gallaudet College students. *Volta Review* 60:316–321.

Harkins, J. E. 1991. *Visual devices for deaf and hard of hearing people: State of the art.* Washington, D.C.: Gallaudet Research Institute, Technology Assessment Program.

Heil, J. J. 1986. *Communication technologies 2000: Do we need a crystal ball?* Proceedings from Life and work in the twenty-first century: The deaf person of tomorrow, National Association of the Deaf Forum, Silver Spring, Maryland.

Hull, R. H. 1992. *Aural rehabilitation,* 2d ed. San Diego, Calif.: Singular Publishing Co.

Kaplan, H., S. J. Bally, and C. Garretson. 1987. *Speechreading: A way to improve understanding,* 2d ed. Washington, D.C.: Gallaudet University Press.

Kos, T. 1989. *Benefits for the hearing impaired,* 2d ed. Rochester, N.Y.: Benefits 4-U Publishing Co.

Kreul, E. J., J. C. Nixon, K. D. Kryter, D. W. Bell, J. S. Lang, and E. D. Schubert. 1968. A proposed clinical test of speech discrimination. *Journal of Speech and Hearing Research* 11:536–552.

National Center for Law and Deafness. 1991. *Legal rights: The guide for deaf and hard of hearing people.* Washington, D.C.: Gallaudet University Press.

Stern, V., and M. R. Redden. 1982. Selected telecommunication devices for hearing impaired persons (background paper no. 2). In *Technology and handicapped people.* Washington, D.C.: Office of Technology Assessment.

Taylor, P. 1988. Telephone relay service: Rationale and overview. *Gallaudet Research Institute Monographs,* series B:2.

Telecommunications for the Deaf, Inc. 1994. *What's in a name?* Silver Spring, Md.: Telecommunications for the Deaf, Inc.

Trammell, J. L., C. Farrar, J. Francis, S. L. Owens, D. E. Schepard, R. P. Witlen, and L. H. Faist. 1976. *Test of Auditory Comprehension.* North Hollywood, Calif.: Foreworks.

Wallber, M. J., D. J. MacKenzie, and W. E. Clymer. 1987. *Telecoil evaluation procedure.* St. Louis, Mo.: Auditec.

13

Case Studies

Mary June Moseley, Susanne M. Scott, and Scott J. Bally

■　■　■　■

Three case studies are included in this chapter to demonstrate the application of the integrated therapy approach to the communication therapy process. Discussion will focus on three different types of clients: a culturally Deaf university student, a university student interested in maintaining oral/aural skills, and an older adult with a progressive loss attributed to presbycusis.

Gert *(Mary June Moseley)*

Information Gathering Interview

Gert is an eighteen-year-old Deaf college student who expressed a desire to enter communication therapy so that she can maintain and enhance her communication skills with the hearing population. Gert has a congenital hearing loss, as do both her parents and her brother. Audiological evaluations indicated that Gert has a profound, bilateral sensorineural hearing loss with no measurable hearing above 1000 Hz in the better ear. The audiological evaluation further indicated no word recognition ability, and an SRT could not be established. Gert has a right ear level hearing aid, but reported she rarely wears it. She indicates inconsistency with benefit from the aid, with only some awareness of environmental sounds and at times no reception of auditory input.

Gert primarily communicates both receptively and expressively with American Sign Language (ASL). She indicates that she sometimes uses simultaneous communication with hearing teachers and friends. She considers herself a part of the Deaf community and socializes, at college, almost exclusively with other Deaf individuals. Gert attended residential schools through junior high school, then transferred to a public school where she was mainstreamed with an interpreter. Gert expressed an interest in working on her English skills in communication therapy so that she could continue to interact with her hearing friends from the mainstream placement.

Gert is an outgoing and friendly person and appeared to be motivated to become involved in communication therapy. She had no specific goals for herself other than "better" communication. After some discussion with the clinician, Gert indicated an interest in working on vocabulary, figurative language, and written language. A dual major in business and art, she would like to have her own interior design business sometime in the future. Her interests include interacting with friends (e.g., eating out, shopping, going to the ballet) and reading for fun, especially mystery stories.

Evaluation of Skills and Abilities

Auditory Skills Gert's previous audiogram indicated no word recognition scores because of severity of loss. No additional word recognition was attempted. In addition, hearing aid evaluations had been recommended in the past, but Gert did not follow through on those recommendations. Gert reported that she uses a TTY for telephone communication.

Personal adjustment and understanding of loss. Gert filled out the Gallaudet University Aural Rehabilitation Questionnaire and discussed her hearing status with the clinician. Gert appears to understand the nature of her hearing loss and to accept her deafness.

Strategies. During conversational interaction with the clinician during the therapy session, Gert depended consistently on the strategy of repetition when she needed clarification. She was, however, able to describe the use of additional strategies that were not observed during conversation.

Expressive Skills *Intelligibility.* Gert's speech was rated at 3.5 for reading ("Rainbow Passage") and spontaneous speech on the Gallaudet University Intelligibility Scale. This indicated the student's speech would be difficult for the general public to understand; however, family and friends would understand because they have adjusted to "deaf speech." The clinician rated the influence of articulation, voice, and pronunciation on intelligibility as moderate. No formal articulation, voice or pronunciation measures were performed at this time.

Written language. A screening for written language was administered by having the student write a story about a group of sequenced pictures. Sequencing was adequate although syntax errors were noted. Formulation of the written story (i.e., time it took to write) was slow. The written story was unclear to the clinician, indicating some difficulty with formulating an effective message. Because formulation appeared difficult, further evaluation was done with taking the receiver's perspective (discussed in chapter 11 of this book).

Taking the receiver's perspective. Gert was asked to write a description of a recent event with the intent of sharing this description with a friend. Gert chose to write about purchasing a new dress for the homecoming dance. In the written description, she demonstrated basic difficulty with directionality and with giving enough information to the reader to convey a message. Written syntax indicated difficulty with determiners, subject-verb agreement, and the use of relative clauses. Gert had expressed an interest in continuing to use simultaneous communication skills with her hearing friends. Therefore, using simultaneous communication, the clinician discussed the written description of the homecoming dress with Gert. During the dialogue, Gert demonstrated inconsistent contingent responses to questions, limited expressive strategies when clarification was needed, and consistent need for clarification by the receiver, resulting in an excessive number of turns to convey the information.

Receptive Skills *Single word vocabulary.* Vocabulary was evaluated using the Peabody Picture Vocabulary Test (PPVT). The student scored in the fifth percentile, a moderately low score in comparison to hearing peers. (This edition of the PPVT was not standardized for deaf students.)

Figurative Language Evaluation. The Gochnour Idiom Screening indicated that this student was slightly above average in comparison to Deaf peers, below average in comparison to hearing peers. Gert experienced most difficulty with complex phraseological idioms. Two subtests of the Test of Language Competence (TLC) were administered to the client. Subtest One investigated the understanding of ambiguous sentences (e.g., "The elephant was ready to lift"). Gert correctly understood 64 percent of the ambiguous sentences, indicating some understanding of nonliteral language. Subtest Four, Understanding Metaphoric Expressions, asked the client to give a verbal/written explanation of idioms as well as to match idioms from a closed set. Gert understood 33 percent of the idioms presented, showing no preference for explaining or matching.

Primary Communication Therapy Design

Goals for therapy were set jointly by Gert and the clinician, after the results of testing were explained to Gert. The following goals were established for a one-semester period of time (three months):

Auditory A hearing aid evaluation was recommended because Gert still has her aid, but feels that the aid is not always beneficial.

Receptive Figurative Language Gert practiced identifying literal and figurative expressions found in daily living—newspaper, magazines, conversation with friends or in classes. An analytical approach was used in deciphering idiomatic expressions. The analytical approach involved discussion between Gert and the clinician, with strong emphasis on analyzing the context of the figurative expression used.

Expressive Skills *Written English.* Gert focused on the use of cohesive devices in writing—determiners, subject-verb agreement, and relative clauses. Both a linguistic and a visual/conceptual approach were used (see chapter 11).

Vocabulary. This area was integrated with written language and the use of cohesive devices. Gert chose vocabulary from daily life activities. Definitions were discussed during therapy; synonyms were generated and used in written activities.

Clarification strategies with simultaneous communication. Gert learned two new strategies for clarification: rephrase and confirm (see chapter 3). The rephrasing strategy was integrated with the use of new vocabulary. The confirming strategy was chosen to help Gert understand and specify new information in a timely manner, leading to less need for the clinician to ask for clarification.

Sample Therapy Session

In previous sessions, Gert and the clinician had discussed the use of determiners in writing to express new or old information, and had worked on the use of relative clauses to describe information. In this particular session, the goal was to integrate the use of those cohesive devices into writing a descriptive account of an event. The task was to write a description of two pictures of ballet dancers in such a way that a receiver could clearly distinguish between the two pictures. Both ballet pictures showed two dancers at the bar in a practice room. Ballet pictures were chosen because ballet was one of Gert's major interests. The visual/conceptual approach was used—identifying the similarities between the two pictures and establishing the topic of the pictures. The following types of questions and directions were posed: *What are they doing? What is the main idea of both pictures? What is the topic of both pictures? What's the same in these two pictures? Describe the women in the pictures—emotions, height, hair color and length, age, clothing (leotard, sleeve length), position of arms, legs, hands, location of the picture (inside or outside), size of the room, light in the room, type of floor, angle of the camera taking the picture (aerial or lateral).*

The clinician and Gert then discussed the differences between the two pictures, generating as many descriptors as possible and using the descriptors in relative clauses. Gert then wrote a description of the picture, correctly using relative clauses and the determiners. She and the clinician then evaluated the writing: it was clear and succinct; relative clauses were used to describe and give information; and determiners were used correctly. Gert showed the pictures to three friends outside the therapy session, all of whom could easily identify the proper pictures with no clarification needed.

Vocabulary about ballet was integrated at a later date with the written descriptions and figurative language relevant to ballet (e.g., "on point," "run like the wind").

Other similar activities, chosen by Gert and related to her interests, were used throughout the therapy sessions.

Summary

Gert did not follow through with scheduling a hearing aid evaluation during the semester. She indicated she intended to do it at a later date.

Evaluation of the integrated therapy sessions during the semester was accomplished by informally testing Gert's use of all the vocabulary and figurative language expressions she had learned during the semester (e.g., asking for explanation and answering written multiple-choice questions). Written language was evaluated by having Gert write another description of an event and by examining correct use of determiners and relative clauses as well as formulation time. Gert demonstrated increased knowledge in all the goal areas.

Gert indicated that, after she had completed therapy, two of her hearing friends, whom she saw at Christmastime, commented that it seemed much "easier" to communicate with her and that they didn't have to ask her so many questions. Gert expressed satisfaction in developing communicative skills that had previously been difficult for her. In addition, approximately a year later, the clinician received a letter from Gert, describing her upcoming wedding in succinct and clear terms. Gert also indicated that she had composed the full letter by using a method learned in communication therapy: writing descriptive phrases about her wedding (describing clothes, church, emotions, location) and then incorporating those phrases into the complete letter.

Jim *(Susanne M. Scott)*

Information Gathering Interview

Jim Smith is an eighteen-year-old college freshman enrolled in his first semester of communication therapy. He has no measurable hearing bilaterally as a result of spinal meningitis contracted when he was two years old. Four years ago, Jim was implanted with a Nucleus 22-Channel Cochlear Implant System. Prior to his implant he used conventional hearing aids, but reported no benefit. Jim is very satisfied with his implant. He reported that while using his implant he is aware of conversational speech and is able to monitor his own speech better. Jim uses his implant during all waking hours.

Jim attended public schools in special classes for deaf and hard of hearing children through elementary and middle school. The mode of communication used for instruction was contact sign language (spoken English and sign). During high school, Jim was mainstreamed in a public high school program with a sign language interpreter. Jim received speech/language services throughout school. He reported that the therapy he received helped him develop the speech skills he has. He indicated that following the extensive "mapping" of his cochlear implant, the speech therapy he received in high school helped him make better use of what he "heard" with his implant.

Jim's communication with other deaf and hard of hearing people consists of the use of American Sign Language and speech with sign language. With non-signers, Jim uses speech with sign language, speechreading, and writing. When asked how well people understand his speech, Jim reported that familiar listeners tend to understand most of what he says, but unfamiliar listeners have more difficulty.

Jim's primary interest in communication therapy was to maintain his oral/aural skills. He felt his pronunciation errors and voice quality interfered with his speech intelligibility. Jim also wanted to fine-tune his listening skills. He reported difficulty tuning out background noise while wearing his implant and while trying to speechread. Jim is majoring in psychology and hopes to pursue a career as a clinical psychologist. He reported that he wants the flexibility of being able to communicate with nonsigners without the use of an interpreter.

Evaluation of Skills and Abilities

Based on Jim's stated communication concerns and areas he is interested in improving, the following assessments were completed.

Receptive Skills *Speechreading.* Jim's speechreading skills were assessed using the CID Everyday Sentences (CHABA). The first list of sentences was presented while Jim wore his implant. He scored 62 percent, indicating he is able to understand most of the content of the message. The second list was presented without the use of his implant. He scored a 48 percent, indicating that he understands with difficulty about one half of the message. These results indicate that Jim does receive some benefit from his implant while speechreading.

Auditory Functioning. The Test of Auditory Comprehension was used to assess Jim's auditory skills while using his implant. He successfully completed subtests one and two. Subtest one assesses the ability to discriminate auditorily between linguistic and nonlinguistic stimuli. Subtest two assesses the ability to discriminate auditorily among linguistic, human nonlinguistic, and environmental stimuli. He was unable to complete successfully the third and fourth subtests. Subtest three assesses the ability to interpret stereotypic messages auditorily. Subtest four assesses the ability to comprehend auditorily single-element, core noun vocabulary from a selection of picture stimuli. These results indicate that Jim is able to detect the presence of speech and identify it as such and to distinguish speech from other environmental sounds. However, he does not glean linguistic meaning from speech without the aid of visual cues.

The screening tests from the *Mini System 22 Rehabilitation Manual* were administered to determine the appropriate level of activities to be used in therapy. Four screening tests were presented to determine Jim's level of skill: (level A) detect sound and discriminate durational cues; (level B) discriminate and identify sentences based on supersegmental cues; (level C) discriminate second formant information; and (level D) recognize open-set speech. Jim was able to meet criterion for level A and B screening tests, but was unable to meet criterion (scored less than 8) on the level C screening test. Activities for therapy were thus to begin with level B.

Expressive Skills *Voice/Intelligibility.* Jim's voice production characteristics and intelligibility were rated using the NTID Speech and Voice Diagnostic Form. Jim was first asked to engage in a nonsigned conversation with the clinician and then to read aloud the "Rainbow Passage." His overall intelligibility rating of 3 indicated "typical deaf speech." His speech was difficult to understand; however, the gist of the conversation could be understood. Intelligibility may improve after the listener becomes accustomed to Jim's speech. Jim's pitch register and pitch control were within normal limits, but judged to be monotone. His loudness was judged to be slightly below appropriate levels, but he demonstrated the ability to control his loudness across utterances. His rate was appropriate, but he experienced some difficulty using appropriate stressing of syllables. Jim's vocal quality was evidenced by slight breathiness and tenseness. He demonstrated slight prevocal air wastage and moderate deficiency of air expenditure during speech. Jim was able to sustain /s/ for 12 seconds, /a/ for 16 seconds, and count to 25 on one breath. Jim exhibited moderate hypernasality and severe pharyngeal resonance. These results indicated that Jim's vocal quality has a significant impact upon his intelligibility.

Articulation. The Fisher-Logemann Test of Articulation Competence Sentence Test was administered to assess Jim's articulation. The only error noted was s/z in the final position.

Pronunciation. The Pronunciation Skills Inventory was administered to assess Jim's knowledge of English pronunciation rules. Jim's overall score was a 90.8 percent, indicating excellent pronunciation skills. One area with a significantly lower score (40 percent) was stress patterns. This score indicates the need for Jim to focus on rate and prosody of speech, particularly stress patterns in multisyllabic words and utterances.

Communication Strategies A tracking activity was utilized to assess Jim's use of receptive communication strategies. The clinician read from a passage, and Jim repeated verbatim what was said. A reverse tracking activity was utilized to assess Jim's use of expressive communication strategies. Jim read from a passage, and the clinician (without the aid of speechreading Jim) repeated verbatim what was said. Jim's only strategy (both receptive and expressive) was to ask for repetition of entire phrases or to repeat entire phrases upon request. This indicated the need for presentation of a wider repertoire of communication strategies for use in various contexts.

Recommendations

Based on the above assessment results and conversations with Jim, the clinician concluded that, overall, Jim had very good communication skills. The assessment results were shared and discussed with Jim. Jim noted that the results were in agreement with his previously stated areas of concern. However, Jim was not familiar with the use of communication strategies and how effective use of strategies could improve his overall communicative effectiveness. Jim's goal is to be flexible and independent in his communication with nonsigners. The clinician and Jim discussed realistic expectations for the outcome of therapy (for example, Jim is now a young adult and changes in vocal quality may be limited). Following this discussion and negotiation, Jim and the clinician mutually agreed upon the following areas to focus on in therapy:

1. Intelligibility (stress patterns and intonation)

2. Speechreading and listening (while using the cochlear implant)

3. Appropriate use of expressive and receptive communication strategies

Integrated Therapy

Initially, therapy sessions focused on teaching and reviewing the following concepts:

1. Syllabification and stress rules using the dictionary

2. Components of speechreading (for example, viseme groups, situational clues, linguistic factors)

3. Communication strategies: anticipatory, maintenance, and repair

4. Discrimination and identification exercises taken from level B of the *Mini System 22 Rehabilitation Manual* (Cochlear Corporation):

   a. Identify words, phrases, and sentences of various lengths

   b. Identify words, phrases, and sentences highly contrasted for F2 pattern information

   c. Identify rising and falling intonation patterns

Some sample therapy activities demonstrating integration of the goal areas were as follows:

Given the role play situation of a job interview (as a teaching assistant in the

Table 13.1 Receptive Constellation Job Interview for a Teaching Assistant Position

1. What can you tell me about yourself?

2. What are your educational goals for the future?

3. Name 3 things that you've learned in school that can be used on this job.

4. Does your grade point average reflect your work ability?

5. Do you like to work with people?

6. What teaching experience do you have?

7. What do you think you do best?

8. Are you interested in research?

9. Why should we choose you for this position?

10. Do you have any questions?

department of psychology), Jim generated a receptive constellation (statements and questions that might be said to him) and an expressive constellation (statements and questions that he might have to say). Upon random presentation of the statements/questions listed in the receptive constellation (table 13.1), Jim was able to speechread with 100 percent accuracy. Jim had to then produce statements/questions from his expressive constellation (table 13.2). The clinician listened to Jim's production (without watching him) and noted the following errors: pronunciation of /s/z/ in plurals and a monotone voice quality resulting in the clinician being unable to determine if a question or statement was being produced. Jim had to use a dictionary to pronounce correctly the following words: psychology, clinical, effective, and organizational.

These therapy activities demonstrate integration of goal areas. Jim used the anticipatory strategy of generating constellations for a given communication situation. He then worked on speechreading and listening using the sentences generated in the receptive constellation and on pronunciation, intonation, and stress using the sentences generated in the expressive constellation.

Jim and the clinician then role played the situation with the clinician as the interviewer. Background noise (an audiotape of cafeteria noise) was used to make it more challenging for both the clinician and Jim. The dialogue between Jim and the clinician incorporated, but was not limited to, the language used in Jim's constellations. Jim needed to use appropriate receptive and expressive repair strategies if and when there was communication breakdown.

Table 13.2   Expressive Constellation Job Interview for a Teaching Assistant Position

1. I'm majoring in clinical psychology.
   I'm a self-starter, highly motivated, and energetic.

2. I want to eventually get a Ph.D. in Clinical Psychology.

3. Study Skills, Organizational Skills, How to relate to others.

4. My grades are above average to excellent, and I think my previous work record has been the same.

5. Yes, I've always worked well with others.

6. I have had no formal teaching experience, but I've tutored small groups of students for the past three years.

7. I'm very organized and relate well to others.

8. Yes, I'm very interested in research in this field.

9. I know I can do a great job and be a very effective teaching assistant.

10. Yes. What are my job responsibilities?
    How many hours a week must I commit to this job?
    Will I get a tuition waiver or a stipend?

The role play was videotaped and later reviewed and evaluated by both Jim and the clinician. Jim used the following receptive communication strategies: repeating parts of sentences, rephrasing, oral spelling, and asking a specific question. He used the following expressive strategies: repeating words/phrases, oral spelling of words, rephrasing (he would use a different word with the same meaning if he was unable to pronounce a word). Jim and the clinician discussed the effectiveness of his strategy use. Both felt that Jim's strategies were very appropriate for the situation. Jim was asked to make a list of the words he "rephrased" in order to review their pronunciation. After the correct pronunciation of those words was modeled for him, Jim was able to self-correct with 80 percent accuracy.

Summary

Jim was enrolled in communication therapy on a twice per week basis for fifty-minute sessions. He was able to meet established criterion levels for most goal areas. Jim had the most difficulty meeting criteria for speechreading in the presence of background noise. The presence of background noise also had an impact on how well he was understood by the listener. The clinician and Jim discussed the importance of appropriate communication strategy use in noisy communication situations. Jim stated that he felt successful during therapy sessions. He reported that, outside of the therapy setting, he felt more confident in his communication with nonsigners. Jim will continue to use his cochlear implant and continue to participate in therapy throughout his undergraduate experience. He wants therapy to focus on improving his intelligibility and on increasing his use of appropriate strategies in the presence of background noise.

Elsie *(Scott J. Bally)*

Information Gathering Interview

Elsie, age 59, came to a university-based Hearing and Speech Center to explore the possibility of speechreading classes. She also wanted to explore the possibility of a cochlear implant because a friend had read about it and she thought it might "cure" her hearing loss. She reported that her physician had told her she had "nerve deafness," and nothing could be done about it. She also mentioned that she thought some sign language lessons might be helpful.

Elsie was accompanied by her daughter at the encouragement of several family members. Previous clinical records reflected a progressive, bilateral, moderately severe-to-profound sensorineural loss, attributed to presbycusis. Elsie's most recent and only testing occurred when she was 55, but she reported being aware of her loss since age 50. She brought along her three-year-old behind-the-ear aids in her purse and was not sure if they were working.

An intake interview revealed the following information regarding Elsie: At 59, Elsie had been widowed for a year and a half, after forty years of marriage and five children. She continued to live alone in a large condominium where she and her husband had resided for the last twenty-one years. Four of her five children lived in the general area with their families.

Elsie was a professional in marketing for a large manufacturing firm, but was given early retirement at age 56. She reported that "it probably was related to my hearing loss, but I was making a lot of mistakes on the telephone, so I went peacefully."

During her most recent work years she had been fairly active. She took both professionally related and "fun" courses at the local community college, played bridge and golf with other couples, traveled extensively, and had several theater subscriptions. She reported that she stopped taking classes because she couldn't understand the classroom discussion and experienced some embarrassment when her comments resulted in questioning stares from the other students. The other activities dwindled after her retirement and stopped after her husband died.

Since retirement, Elsie has been doing volunteer work a few hours each week at the information desk of a small local museum. However, she reported that she is thinking about changing to the textile care unit at the museum because it requires less interaction with people.

Currently, she is on the condominium board of directors, but plans to resign. She spends her time working on family photo albums and has a ballet subscription with a friend. She occasionally lunches with individual family members but avoids family gatherings because they are "too frustrating."

Elsie reported attending a few speechreading classes several years before, but stopped because she didn't have a practice partner. She reported that she was thinking about taking a sign language class at the "Y."

When asked about her hearing aids, Elsie reported that she hadn't worn them much after she picked them up at the hearing aid dealer. She found them "too noisy" and they made her ears feel "stuffed up." She was unable to identify the use of the "M-T-O" switch, and a cursory look showed corroded batteries in the aids. She noted that she had a telephone amplifier, but still had difficulty hearing numbers and unfamiliar names when she used it. She noted that she never initiated phone calls unless it was absolutely necessary.

At Elsie's request, her daughter, Arlene, attended the initial sessions. Arlene corroborated Elsie's report, noting that Elsie often smiled and nodded when she, in fact, did not understand what was being said. She also reported the family's concern that Elsie was living alone because, along with her hearing problem, she seemed forgetful. She acknowledged that the doctor had given Elsie a clean bill of health, but the family was still worried.

Based on the interview, Elsie was referred for diagnostic evaluations, including audiologic testing, and for aural rehabilitation.

Evaluation of Skills and Abilities

Audiologic testing confirmed previous test results and reflected less than a 5 dB decrease in pure tone responses since her previous testing. Pure Tone averages were at 85 dBHL bilaterally. Speech Recognition scores were 67 percent at 60 dBHL bilaterally. Impedance testing showed normal middle ear pressure. Acoustic reflexes were consistent with the type and degree of loss. Elsie's hearing aids were deemed to be appropriate, pending adjustment, and were sent to the manufacturer for cleaning and new terminals in the battery chamber. New vented earmolds were recommended and made two weeks later after a visit to her physician for an ear check. She was scheduled for a return visit for fitting pending the return of the aids and was advised that the aural rehabilitationist would help her to understand them and learn how to use them more effectively.

An aural rehabilitation evaluation included further interview, the Communication Scale for Older Adults (CSOA), and continuous discourse tracking (both receptive and expressive) to examine communication attitudes and use of communication strategies. The Binnie Lipreading Test and the Central Institute for the Deaf (CID) Everyday Sentences were used to assess speechreading. The Test of Auditory Comprehension (TAC) was administered to establish a baseline for auditory skills, although it was recognized that it was not normed on populations in her age range. Other than a receptive tracking procedure, no other expressive testing was deemed necessary. It was noted that Elsie occasionally had some difficulty keeping the volume of her voice at an appropriate level.

Elsie's results on the Communication Scale for Older Adults reflected poor use of communication strategies, extensive use of maladaptive strategies, a lack of acceptance of hearing loss, and withdrawal from social activities as a result. Elsie scored 72 percent on the Binnie Lipreading Test, reflecting good lipreading ability. When she made errors, they were usually within visemes. She achieved an 82 percent score on the CHABA sentences without voice and a 98 percent with voice. When competing noise was introduced, her scores dropped below 40 percent. Her initial score on the Continuous Discourse tracking procedure was 48 words in five minutes. Strategy use was limited to asking for repetition and slowing the rate of speech. Scores on the expressive or reverse tracking procedure reflected a 100 percent intelligibility for all utterances by the clinician. On the Test of Auditory Comprehension, Elsie was able to complete the first five subtests with high scores and the next four with moderate scores. Scores dropped dramatically when competing noises were introduced.

Further interviewing was based on responses on the CSOA. When asked to discuss some of her responses, her comments reflected a frustrated and lonely individual who felt that her family did "not understand what I've been going through." She commented that she felt she could not "make any further contributions to her family or friends given her hearing loss" and that it "was not fair to waste their time with my handicap." She explained that she had resigned herself to "growing old gracefully" and not burdening her family and friends. Further, she felt that she had made the best adjustments to her hearing loss possible with "respect to my family and friends."

Recommendations

1. Referral for counseling to social work or other professionals with experience working with persons with hearing loss

2. Informational counseling to discuss realistic expectations and therapy options (including cochlear implants and sign language)

3. Hearing aid orientation, assistive devices evaluation, and auditory training

4. Integrated program of aural rehabilitation to include

   a. speechreading

   b. auditory training

   c. communication strategies (including the elimination of counterproductive strategies)

Integrated Therapy

The test results were explained to Elsie, and she received informational counseling regarding cochlear implants (not recommended), sign language classes (of limited benefit because no one she knew signed), and hearing aid orientation ("a revelation!"). Therapy options were presented, and her priorities were integrated in an aural rehabilitation program that focused on receptive communication skills. Four elements of speechreading training included analytic and synthetic skills, auditory training, and the use of receptive and expressive communication strategies. Further, Elsie herself broached the subject of counseling, noting that she didn't feel she was coping as effectively as possible with the death of her husband or the compounding frustration of her hearing loss. Elsie and the clinician discussed counseling options, and a referral was made. An integrated and interdisciplinary approach to communication therapy was defined. Elsie signed release of information forms so that the social worker she had selected and the aural rehabilitationist were able to work cooperatively.

The social worker directed her efforts toward helping Elsie understand the impact of both her hearing loss and widowhood on her life. Further, she helped Elsie develop coping strategies for dealing with the stress and isolation of both. Family issues were explored. In addition, Elsie was given some assertiveness training to help her in difficult communication situations as well as in dealing with some family members and with "a few aggressive and opinionated friends."

Aural rehabilitation was initiated after her reconditioned aids were returned and was started with hearing aid orientation and a structured program that fostered more extensive hearing aid use. Analytic training focused on identification of phonemes within viseme groups. Synthetic training focused on the use of linguistic knowledge to help Elsie understand associated words, phrases, and sentences within contexts that she identified as being problematic. Auditory training focused on communication in groups in which some elements of competing noise were present. An evaluation of routine communication environments ensued.

The use of communication strategies focused on the effective selection and use of appropriate anticipatory, maintenance, and repair strategies as well as on the reinforcement of effective assertive approaches in order to create better overall communication. During the course of therapy, the clinician helped Elsie to analyze problem communication situations in her daily life. The multiple causes of communication breakdown were identified, and she learned to identify a range of strategies that resolved interpersonal, language, and environmental problems. Communication situations such as her volunteer job at the information desk, family interactions, and condo board meetings were addressed, and Elsie reconsidered her participation in all three. She was realistic enough to realize that communication in these situations could be improved but would still be difficult.

Summary

After six months of therapy, Elsie reported that she is much happier with her hearing aids and wears them most of the time, except in especially noisy situations. She was immediately pleased with her new vented earmolds, which she said reduced the stuffy feeling in her ears. With amplification and increased comfort using communication strategies, she felt she was "back in touch with the world."

She is planning to participate in some of the activities of a local senior activities center, including their day trip program and some short courses of interest to her. Relative to such participation, she has been referred for an assistive devices assessment.

After a period of auditory training, Elsie's scores on the TAC improved only marginally, but her confidence improved enormously. She made dramatic gains on her continuous discourse tracking scores, demonstrated significant improvements in strategy use in spontaneous conversations with the clinician, and reported a studied use of strategies outside the clinical setting. She succeeded in persuading two of her daughters to attend partner training sessions. Together, the three of them had been making inroads in improving some of the communication behaviors of some other family members.

Counseling revealed problems relative to her self-esteem—"I'm only half a couple"—and family situations that were only exacerbated by her hearing loss. She felt that the family had "written her off" after her husband's death. As a result of her family attitude and as part of her grieving process, she had subconsciously withdrawn from them. She confided that she didn't like the way they were treating her ("like some old senile woman!") and felt they wanted to put her in "a home." Counseling helped her to assess her family relations, and she has been working toward helping her family understand her need for independence as well as equitable family relations. She has continued her one-on-one lunches with various family members and is using these opportunities to talk through some of her concerns with them. Jointly, they worked out a system of regular communication so they are less concerned about Elsie's safety. Elsie conceded that she would consider moving if and when her health status warranted it. (She confided in the counselor that she wouldn't rule out remarrying if the right man came along. "My family would have a cow!" she added.)

Elsie came to realize that her hearing loss and her efforts to conceal it may have been responsible for the impression that she was becoming forgetful. In both counseling and aural rehabilitation she has diminished her use of counterproductive strategies: "At my age, it's hard to break bad habits, but I'm trying."

Elsie has started to attend family gatherings again, as a self-appointed family historian. At the get-togethers, she establishes herself in one of the smaller rooms of a family member's house where individuals visit her in small groups for family updates. Family members have started bringing photographs of their activities to give to her for the family album. She "takes five" between groups because, although communication is better, it is still tiring. Nevertheless, Elsie feels that she is now closer to her family and that their collective attitude has improved enormously.

Elsie has decided to complete her term on the condo board. Of her own volition, she composed a letter to the board members, expressing her commitment to the board and her concern and frustration regarding her inability to follow meetings. The topic was put on the agenda, there was an open discussion about it at a Board meeting, and she is chairing a small task force that will draw up some communication guidelines and explore the possibilities of acquiring a group amplification system for the activities room. Such a system would need to be multifunctional, serving not only the board meeting, but other community activities. Once her term is up, Elsie has decided not to run for reelection, but to participate actively on committees of interest to her, in which the groups would be smaller and communication more manageable, especially with her new strategies. She notes that although things have improved in the board meeting, people forget and retreat into their old habits.

Elsie did elect to retire from the information desk at the museum. She noted that because the entrance way to the museum was "an acoustical nightmare" (with no budget for modifications), it had become too stressful and "not much fun." Elsie has also been attending meetings of her local SHHH chapter and has already accepted a committee membership. She feels her work experience may help the publicity committee to attract more people to activities and increase membership.

Finally, Elsie hesitatingly approached her clinician to say she would be transferring to the group speechreading class that the SHHH chapter was forming. The clinician smiled and nodded because, unbeknownst to Elsie, she had been contracted to teach the course.

Clinician's note: Elsie's daughter, Arlene, made an appointment to have her own hearing checked and a mild to moderate loss was identified. A communication practice partner for Elsie?

Index

■ ■ ■ ■

A t following a page number indicates a table; an f following a page number indicates a figure.